Bladder Diseases: Diagnosis and Treatment

Bladder Diseases: Diagnosis and Treatment

Edited by Phoebe Cameron

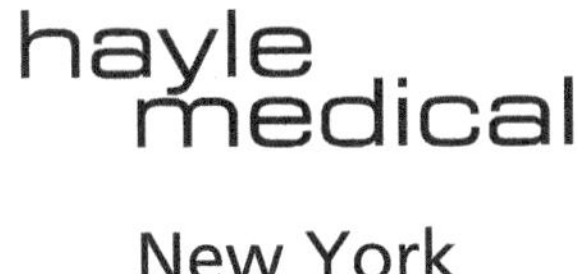

New York

Hayle Medical,
750 Third Avenue, 9th Floor,
New York, NY 10017, USA

Visit us on the World Wide Web at:
www.haylemedical.com

ISBN: 978-1-63241-917-0

Cataloging-in-Publication Data

Bladder diseases : diagnosis and treatment / edited by Phoebe Cameron.
p. cm.
Includes bibliographical references and index.
ISBN 978-1-63241-917-0
1. Bladder--Diseases. 2. Bladder--Diseases--Diagnosis. 3. Bladder--Diseases--Treatment.
I. Cameron, Phoebe.
RC919 .B53 2020
616.62--dc23

Table of Contents

Preface

The urinary bladder can be affected by a number of conditions such as cystitis, urinary incontinence, bladder cancer, interstitial cystitis and overactive bladder. These conditions are together referred to as bladder disease. Such diseases can be diagnosed through X-ray imaging, urine tests and bladder examination using cystoscope. Bladder obstruction is the condition when there is a heavy blood clot formation within the bladder outlet. It generally arises due to bladder cancer and requires surgery. This book discusses the fundamentals as well as modern approaches in the diagnosis and treatment of bladder diseases. It will also provide interesting topics for research which interested readers can take up. Coherent flow of topics, student-friendly language and extensive use of examples make this book an invaluable source of knowledge.

This book is a comprehensive compilation of works of different researchers from varied parts of the world. It includes valuable experiences of the researchers with the sole objective of providing the readers (learners) with a proper knowledge of the concerned field. This book will be beneficial in evoking inspiration and enhancing the knowledge of the interested readers.

In the end, I would like to extend my heartiest thanks to the authors who worked with great determination on their chapters. I also appreciate the publisher's support in the course of the book. I would also like to deeply acknowledge my family who stood by me as a source of inspiration during the project.

Editor

1

Long term follow-up in patients with initially diagnosed low grade Ta non-muscle invasive bladder tumors: tumor recurrence and worsening progression

Hiroaki Kobayashi[1], Eiji Kikuchi[1*], Shuji Mikami[2], Takahiro Maeda[1], Nobuyuki Tanaka[1], Akira Miyajima[1], Ken Nakagawa[1] and Mototsugu Oya[1]

Abstract

Background: We evaluated the clinical outcome of low grade Ta bladder cancer followed-up for a long period using the 2004 WHO grading system.

Methods: We retrospectively reviewed 190 patients with primary, low grade Ta bladder cancer. We defined worsening progression (WP) as confirmed high grade Ta, all T1 or Tis/concomitant CIS of bladder recurrence, upper urinary tract recurrence (UTR), or progression to equal to or more than T2. The associations between clinicopathological factors and tumor recurrence as well as WP pattern were analyzed. We also evaluated the late recurrence of 76 patients who were tumor-free for more than 5 years.

Results: Tumor recurrence and WP occurred in 82 (43.2%) and 21 (11.1%) patients during follow-up (median follow-up: 101.5 months), respectively. WP to high grade Ta, all T1 or Tis/concomitant CIS was seen in 17 patients, and UTR and progression to equal to or more than T2 were seen in 2 and 2 patients, respectively. Multivariate analyses demonstrated that multiple tumor ($p < 0.001$, HR: 2.97) and absence of intravesical instillation (IVI) ($p < 0.001$, HR: 2.88) were significant risk factors for tumor recurrence while multiple tumor was the only risk factor for WP ($p = 0.001$, HR: 5.26). After a 5-year tumor-free period, 9 patients experienced late recurrence in years 5 and 10 and were diagnosed at a follow-up cystoscopy, however, only 2 patients recurred beyond 10 years and were found by gross hematuria. There were no significant risk factors of late recurrence.

Conclusions: Multiple tumor was a risk factor for both tumor recurrence and WP while IVI did not affect the occurrence of WP. Our results suggest that routine follow-up of patients with low grade Ta bladder cancer is needed up to 10 years from the initial diagnosis.

Keywords: Bladder cancer, Intravesical instillation, Recurrence, Progression

Background

Approximately 50 % of newly diagnosed cases of bladder cancer are low grade, noninvasive and papillary tumors [1]. The standard treatment for non-muscle invasive bladder cancer (NMIBC) is transurethral resection of the bladder tumor (TUR-BT) with or without adjuvant intravesical instillation (IVI) of chemotherapy or Bacillus Calmette-Guerin (BCG) therapy [2]. The most important problems associated with NMIBC are that they have high rates of recurrence and risk of progression. Approximately 50% to 70% of NMIBC have a recurrence within 5 years, and 5% to 20% progress to invasive tumors [3]. To the best of our knowledge, there have been no reports with longer follow-up data focusing on the effects of IVI on tumor recurrence and progression in patients with low grade Ta tumors based on the 2004 WHO classification [4,5]. Also, there are few published studies in which a large number of patients were

* Correspondence: eiji-k@kb3.so-net.ne.jp
[1]Department of Urology, Keio University School of Medicine, 35 Shinanomachi, Shinjuku-ku, Tokyo 160-8582, Japan
Full list of author information is available at the end of the article

followed for more than 5 years after the initial diagnosis. Only two papers provide information on the risk of recurrence and progression after a long tumor-free period [6,7]. Although some long follow-up studies also showed most tumors recurred or progressed within 5 years, recent data support the need for long term follow-up for more than 10–15 years in such patients even after an initial response to BCG therapy and a recurrence-free period for more than 5 years [6].

In this study, we analyzed the clinical outcome of initially diagnosed low grade Ta tumors after re-assessing all pathological specimens according to the 2004 WHO classification, with a special focus on tumor recurrence and worsening progression (WP) pattern and discuss the need for longer follow-up.

Methods

We reviewed the medical records of 242 patients (male: 199, female: 43) who underwent TUR-BT with complete tumor resection for the past 30 years at Keio University Hospital for an initially diagnosed TaG1-2 tumor. We excluded 44 patients who had already undergone TUR-BT at another hospital or who had a history of upper tract urothelial cancer. After re-evaluation of all pathological specimens by a dedicated uro-pathologist, with a special focus on the 2004 WHO grading system, 8 patients with G2 tumors were re-classified as high grade. The remaining 190 NMIBC patients (male: 156, female: 34) who were initially diagnosed with a tumor that was low grade Ta were included in the current analysis. All of the tumors were histologically confirmed as urothelial carcinoma.

These patients were followed by urine cytology and cystoscopy at 3-month intervals during the initial year, every 6 months for the next 5 years, and then yearly thereafter. Intravenous urography, ultrasonography, and/or CT scanning were used to evaluate distant metastasis and upper urinary tract recurrence (UTR) every 1 or 2 years for 5 years. Recurrence was defined as the occurrence of a new tumor in the bladder. Worsening progression (WP) was defined as confirmed (1) high grade Ta, all T1, or Tis/concomitant CIS of bladder recurrence, (2) UTR, or (3) progression to equal to or more than T2.

The use of adjuvant therapies including intravesical BCG or mitomycin (MMC) instillation depended primarily on the discretion of the attending physician. In the overall patient population, BCG and MMC therapies were performed in 71 patients (37.4%) and 12 patients (6.3%), respectively. This study was approved by Keio university hospitals ethical committee. We obtained the patient's informed consent including their approval for potential use of their anonymized medical data from our data base for research and audit purposes.

The following were analyzed for each individual patient: age, gender, multiplicity and smoking status. Smoking status was classified as 1) nonsmokers; those who had never smoked during their lifetime, 2) ex-smokers; those who had quit smoking before the diagnosis and 3) current smokers; those who still smoked regularly at the initial TUR-BT. Recurrence-free survival rate curves were constructed using the Kaplan-Meier method, and were compared using the log-rank test. Differences among groups were regarded as significant when $p < 0.05$. Univariate and multivariate analyses of data were performed using the Cox proportional hazards model with stepwise forward selection. These analyses were performed with a statistical software package (SPSS, version 19.0).

Results

Tumor recurrence and worsening progression rate in entire patient population

The mean age of the patients was 62.9 years (range, 22–89) and the median follow-up interval was 101.5 months (range, 11.1 to 298.2). Solitary/multiple tumors were seen in 114/76 patients, respectively. Tumor recurrence occurred in 82 patients (43.2%). Most patients who had tumor recurrence could be diagnosed by the routine follow-up cystoscopic examination except for 3 patients (3.7%) who were detected due to gross hematuria. When we divided the patients into two groups, those with or without tumor recurrence, there were no significant differences in age, gender, IVI or smoking status between the two groups (Table 1). The recurrence rate in multiple tumors (53.9%) was significantly higher than that in solitary tumors (36.0%). Univariate and multivariate analyses demonstrated that multiple tumor and absence of IVI were significant risk factors for tumor recurrence (Table 2). Kaplan-Meier curves demonstrated that the 5-year recurrence free survival rate for solitary tumors (68.0%) was significantly higher than that for multiple tumors (45.9%, $p = 0.001$) (Figure 1A), and also higher for patients receiving intravesical instillation (71.3% vs. 50.3% without IVI, $p = 0.007$) (Figure 1B).

Overall WP occurred in 21 patients (11.1%) and the average time to WP was 82.4 months (range, 5.6-298.2). WP to high grade Ta, all T1, or Tis/concomitant CIS of bladder recurrence was seen in 4, 8 and 5 patients, respectively, UTR was seen in 2 patients (1.1%), and progression to equal to or more than T2 was observed in 2 patients (1.1%). Also, there were various types of timing and intervals for WP. Twenty of 21 patients (95.2%) experienced WP until the 2nd recurrence and 12 patients (57.1%) experienced WP on the 1st recurrence. All 8 patients who experienced WP on the 2nd recurrence had a low grade Ta type tumor on the 1st recurrence, and the average time between the 1st and 2nd recurrence was

Table 1 Clinical characteristics of all 190 patients

		Total	Recurrence (+)	Recurrence (−)	*p* value	WP (+)	WP (−)	*p* value
N		190	82	108		21	169	
Age (y)	Mean Range	62.9	63.0	62.9		64.9	62.7	
		22-89	26-83	22-89		47-83	22-89	
	≤70	128	56	72	NS	14	114	NS
	>70	62	26	36		7	55	
Gender	Male	156	72	84	NS	19	137	NS
	Female	34	10	24		2	32	
Multiplicity	Solitary	114	41	73	0.017	7	107	0.016
	Multiple	76	41	35		14	62	
IVI	Yes	83	29	54	NS	11	72	NS
	No	107	53	54		10	97	
Smoking	None	100	40	60	NS	10	90	NS
	Current	56	29	27		9	47	
	Ex-smoker	27	10	17		2	25	
	Unknown	7	3	4		0	7	

IVI intravesical instillation, *WP* worsening progression, *NS* non-significant.

22.9 months. An exception was one patient who experienced minor recurrences three times and WP occurred on the 4th recurrence. The three recurrences were all low grade Ta, and in the end WP to high grade T1 occurred although intravesical chemotherapy and BCG instillations were performed after every TUR-BT.

When we divided the patients into two groups, those with or without WP, there were no significant differences in age, gender, IVI or smoking status between the two groups (Table 1). WP occurred more often in the multiple tumor group (18.4%) than in the solitary tumor group (6.1%) and the difference was significant (p = 0.016). Univariate and multivariate analyses demonstrated that multiple tumor was the only significant risk factor for WP (Table 2). Kaplan-Meier curve demonstrated that the 5-year WP free survival rate for solitary tumors (97.2%) was significantly higher than that for multiple tumors (85.5%, p = 0.003) (Figure 2).

Late recurrence beyond 5-year tumor-free period

We next focused on patients who were tumor-free for more than 5 years from initial TUR-BT to first tumor recurrence and WP, called "late recurrence" and "late WP". We identified 76 patients in this category, among whom adjuvant IVI had been performed in 40 (52.6%) patients (Table 3). The mean age of the patients was 61.1 years (range, 22–84), and solitary/multiple tumors were seen in 53/23 patients, respectively. Eleven patients (14.5%) experienced late recurrence, and of them, 5 patients (6.6%) had late WP (Table 4). There were no significant differences in age, gender, multiplicity, smoking status or adjuvant IVI performed in patients with or without late recurrence, and there were no significant risk factors of late recurrence. The average time to late recurrence and late WP was 103.5 and 104.5 months, respectively. Nine of 11 patients whose cancer recurred in years 5 and 10 in our study were diagnosed at a follow-

Table 2 Univariate and multivariate analyses for tumor recurrence and WP in overall patient population

	Recurrence			WP		
	Univariate	Multivariate		Univariate	Multivariate	
	p value	p value	HR	p value	p value	HR
Age (≤70 vs. >70)	0.465			0.444		
Gender (male vs. female)	0.152			0.412		
Multiplicity (solitary vs. multiple)	0.001	<0.001	2.97	0.003	0.001	5.26
Treatment (IVI vs. observation)	0.007	<0.001	2.88	0.454		
Smoking (nonsmoker vs. smoker)	0.501			0.606		

IVI intravesical instillation, *WP* worsening progression, *smoker*: current smoker + ex-smoker.

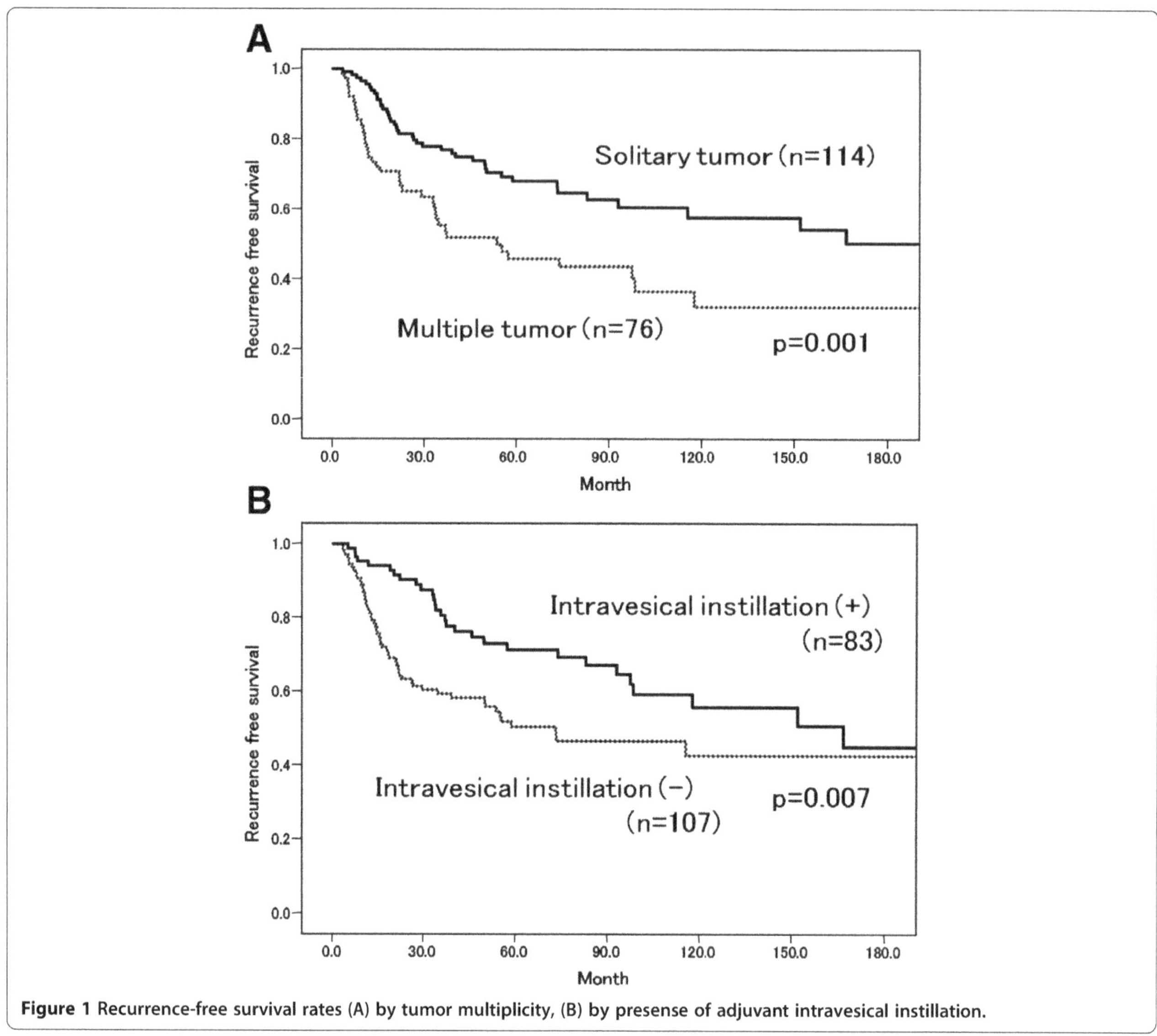

Figure 1 **Recurrence-free survival rates (A) by tumor multiplicity, (B) by presense of adjuvant intravesical instillation.**

up cystoscopy. Meanwhile, recurrence in 2 patients who were tumor-free beyond 10 years was found by gross hematuria. WP to high grade Ta, low grade T1, Tis, UTR, and high grade T3 were observed in one case in each. Also, 4 patients experienced WP on the first late recurrence while only one patient did on the 2nd recurrence.

Discussion

We reviewed 190 patients with primary, low grade Ta NMIBC patients and evaluated whether patient-related factors (age, gender, multiplicity, smoking status and adjuvant treatment) were associated with tumor recurrence and WP. Multivariate analysis demonstrated that multiplicity was a risk factor for both tumor recurrence and WP, and that IVI did not affect the occurrence of WP. While none of the patients died of bladder cancer during follow-up, late recurrence and late WP occurred in 11 and 5 patients, respectively.

Zieger et al. presented the natural history of 212 patients initially diagnosed with TaG1-2 tumors for up to 20 years. Only 14 patients received intravesical instillation in their study. Ten of the 212 (4.7%) developed into TaG3 or CIS, 18 (8.5%) developed into T1, and 23 (10.8%) showed muscle invasion or distant metastases 8]. According to our definition of WP, WP was seen in 24.1% in their study, which was relatively high compared to our study. Similarly, Prout et al. followed 178 patients with TaG1 bladder tumors for up to 10 years. They reported that a change in grade or stage progression occurred in 13 (7.3%) patients, while only 14 patients (7.9%) received intravesical chemotherapy [9]. Akagashi et al. reported no patients initially diagnosed with TaG1-2 tumors progressed to muscle invasive

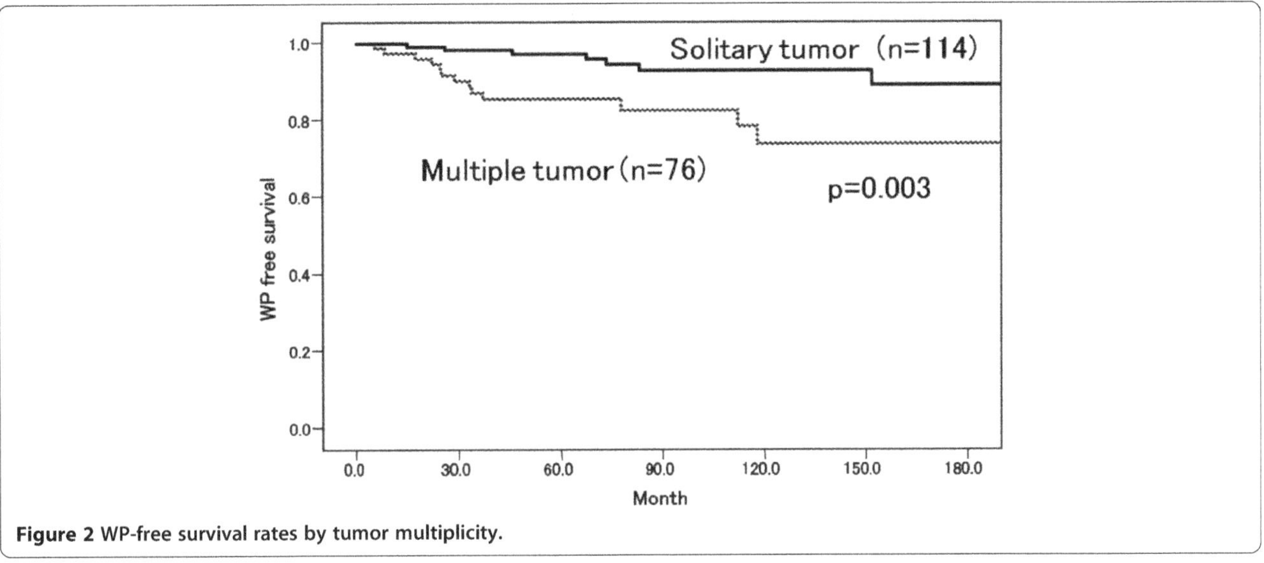

Figure 2 WP-free survival rates by tumor multiplicity.

tumors, while 6 of 62 (9.7 %) patients developed into Tis or T1. One reason for this low percentage of progression was that most of the patients received intravesical chemotherapy for more than 2 years [10]. From these reports, the recurrence rate of initially diagnosed TaG1-2 bladder cancer was 50-60%, and the WP rate was highly variable (between 7% and 24%). In our population of initially diagnosed low grade Ta bladder tumors, the recurrence rate and WP rate were 43.2% and 11.1%, respectively.

We reviewed longer follow-up data for a maximum of 25 years and re-assessed all pathological specimens using the 2004 WHO classification. Only 8 of 198 (4.0%) of G1-2 tumors were re-classified as high grade in our study. Miyamoto et al. evaluated low grade papillary urothelial carcinoma after re-classifying all specimens and reported that 8 of 55 patients (14.5%) were re-classified as having high grade tumors [11]. Pellucchi et al. evaluated tumor recurrence and progression with both the 1973 and 2004 WHO grading systems in patients with primary low grade Ta NMIBC and concluded that the 1973 WHO grading system predicted the risk of recurrence more accurately than the 2004 system and the 2 classifications showed the same accuracy for predicting the risk of progression [12]. The 2013 EAU guideline states that both grading classifications should be used until the 2004 WHO system is validated by more prospective trials [13].

Table 3 Clinical characteristics of 76 patients with a tumor-free period for more than 5 years from initial diagnosis

		Total	Late recurrence (+)	Late recurrence (−)	*p* value
N		76	11	65	
Age (y)	Mean	61.1	64.1	60.6	
	Range	(21.8-84.2)	(56.9-78.1)	(21.8-84.2)	
	≤70	58	9	49	NS
	>70	18	2	16	
Gender	Male	60	10	50	NS
	Female	16	1	15	
Multiplicity	Solitary	53	7	46	NS
	Multiple	23	4	19	
IVI	Yes	40	8	32	NS
	No	36	3	33	
Smoking	None	44	6	38	NS
	Current	23	3	20	
	Ex-smoker	8	1	7	
	Unknown	1	1	0	

Table 4 Clinical data for patients with late recurrence and late WP

Patient no.	Age (yr)	Gender	Smoking status	Multiplicity	Tumor-free period (mo)	Pathology on late rec./WP	Follow up (mo)	Status of last contact
1	57	Male	Current	M	98.4	S, low, Ta	232.6	Alive, NED
2	58	Male	None	M	117.8	M, high, Tis	172.1	Alive, cystectomy performed
3	58	Male	Ex-smoker	M	74.0	S, low, Ta	298.2	Alive, NED
4	59	Female	None	M	97.4	M, low, Ta	118.2	Alive, UTR, NUx performed
5	60	Male	None	S	166.6	S, low, Ta	178.4	Alive, NED
6	61	Male	None	S	73.5	S, low, Ta	273.6	Alive, NED
7	62	Male	Current	S	73.3	S, high, Ta	244.3	Alive, NED
8	67	Male	Unknown	S	92.9	M, low, Ta	134.8	Alive, NED
9	68	Male	Current	S	151.8	M, low, T1	206.4	Alive, NED
10	76	Male	None	S	115.5	S, low, Ta	176.0	Alive, NED
11	78	Male	None	S	83.1	M, high, T3	96.8	Dead of intercurrent disease

M multiple, *S* solitary, *WP* worsening progression, *NED* no evidence of disease, *UTR* upper urinary tract recurrence, *NUx* nephroureterectomy.

Holmang et al. reported the outcomes in patients treated with BCG intravesical therapy who were tumor-free for more than 5 years (N = 204). Of the 204 patients, 110 (53.9%) had a G1 or G2 tumor. They stated that patients with TaG1-2 tumors treated with BCG have a very good long-term prognosis, but late recurrences were observed. Furthermore, as all low grade recurrences were diagnosed at a follow-up cystoscopy and office cystoscopy generally is a simple procedure, they concluded that continuing to follow patients with TaG1-2 for more than 5 years is encouraging [6]. Our results support their findings. All patients in our study who experienced recurrence in years 5 and 10 were diagnosed at a follow-up cystoscopy. Meanwhile, recurrence in 2 patients who had been tumor-free beyond 10 years was found by gross hematuria. These results suggest that follow-up cystoscopy can be discontinued around 10 years from the initial diagnosis in patients with low grade Ta bladder cancer.

Smoking status is a well-known risk factor for poor outcome in bladder cancer and the strong association between smoking and primary NMIBC recurrence was observed in previous studies [14-16]. However, our results revealed that smoking status is not associated with bladder recurrence rate, WP rate, or late recurrence rate. One of the reasons for our negative result is that the relatively lower percentage of smokers and lower amount of smoking in Japanese NMIBC populations. Further studies with a larger population are warranted in order to evaluate the association between smoking status and tumor outcome in low grade Ta NMIBC.

The present study has several limitations. First, it was performed in a retrospective manner with a limited number of patients, thus unknown sources of bias may exist in the findings. However, since we re-reviewed all pathological specimens and reclassified them as absolute low grade tumors, our results represent more reliable data compared to data obtained before re-evaluation. Second, in our database, tumor size/volume was not included routinely because of the inaccuracy of measurements of tumor size by cystoscopic findings. Finally, we did not provide all patients with a single immediate postoperative instillation of chemotherapy within 24 h or any maintenance intravesical therapies, which may have improved the results.

Conclusions

The tumor recurrence rate and WP rate in patients with primary, low grade Ta bladder cancer were 43.2 % and 11.1 %, respectively. Multiple tumor was a risk factor for both tumor recurrence and WP, while IVI did not affect the occurrence of WP. The late recurrence rate and late WP rate were 14.5 % and 6.6 %, respectively. Our results suggest that routine follow-up of patients with low grade Ta bladder cancer is needed up to 10 years from the initial diagnosis.

Competing interests

The authors declare that they have no competing interests.

Authors' contributions

HK, TM and NT formulated database. HK performed the initial analyses and drafted the first manuscript. All authors assisted in the analysis and interpretation of data. EK conceived of the study, and participated in its design and coordination and helped to draft the manuscript. All authors read and approved the final manuscript.

Author details

[1]Department of Urology, Keio University School of Medicine, 35 Shinanomachi, Shinjuku-ku, Tokyo 160-8582, Japan. [2]Division of Diagnostic Pathology, Keio University School of Medicine, 35 Shinanomachi, Shinjuku-ku, Tokyo 160-8582, Japan.

References

1. Greenlee RT, Murray T, Bolden S, Wingo PA: **Cancer statistics, 2000.** *CA Cancer J Clin* 2000, **50**(1):7–33.
2. Hendricksen K, Witjes JA: **Current strategies for first and second line intravesical therapy for nonmuscle invasive bladder cancer.** *Curr Opin Urol* 2007, **17**(5):352–357.
3. Donat SM: **Evaluation and follow-up strategies for superficial bladder cancer.** *Urol Clin North Am* 2003, **30**(4):765–776.
4. MacLennan GT, Kirkali Z, Cheng L: **Histologic grading of noninvasive papillary urothelial neoplasms.** *Eur Urol* 2007, **51**(4):889–897.
5. Epstein JI, Amin MB, Reuter VR, Mostofi FK: **The World Health Organization/International Society of Urological Pathology consensus classification of urothelial (transitional cell) neoplasms of the urinary bladder. Bladder Consensus Conference Committee.** *Am J Surg Pathol* 1998, **22**(12):1435–1448.
6. Holmang S, Strock V: **Should Follow-up Cystoscopy in Bacillus Calmette-Guerin-Treated Patients Continue After Five Tumour-Free Years?** *Eur Urol* 2012, **61**(3):503–507.
7. Matsumoto K, Kikuchi E, Horiguchi Y, Tanaka N, Miyajima A, Nakagawa K, Nakashima J, Oya M: **Late recurrence and progression in non-muscle-invasive bladder cancers after 5-year tumor-free periods.** *Urology* 2010, **75**(6):1385–1390.
8. Zieger K, Wolf H, Olsen PR, Hojgaard K: **Long-term follow-up of noninvasive bladder tumours (stage Ta): recurrence and progression.** *BJU Int* 2000, **85**(7):824–828.
9. Prout GR Jr, Barton BA, Griffin PP, Friedell GH: **Treated history of noninvasive grade 1 transitional cell carcinoma. The National Bladder Cancer Group.** *J Urol* 1992, **148**(5):1413–1419.
10. Akagashi K, Tanda H, Kato S, Ohnishi S, Nakajima H, Nanbu A, Nitta T, Koroku M, Sato Y, Hanzawa T: **Recurrence pattern for superficial bladder cancer.** *Int J Urol* 2006, **13**(6):686–691.
11. Miyamoto H, Brimo F, Schultz L, Ye H, Miller JS, Fajardo DA, Lee TK, Epstein JI, Netto GJ: **Low-grade papillary urothelial carcinoma of the urinary bladder: a clinicopathologic analysis of a post-World Health Organization/International Society of Urological Pathology classification cohort from a single academic center.** *Arch Pathol Lab Med* 2010, **134**(8):1160–1163.
12. Pellucchi F, Freschi M, Ibrahim B, Rocchini L, Maccagnano C, Briganti A, Rigatti P, Montorsi F, Colombo R: **Clinical reliability of the 2004 WHO histological classification system compared with the 1973 WHO system for Ta primary bladder tumors.** *J Urol* 2011, **186**(6):2194–2199.
13. Babjuk M, Burger M, Zigeuner R, Shariat SF, van Rhijn BW, Comperat E, Sylvester RJ, Kaasinen E, Bohle A, Palou Redorta J, *et al*: **EAU guidelines on non-muscle-invasive urothelial carcinoma of the bladder: update 2013.** *Eur Urol* 2013, **64**(4):639–653.
14. Fleshner N, Garland J, Moadel A, Herr H, Ostroff J, Trambert R, O'Sullivan M, Russo P: **Influence of smoking status on the disease-related outcomes of patients with tobacco-associated superficial transitional cell carcinoma of the bladder.** *Cancer* 1999, **86**(11):2337–2345.
15. Lammers RJ, Witjes WP, Hendricksen K, Caris CT, Janzing-Pastors MH, Witjes JA: **Smoking status is a risk factor for recurrence after transurethral resection of non-muscle-invasive bladder cancer.** *Eur Urol* 2011, **60**(4):713–720.
16. Rink M, Furberg H, Zabor EC, Xylinas E, Babjuk M, Pycha A, Lotan Y, Karakiewicz PI, Novara G, Robinson BD, *et al*: **Impact of smoking and smoking cessation on oncologic outcomes in primary non-muscle-invasive bladder cancer.** *Eur Urol* 2013, **63**(4):724–732.

2

Dual-specificity tyrosine phosphorylation-regulated kinase 2 (DYRK2) as a novel marker in T1 high-grade and T2 bladder cancer patients receiving neoadjuvant chemotherapy

Shunichiro Nomura[1*], Yasutomo Suzuki[1], Ryo Takahashi[1], Mika Terasaki[2], Ryoji Kimata[1], Yasuhiro Terasaki[2], Tsutomu Hamasaki[1], Go Kimura[1], Akira Shimizu[2] and Yukihiro Kondo[1]

Abstract

Background: To investigate associations between dual-specificity tyrosine phosphorylation-regulated kinase 2 (DYRK2) expression and survival in T1 high-grade or T2 bladder cancer patients treated with neoadjuvant chemotherapy.

Methods: The cohort under investigation comprised 44 patients who underwent neoadjuvant chemotherapy for pT1 high-grade or pT2N0M0 bladder cancer at our institution between 2002 and 2011. Immunohistochemical analysis was used to determine expression of DYRK2 in bladder cancer specimens obtained by transurethral resection before chemotherapy. Relationships between DYRK2 expression and both response to chemotherapy and survival in these patients were analyzed.

Results: DYRK2 expression was positive in 21 of 44 patients (47.7 %) and negative in 23 patients (52.3 %). In total, 20 of 21 DYRK2-positive cases showed complete response to neoadjuvant chemotherapy, whereas 11 of 23 DYRK2-negative cases did not show complete response. Sensitivity and specificity were 62.5 % and 91.7 %, respectively ($P = 0.0018$). In addition, disease-specific survival rate was significantly higher for DYRK2-positive patients than for DYRK2-negative patients ($P = 0.017$). In multivariate analysis, DYRK2 expression level was identified as an independent prognostic factor for disease-specific survival ($P = 0.029$). We also showed that DYRK2 mRNA expression was significantly higher in DYRK2-positive samples by immunohistochemistry than DYRK2-negative samples ($P = 0.040$).

Conclusions: DYRK2 expression level may predict the efficacy of neoadjuvant chemotherapy for T1 high-grade and T2 bladder cancer.

Keywords: DYRK2, Bladder cancer, Prognostic marker, Chemotherapy

Background

Radical cystectomy is widely performed to treat muscle-invasive bladder cancer. However, radical cystectomy only results in 5-year survival in about 50 % of patients [1–5]. To improve these unsatisfactory results, the use of peri-operative chemotherapy has been explored. More specifically, the benefits of neoadjuvant chemotherapy have been observed in several trials [6–8].

However, some patients with muscle-invasive bladder cancer do not achieve results even from neoadjuvant chemotherapy. To optimize survival, selecting patients with muscle-invasive bladder cancer who are expected to show a good response to neoadjuvant chemotherapy is important. Various pathological factors have been reported as prognostic markers of poor survival in patients with bladder cancer, but are inadequate for predicting survival in bladder cancer patients. Therefore, molecular markers that better predict

* Correspondence: shun1982@nms.ac.jp
[1]Departments of Urology, Nippon Medical School, 1-1-5 Sendagi, Bunkyo-ku, Tokyo 113-8603, Japan
Full list of author information is available at the end of the article

survival in T2 bladder cancer patients treated with neoadjuvant chemotherapy are sorely needed.

Dual-specificity tyrosine phosphorylation-regulated kinases (DYRKs) are a subfamily of protein kinases that catalyze their autophosphorylation on tyrosine residues and the phosphorylation of serine/threonine residues on exogenous substrates [9–11]. DYRKs play key roles in the regulation of cell differentiation, proliferation, and survival [12, 13]. Specifically, DYRK2 is associated with cancer survival. DYRK2 phosphorylates p53 at Ser46 during the apoptotic response to DNA damage, thereby promoting cellular apoptosis after genotoxic stress [14]. The presence of DYRK2 may thus predict response to neoadjuvant chemotherapy that induces DNA damage. This finding led us to hypothesize that DYRK2 might be a novel marker of response to neoadjuvant chemotherapy, including cisplatin, at our institution. The present study therefore examined the association between DYRK2 expression and efficacy of neoadjuvant chemotherapy in clinical practice for patients with T1 high-grade or T2 bladder cancer.

Methods

Patients and samples

The cohort under investigation comprised 44 patients who underwent neoadjuvant chemotherapy for pT1 high-grade or pT2N0M0 bladder cancer at our institution between April 2003 and February 2011. Having been compiled for research purposes, this group represents patients for whom pretreatment, archival paraffin-embedded tissue blocks and data from complete clinical follow-up were available. Diagnostic work-up included initial transurethral resection of bladder tumor (TURBT), pelvic magnetic resonance imaging (MRI), chest and abdominal computed tomography (CT), and bone scintigraphy. Tumors were graded histologically in accordance with World Health Organization (WHO) classifications and were staged as per the TNM staging system of the Union for International Cancer Control (2009). Histological type was urothelial carcinoma in all cases.

Neoadjuvant intra-arterial chemotherapy was performed after complete TURBT, only after the patient consented to therapy based on our recommendation. Written informed consent was obtained from all patients. Anticancer agents administered as neoadjuvant chemotherapy consisted of cisplatin at 100 mg/m^2, methotrexate at 30 mg/m^2, and doxorubicin at 20 mg/m^2. Our therapeutic protocol comprised two courses of neoadjuvant chemotherapy. Following this, a second TURBT was performed to obtain a biopsy specimen. We assessed the efficacy of neoadjuvant chemotherapy using the pathological results of TURBT. Complete response (CR) was defined as T0 (no evidence of tumor), Ta (noninvasive papillary tumor), or Tis (tumor at a site distant from the original tumor), as in RTOG 99–06 [15]. In cases of CR on the second TURBT, the bladder was preserved, while advanced cases and cases with residual invasive bladder tumors were treated by total cystectomy or systemic chemotherapy [16].

After the second TURBT, cystoscopy and urinary cytological examinations were performed every 3 months for 2 years, every 6 months from 3–5 years, and annually thereafter. Chest radiography and pelvic CT were performed every 6 months for 3 years, and annually thereafter. In cases with visible tumors or hyperemic mucosa in the bladder on cystoscopy or pelvic urinary cytological findings, transurethral biopsy was performed to detect disease recurrence.

This study was carried out in accordance with the Declaration of Helsinki and Good Clinical Practice Guidelines. Approval of the protocol was obtained from the Institutional Review Board of Nippon Medical School, Tokyo, Japan.

Immunohistochemical analysis

DYRK2 expression was determined by immunohistochemical (IHC) staining of paraffin-embedded tissue sections from TURBT specimens immediately before neoadjuvant chemotherapy. The 3-μm-thick sections were deparaffinized, rehydrated using xylene and alcohol, and incubated with 0.3 % H_2O_2 to block endogenous peroxidase activity. Before immunostaining, antigen retrieval was performed at 120 °C for 10 min in an autoclave with citrate buffer (pH 6.0). Staining with a polyclonal anti-DYRK2 antibody (AP7534a; dilution, 1:50; Abgent, San Diego, CA, USA) was performed overnight at 4 °C. Histofine Simple Stain Rabbit MAX PO (MULTI; Nichirei, Tokyo, Japan) was used as the secondary antibody in accordance with the manufacturer's instructions. Color was developed using diaminobenzidine with 0.01 % H_2O_2. Hematoxylin was used as a counterstain. Stained tumor tissues were evaluated blindly with respect to clinical patient data. Cytoplasmic staining was considered positive, and staining intensity was scored as 0, 1, 2, or 3, corresponding to no staining, weak, moderate, and strong intensities, respectively (Fig. 1). Percentage scores of cells showing cytoplasmic staining were also counted (0–100 %). Total histochemical score (H-score) was calculated by multiplying the intensity score by the percentage score (0–300). An H-score higher than the median was considered positive. Negative controls were incubated without the primary antibody.

Analysis of real-time quantitative reverse-transcriptase polymerase chain reaction

Total RNA from formalin-fixed paraffin-embedded tissues was isolated using an Allprep DNA/RNA kit (Qiagen, Tokyo, Japan). The quantity and quality of RNA were evaluated by spectrophotometry. Reverse transcription of RNA to cDNA was achieved using a

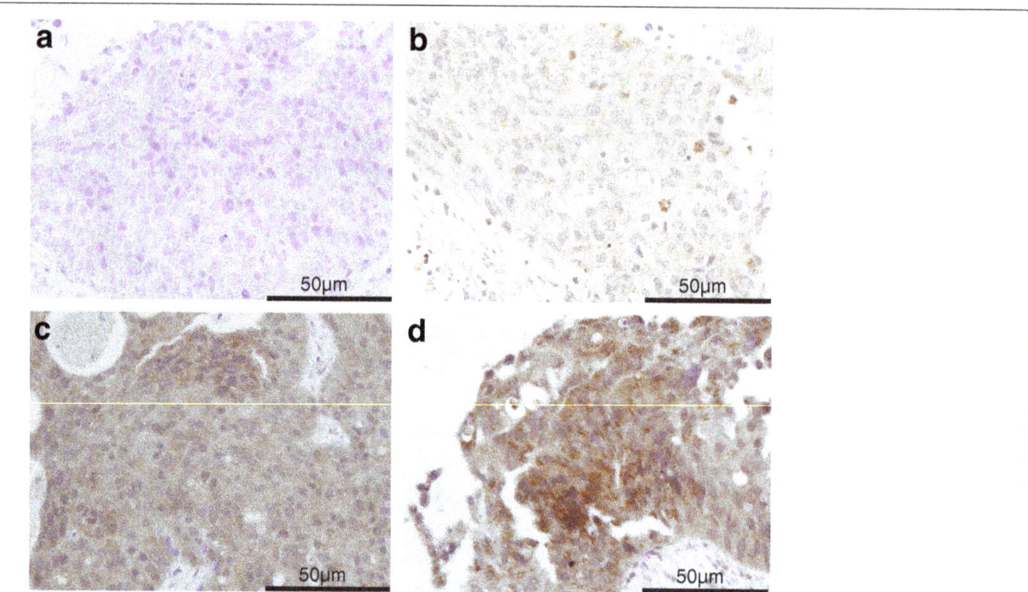

Fig. 1 Immunohistochemical staining of paraffin-embedded sections immediately before neoadjuvant chemotherapy with an anti-DYRK2 antibody. DYRK2 protein expression was localized within the cytoplasm. Magnification × 600. **a** DYRK2-negative staining pattern (no staining: score 0). **b** DYRK2-negative staining pattern (weak: score 1). **c** DYRK2-positive staining pattern (moderate: score 2). **d** DYRK2-positive staining pattern (strong: score 3)

High-Capacity cDNA Reverse Transcription kit (Applied Biosystems, Foster City, CA, USA). Quantitative gene expression was determined for DYRK2 (Hs00705109_s1) and 18 s (Hs03928990_g1) using gene-specific probes (Applied Biosystems) using TaqMan Fast Advanced Master Mix and the 7900HT Fast Real-time PCR system (Applied Biosystems). PCR conditions were: 5 °C for 2 min and 95 °C for 20 s, followed by 45 cycles at 95 °C for 1 s and 60 °C for 20 s. Data were then quantified using the comparative Ct method for relative gene expression compared with 18S as an endogenous control.

Statistical analysis

Associations between DYRK2 expression and clinicopathological factors were analyzed using the Fisher's exact test. Disease-specific survival rates were calculated using the Kaplan–Meier method and differences in survival among groups were compared using log-rank testing. We used Cox proportional hazards regression analysis to assess DYRK2 expression and sex for disease-specific survival. Differences in DYRK2 mRNA between DYRK2-positive and -negative tumors by IHC analysis were determined using the paired *t*-test. *P*-values < 0.05 were considered statistically significant. All statistical analyses were performed using SPSS version 21.0 statistical software (IBM Corp, Armonk, NY, USA).

Results

Patient characteristics

Baseline characteristics for all 44 patients are shown in Table 1. The mean age of patients at first TURBT was 70 years (range, 43–84 years) and only eight patients were female. Of the 44 patients, 14 (32 %) showed pT1 high-grade and 30 (68 %) had pT2. Cystectomy was performed after intra-arterial chemotherapy in four patients (9.1 %). With a median follow-up of 47 months, the 5-year survival rate was 82.7 % for all patients. At the time of analysis, 36 patients (81.8 %) were alive and 8 patients (18.2 %) had died of bladder cancer. Overall and disease-specific survival were thus similar.

Immunohistochemical assessment of DYRK2 expression

DYRK2 was localized in the cytoplasm of bladder tumor cells. Representative cases for the different staining levels (0, 1, 2, and 3) are presented in Fig. 1. Median H-score was 10 (range, 0–230). Therefore, tumors with H-score >10 were deemed DYRK2-positive. Twenty-three specimens (52.3 %) showed low DYRK2 expression, whereas 21 specimens showed high expression (47.7 %).

The relationship between DYRK2 expression and clinicopathological factors is summarized in Table 1. No significant association was observed between DYRK2 expression and the following clinicopathological factors: age, sex, pathological T stage, histological grade, concurrent CIS, or lymphovascular invasion (*P* > 0.05).

Table 1 Clinicopathological factors of bladder cancer and associations with DYRK2 expression

	Patients (%)	DYRK2 expression		
		Negative	Positive	P
All patients	44	23	21	
Age				0.35
<70 years	17 (39 %)	7	11	
≥70 years	27 (61 %)	16	10	
Sex				0.70
Male	36 (82 %)	18	18	
Female	8 (18 %)	5	3	
Pathological T stage				0.27
1	14 (32 %)	5	9	
2a	20 (46 %)	11	9	
2b	10 (23 %)	7	3	
Histological grade				
Low	3 (7 %)	1	2	0.60
High	41 (93 %)	22	19	
Concurrent CIS				0.23
Yes	7 (16 %)	2	5	
No	37 (84 %)	21	16	
Lymphovascular invasion				1.00
Yes	3 (7 %)	2	1	
No	41 (93 %)	21	20	

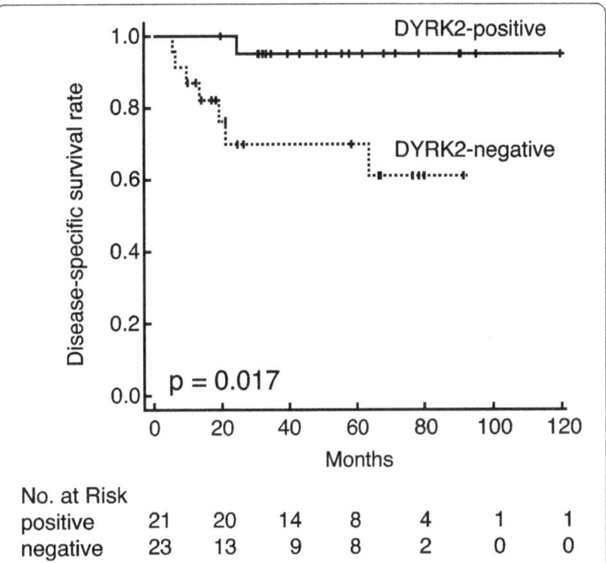

Fig. 2 Kaplan–Meier survival analysis in patients positive and negative for DYRK2 expression. Differences in disease-specific survival between subgroups were analyzed by log-rank test. Disease-specific survival was significantly longer for DYRK2-positive patients than for DYRK2-negative patients ($P = 0.017$)

DYRK2 expression and response to Neoadjuvant chemotherapy

Overall, 20 of the 21 DYRK2-positive cases showed CR after neoadjuvant chemotherapy, whereas 11 of the 23 DYRK2-negative cases showed non-CR. The efficacy of neoadjuvant chemotherapy as determined by DYRK2 expression had a sensitivity of 62.5 % and specificity of 91.7 % ($P = 0.0018$, Table 2).

DYRK2 expression and survival

Disease-specific survival was significantly longer for DYRK2-positive patients than for DYRK2-negative patients ($P = 0.017$; Fig. 2). In T2 bladder cancer patients only, DYRK2 expression was associated with increased disease-specific survival ($P = 0.036$). In T1 high-grade bladder cancer patients only, no significant association was observed between DYRK2 expression and disease-specific survival ($P = 0.157$).

Multivariate analysis was performed to evaluate the influence of DYRK2 on disease-specific survival after adjusting for possible confounding factors. From the results shown in Table 1, no clinicopathological factors were significantly correlated with DYRK2. From the results of the univariate analysis, however, DYRK2 and sex significantly correlated with disease-specific survival. Therefore, only DYRK2 and sex were included in the Cox proportional hazards model. DYRK2 expression remained statistically significant ($P = 0.029$), and the hazard ratio (HR) was 11.5 (95 % confidence interval [CI]: 1.29–102; Table 3).

Table 2 DYRK2 immunohistochemical staining and clinical response (Fisher's exact test: $P = 0.0018$)

DYRK2	Clinical response	
Immunoreactive	CR	Non-CR
Positive	20	1
Negative	12	11

CR complete response

DYRK2 mRNA expression in bladder cancer tissue

DYRK2 mRNA expression was assessed in 39 samples. We detected levels of DYRK2 mRNA in DYRK2-positive and DYRK2-negative samples by IHC analysis. Relative mRNA levels of the DYRK2 gene (DYRK2 per 18S, mean ± standard deviation) differed significantly between DYRK2-positive (mRNA 3.82 ± 2.10) and DYRK2-negative patients (mRNA 2.65 ± 1.23). Paired *t*-test showed that mRNA levels were significantly higher in DYRK2-positive patients than in DYRK2-negative patients ($P = 0.040$; Fig. 3).

Discussion

The present study revealed a significant association between DYRK2 expression and efficacy of neoadjuvant

Table 3 Univariate and multivariate analysis for disease-specific survival

	Disease-specific survival		
	Univariate analysis	Multivariate analysis	
Characteristics	*P*	HR (95 % CI)	*P*
Age (<70 years vs. ≥70 years)	0.37		
Sex (male vs. female)	0.034	0.15 (0.03-0.79)	0.025
Pathological T stage (T1 vs. T2)	0.18		
Histological grade (low vs. high)	0.38		
Concurrent CIS (Yes vs. No)	0.18		
Lymphovascular invasion (Yes vs. No)	0.35		
DYRK2 expression (positive vs. negative)	0.017	11.5 (1.29-102)	0.029

chemotherapy for T1 high-grade and T2 bladder cancer patients. High levels of DYRK2 expression was associated with increased disease-specific survival time in T1 high-grade and T2 bladder cancer patients treated with neoadjuvant chemotherapy. In multivariate analysis, DYRK2 expression levels emerged as independent prognostic markers of survival. DYRK2 may therefore predict prognosis independent of common prognostic factors, such as clinical T stage and histological grade. Moreover, we showed that DYRK2 mRNA expression was significantly higher in DYRK2-positive samples by IHC than DYRK2-negative samples.

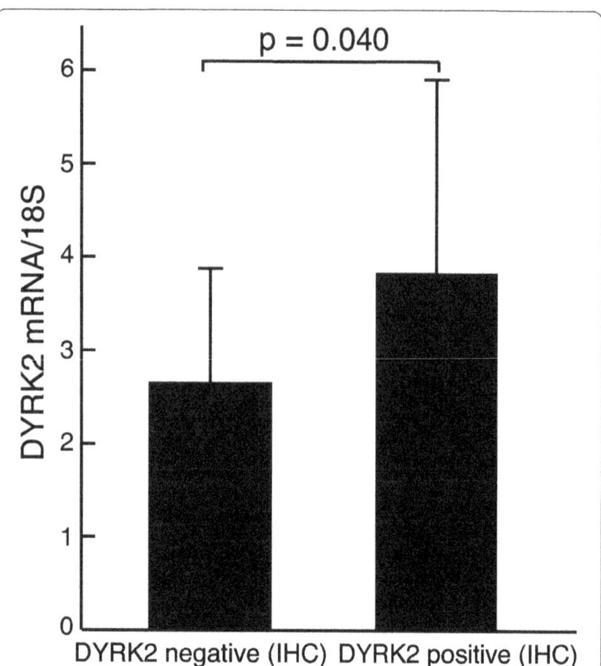

Fig. 3 Relative levels of DYRK2 mRNA in DYRK2-positive and -negative cases by IHC analysis. DYRK2 mRNA levels were significantly higher in DYRK2-positive patients than in DYRK2-negative patients ($P = 0.040$)

DYRK2 is an important factor in cellular apoptosis after genotoxic stress. Taira et al. reported that knock down of DYRK2 function attenuates the apoptosis elicited by DNA damage induced by doxorubicin in vitro [14]. Yamashita et al. reported that DYRK2 may predict progression-free survival in patients with recurrent non-small-cell lung cancer treated using platinum-based chemotherapy [17]. DYRK2 can thus predict response to different chemotherapies, including doxorubicin and cisplatin. As our regimen includes both cisplatin and doxorubicin, DYRK2 may therefore be a useful marker of sensitivity to neoadjuvant chemotherapy at our institution. Furthermore, one of the most popular neoadjuvant chemotherapy regimens includes methotrexate, vinblastine, doxorubicin, and cisplatin (M-VAC), while another popular neoadjuvant chemotherapy regimen consists of gemcitabine and cisplatin (GC). Thus, DYRK2 may predict response to M-VAC and GC. Therefore, trials with M-VAC and GC are needed to confirm this hypothesis.

Few genetic markers have been confirmed to predict survival in bladder cancer patients treated with chemotherapy. Bellmunt et al. reported that excision repair cross-complementing 1 (ERCC1) gene expression may predict survival in patients with bladder cancer treated with platinum-based therapy [18]. Moreover, Font et al. reported that bladder cancer susceptibility 1 (BRCA1) gene expression may predict the efficacy of cisplatin-based neoadjuvant chemotherapy [19]. Finally, Hoffmann et al. reported that high multidrug resistance 1 (MDR1) gene expression was associated with inferior outcomes after cisplatin-based adjuvant chemotherapy for locally advanced bladder cancer [20]. We have also previously reported that Snail expression may predict poor outcomes in bladder cancer patients treated with neoadjuvant chemotherapy [21]. Thus, Use of ERCC1, MDR1, BRCA1, and Snail in combination with DYRK2 may further improve the accuracy of predicting survival in bladder cancer patients treated with neoadjuvant chemotherapy.

We have previously reported that CYFRA 21–1 may be a useful marker for monitoring neoadjuvant chemotherapy [16]. However, this marker cannot predict the efficacy of neoadjuvant chemotherapy prior to administration. The results of the present study indicate that DYRK2 can help identify patients with T1 high-grade and T2 bladder cancer that will respond to neoadjuvant chemotherapy. Therefore, a selective approach using this information could result in patients with high DYRK2 expression receiving neoadjuvant chemotherapy, while those with low DYRK2 expression would undergo radical cystectomy. Prospective studies applying this approach are needed in the future.

In T2 bladder cancer patients only, DYRK2 expression was associated with increased disease-specific survival time ($P = 0.036$). However, no significant association was observed between DYRK2 expression and disease-specific survival in only T1 high-grade bladder cancer patients ($P = 0.157$). However, a trend toward longer disease-specific survival was observed. Further studies with a large cohort of T1 high-grade bladder cancer patients are warranted to confirm this result.

One limitation of the present study is that we have not shown a direct role of DYRK2 in bladder cancer. However, our DYRK2 staining results with clinical samples suggest that the abundance of DYRK2 is associated with the response to neoadjuvant chemotherapy. Other limitations of this study include that the sample size for DYRK2 immunohistochemical analysis was very small, the study was retrospective, and our regimen does not represent standard chemotherapy. More detailed studies are needed to address these limitations.

Conclusions

Although the sample size of this study was small, our results indicate that DYRK2 might represent a new molecular marker for predicting the efficacy of neoadjuvant chemotherapy in T1 high-grade and T2 bladder cancer. Further careful study is needed to confirm our preliminary results.

Abbreviations

CI: Confidence interval; RTOG: Radiation Therapy Oncology Group; CIS: Carcinoma *in situ*.

Competing interests

The authors declare that they have no competing interests.

Authors' contributions

SN evaluated immunohistochemical staining, performed the statistical analyses, and drafted the manuscript. YS assisted with the statistical analysis and helped draft the manuscript. RT collected clinical data and revised the manuscript. MT participated in the data interpretation and revision of the manuscript. RK performed data acquisition. YT revised the manuscript. TH revised the manuscript. GK conceived the study, evaluated the immunohistochemistry, and helped draft the manuscript. AS performed data acquisition. YK participated in the study conception and design, data analysis, interpretation, drafting, and final approval of the manuscript. All authors have read and approved the final manuscript.

Acknowledgments

Takashi Arai, Kyoko Wakamatsu, and Naomi Kuwabara provided technical support.

Author details

[1]Departments of Urology, Nippon Medical School, 1-1-5 Sendagi, Bunkyo-ku, Tokyo 113-8603, Japan. [2]Analytic Human Pathology, Nippon Medical School, 1-1-5 Sendagi, Bunkyo-ku, Tokyo 113-8603, Japan.

References

1. Bassi P, Ferrante GD, Piazza N, Spinadin R, Carando R, Pappagallo G, et al. Prognostic factors of outcome after radical cystectomy for bladder cancer: a retrospective study of a homogeneous patient cohort. J Urol. 1999;161(5):1494–7.
2. Dalbagni G, Genega E, Hashibe M, Zhang ZF, Russo P, Herr H, et al. Cystectomy for bladder cancer: a contemporary series. J Urol. 2001;165(4):1111–6.
3. Ghoneim MA, el-Mekresh MM, el-Baz MA, el-Attar IA, Ashamallah A. Radical cystectomy for carcinoma of the bladder: critical evaluation of the results in 1,026 cases. J Urol. 1997;158(2):393–9.
4. Stein JP, Lieskovsky G, Cote R, Groshen S, Feng AC, Boyd S, et al. Radical cystectomy in the treatment of invasive bladder cancer: long-term results in 1,054 patients. J Clin Oncol. 2001;19(3):666–75.
5. Stein JP, Skinner DG. Radical cystectomy for invasive bladder cancer: long-term results of a standard procedure. World J Urol. 2006;24(3):296–304.
6. Grossman HB, Natale RB, Tangen CM, Speights VO, Vogelzang NJ, Trump DL, et al. Neoadjuvant chemotherapy plus cystectomy compared with cystectomy alone for locally advanced bladder cancer. The New England Journal of Medicine. 2003;349(9):859–66.
7. Sherif A, Holmberg L, Rintala E, Mestad O, Nilsson J, Nilsson S, et al. Neoadjuvant cisplatinum based combination chemotherapy in patients with invasive bladder cancer: a combined analysis of two Nordic studies. European Urology. 2004;45(3):297–303.
8. Winquist E, Kirchner TS, Segal R, Chin J, Lukka H. Neoadjuvant chemotherapy for transitional cell carcinoma of the bladder: a systematic review and meta-analysis. J Urol. 2004;171(2 Pt 1):561–9.
9. Becker W, Joost HG. Structural and functional characteristics of Dyrk, a novel subfamily of protein kinases with dual specificity. Progress in Nucleic Acid Research and Molecular Biology. 1999;62:1–17.
10. Campbell LE, Proud CG. Differing substrate specificities of members of the DYRK family of arginine-directed protein kinases. FEBS Lett. 2002;510(1–2):31–6.
11. Himpel S, Panzer P, Eirmbter K, Czajkowska H, Sayed M, Packman LC, et al. Identification of the autophosphorylation sites and characterization of their effects in the protein kinase DYRK1A. The Biochemical Journal. 2001;359 (Pt 3):497–505.
12. Aranda S, Laguna A, de la Luna S. DYRK family of protein kinases: evolutionary relationships, biochemical properties, and functional roles. FASEB J. 2011;25(2):449–62.
13. Park J, Song WJ, Chung KC. Function and regulation of Dyrk1A: towards understanding Down syndrome. Cell Mol Life Sci. 2009;66(20):3235–40.
14. Taira N, Nihira K, Yamaguchi T, Miki Y, Yoshida K. DYRK2 is targeted to the nucleus and controls p53 via Ser46 phosphorylation in the apoptotic response to DNA damage. Mol Cell. 2007;25(5):725–38.
15. Kaufman DS, Winter KA, Shipley WU, Heney NM, Wallace 3rd HJ, Toonkel LM, et al. Phase I-II RTOG study (99–06) of patients with muscle-invasive bladder cancer undergoing transurethral surgery, paclitaxel, cisplatin, and twice-daily radiotherapy followed by selective bladder preservation or radical cystectomy and adjuvant chemotherapy. Urology. 2009;73(4):833–7.
16. Takahashi R, Kimata R, Nomura S, Matsuzawa I, Suzuki Y, Hamasaki T, et al. The role of serum cytokeratin 19 fragment in transarterial infusion against invasive bladder cancer. Open J Urol. 2013;3(3):160–4.
17. Yamashita S, Chujo M, Moroga T, Anami K, Tokuishi K, Miyawaki M, et al. DYRK2 expression may be a predictive marker for chemotherapy in non-small cell lung cancer. Anticancer Res. 2009;29(7):2753–7.
18. Bellmunt J, Paz-Ares L, Cuello M, Cecere FL, Albiol S, Guillem V, et al. Gene expression of ERCC1 as a novel prognostic marker in advanced bladder cancer patients receiving cisplatin-based chemotherapy. Ann Oncol. 2007;18(3):522–8.
19. Font A, Taron M, Gago JL, Costa C, Sanchez JJ, Carrato C, et al. BRCA1 mRNA expression and outcome to neoadjuvant cisplatin-based chemotherapy in bladder cancer. Annals Oncol. 2011;22(1):139–44.
20. Hoffmann AC, Wild P, Leicht C, Bertz S, Danenberg KD, Danenberg PV, et al. MDR1 and ERCC1 expression predict outcome of patients with locally advanced bladder cancer receiving adjuvant chemotherapy. Neoplasia (New York, NY). 2010;12(8):628–36.
21. Nomura S, Suzuki Y, Takahashi R, Terasaki M, Kimata R, Hamasaki T, et al. Snail expression and outcome in T1 high-grade and T2 bladder cancer: a retrospective immunohistochemical analysis. BMC Urol. 2013;13(1):73.

Expression of parathyroid hormone/parathyroid hormone-related peptide receptor 1 in normal and diseased bladder detrusor muscles

Nobuyuki Nishikawa[1,2], Rie Yago[3], Yuichiro Yamazaki[4], Hiromitsu Negoro[1], Mari Suzuki[3], Masaaki Imamura[1,5], Yoshinobu Toda[6], Kazunari Tanabe[3], Osamu Ogawa[1] and Akihiro Kanematsu[7*]

Abstract

Background: To investigate the expression of parathyroid hormone (PTH)/PTH-related peptide (PTHrP) receptor 1 (PTH1R) in clinical specimens of normal and diseased bladders. PTHrP is a unique stretch-induced endogenous detrusor relaxant that functions via PTH1R. We hypothesized that suppression of this axis could be involved in the pathogenesis of bladder disease.

Methods: PTH1R expression in clinical samples was examined by immunohistochemistry. Normal kidney tissue from a patient with renal cancer and bladder specimens from patients undergoing ureteral reimplantation for vesicoureteral reflux or partial cystectomy for urachal cyst were examined as normal control organs. These were compared with 13 diseased bladder specimens from patients undergoing bladder augmentation. The augmentation patients ranged from 8 to 31 years old (median 15 years), including 9 males and 4 females. Seven patients had spinal disorders, 3 had posterior urethral valves and 3 non-neurogenic neurogenic bladders (Hinman syndrome).

Results: Renal tubules, detrusor muscle and blood vessels in normal control bladders stained positive for PTH1R. According to preoperative urodynamic studies of augmentation patients, the median percent bladder capacity compared with the age-standard was 43.6% (range 1.5–86.6%), median intravesical pressure at maximal capacity was 30 cmH_2O (range 10–107 cmH_2O), and median compliance was 3.93 ml/cmH_2O (range 0.05–30.3 ml/cmH_2O). Detrusor overactivity was observed in five cases (38.5%). All augmented bladders showed negative stainings in PTH1R expression in the detrusor tissue, but positive staining of blood vessels in majority of the cases.

Conclusions: Downregulation of PTH1R may be involved in the pathogenesis of human end-stage bladder disease requiring augmentation.

Keywords: Parathyroid hormone-related peptide, Parathyroid hormone 1 receptor, Bladder compliance, Smooth muscle

Background

Relaxation of the detrusor muscle is a fundamental requirement for normal bladder storage function. Severe failure of this relaxation mechanism causes upper urinary tract deterioration as a result of abnormal elevation of intravesical pressure [1]. Such extreme pathology is termed low-compliance bladder, and is typically seen in paediatric cases with congenital spinal disorders, posterior urethral valves, and also in rare forms of severe non-neurogenic neurogenic bladder (Hinman syndrome). The primary goal in treating such patients is to prevent urinary tract damage by maintaining low-pressure storage and effective bladder evacuation [2]. This is usually achieved through medical therapy using antimuscarinic drugs combined with clean intermittent catheterization. However,

* Correspondence: aqui@hyo-med.ac.jp
[7]Department of Urology, Hyogo College of Medicine, Nishinomiya, Japan
Full list of author information is available at the end of the article

if these conservative therapies fail, bladder augmentation using the digestive tract is indicated, though such surgery may lead to various long-term complications, including metabolic acidosis, bowel dysfunction, rupture, and risk of secondary malignancies [3,4]. However, despite these clinical problems, the molecular mechanisms underlying low-compliance end-stage bladder disease have not yet been thoroughly investigated [4].

Parathyroid hormone-related peptide (PTHrP) was originally identified as a cause of hypercalcemia in paraneoplastic syndrome, [5] and has since been found to be expressed in most systemic tissues, with diverse physiological roles [6,7]. We previously reported that PTHrP acted as a stretch-induced endogenous relaxant of detrusor muscle [8]. PTHrP functions via the PTH/PTHrP receptor 1 (PTH1R), which is expressed in detrusor muscle but not in urothelium. In rat experiments, PTHrP peptide potently suppressed spontaneous contraction of detrusor muscle strips, and intravenous administration of PTHrP peptide increased bladder compliance [8]. These results suggest that endogenous PTHrP may inhibit the abnormal decrease in bladder compliance by bladder distention. We hypothesized that PTH1R should also be expressed in human bladder detrusor muscle, and that suppression of this axis could be involved in the pathogenesis of end-stage low-compliance bladder.

In this study, we therefore investigated the expression of PTH1R in clinical specimens from patients with normally functioning bladder and those undergoing bladder augmentations, to explore the involvement of the PTHrP-PTH1R axis in normal and diseased bladder detrusor muscle.

Methods

Clinical specimens

This study was authorized by the Institutional Review Board of Kyoto University (G279) and Tokyo Women's Medical University (2089), and written informed consents for participation in the study were obtained from participants or parents. Normal kidney tissue, as a positive control of PTH1R, was obtained from a nephrectomy specimen from a patient with renal cell carcinoma without paraneoplastic hypercalcemia, and was used as a positive control for the staining procedure. Bladder specimens were obtained from the bladder dome by sagittal section in following patients. In total, 3 normal control bladder tissues were obtained during cystotomy for ureteral reimplantation for vesicoureteral reflux in two patients, and partial cystectomy for urachal cyst in one patient, who all underwent surgery at the Department of Urology, Kyoto University Hospital. These three patients had no symptoms of abnormal bladder storage or emptying. The clinical backgrounds of the control patients are summarized in Table 1. Data are expressed as mean ± S.D.

In total, 13 diseased bladder tissues were obtained from patients who underwent bladder augmentation at the Department of Urology, Tokyo Women's Medical University. The clinical backgrounds of the patients are summarized in Table 2. The median age of the patients was 15 years (range 8–31 years, mean 17.8 ± 8.8 years), and included 9 males and 4 females. Seven patients had spinal disorders, three had posterior urethral valves and three had Hinman syndrome. All the patients underwent preoperative urodynamic studies combined with cystography. Bladder augmentation was indicated for low-compliance bladder and/or incontinence, despite aggressive anti-cholinergic regimens. The bladder capacity was presented as the percentage of the reported age-standard capacity for Japanese children, calculated by the formula 25 × (age in years + 2) for patients younger than 12 years, and 350 ml was defined as 100% for patients older than 12 years [9].

Immunohistochemistry

The specimens were fixed in formalin and paraffin-embedded. Sections were mounted on glass slides and used for immunohistochemical detection of PTH1R. Incubation and washing procedures were carried out at room temperature, unless otherwise specified. Deparaffinization and antigen retrieval were carried out in a microwave, as described previously, [10] and endogenous peroxidase activity was then blocked with 0.3% H_2O_2 in methyl alcohol for 30 min. The glass slides were washed six times in phosphate-buffered saline (PBS) for 5 min each, and mounted with 1% horse normal serum in PBS for 30 min for pre-blocking. Primary antibody against PTH1R (3D1.1, Santa Cruz Biotechnology, Dallas, TX, USA; 1:100) was then applied overnight at 4°C, followed by incubation with biotinylated horse anti-mouse serum (second antibody) (ABC-Elite, Vector Laboratories, Burlingame, CA, USA) diluted 1:300 in PBS for 40 min, followed by six washes in PBS (5 min each). Avidin-biotin-peroxidase complex (ABC-Elite, Vector Laboratories, Burlingame, CA) was applied for 50 min at a dilution of 1:100 in bovine serum albumin. After washing six times in PBS (5 min each), a coloring reaction was carried out using diaminobenzidine, with a uniform reaction time for all specimens. Nuclei were counterstained with haematoxylin. PTH1R protein-expression intensity was classified as negative or positive by two independent examiners, with reference to renal tubules as a positive immunostaining control.

Results

Immunostaining study with PTH1R of a kidney and normal control bladders

In the kidney specimen, the tubules stained positive for PTH1R, in contrast to the glomeruli, which stained faint, as reported previously (Figure 1A) [11]. In the normal

Table 1 Clinical background and immunostaining result of the control tissue

Sample	Underlying disease	Gender	Age	IHC-PTH1R	
				Detrusor	Blood vessels
Normal Kidney	Renal Cell Carcinoma	M	54	N/A	+
Normal bladder-1	Urachal cyst	F	57	+	+
Normal bladder-2	Vesicoureteral reflux	F	1	+	+
Normal bladder-3	Vesicoureteral reflux	F	12	+	+

IHC, immunohistochemistry.

control bladder specimens, both the detrusor tissue and blood vessel stained positive for PTH1R. Staining in the detrusor tissue was mainly observed in the cytosol (Figure 1B).

Preoperative urodynamic study

Preoperative urodynamic study revealed that the bladders in all patients undergoing bladder augmentation had deteriorated storage function. The median bladder capacity was 146 ml (range 5–303 ml, mean 153.6 ± 84.0 ml), median percent capacity of age-standard was 43.6% (range 1.5–86.6%, mean 46.9 ± 23.2%), median intravesical pressure at maximal capacity was 30 cmH_2O (range 10–107 cmH_2O, mean 38.8 ± 23.3cmH_2O), and the median compliance was 3.93 ml/cmH_2O (range 0.05–30.3 ml/cmH_2O, mean 6.6 ± 7.8 ml/cmH_2O). Detrusor overactivities were noted in five patients and vesicoureteral reflux in eight patients (Table 2).

Immunostaining study with PTH1R of low compliance bladder

All of the bladder-augmentation specimens showed negative PTH1R staining in detrusor smooth muscle cells in the bladder wall, in contrast to the positive staining seen in normal control bladder specimen. However, blood vessels stained positive for PTH1R in seven out of 13 augmentation cases (53.8%), indicating that the negative staining was not the result of a technical failure, but rather reflected downregulation of PTH1R expression in these bladders (Figure 2).

Discussion

This paper demonstrated the expression of PTH1R in normal bladder tissue and its downregulation in end-stage low-compliance bladders requiring augmentation. Combined with the potent relaxant effect of PTHrP peptide in rat bladder reported in our previous study, [8] these findings suggest the functional involvement of this axis in normal human bladder physiology, and its loss in severely diseased bladders with decreased compliance.

The relaxant effect of PTHrP in the bladder has been reported previously [12,13] Yamamoto et al. focused on stretch-induced upregulation of PTHrP in the bladder in vivo, [12] which effect was replicated in cultured smooth muscle cells under stretch by Steers et al [13]. However, PTHrP showed only modest suppression of carbachol-induced contraction of bladder strips in those

Table 2 Clinical background and staining results of the diseased bladder

	Gender	Age	Maximal Bladder Capacity		Intravesical Pressure at Maximal Capacity (cmH_2O)	Compliance (ml/cmH_2O)	DO	VUR	Leak Point Pressure (cmH_2O)	IHC-PTH1R	
			Maximal Capacity (ml)	Percent capacity of age standard						Detrusor	Blood vessels
Myelomeningocele-1	M	14	60	17.1	40	1.5	-	-	Incontinent	-	-
Myelomeningocele-2	F	15	117	33.4	53	2.21	-	+	>60	-	+
Myelomeningocele-3	M	20	250	71.4	24	10.4	-	-	25	-	-
Myelomeningocele-4	F	27	147	42.0	30	4.9	-	+	22.5	-	-
Myelomeningocele-5	F	29	212	60.6	23	9.22	+	+	25	-	-
Sacral agenesis-1	M	30	146	41.7	30	4.87	-	+	NA	-	+
Sacral agenesis-2	F	31	266	76.0	30	8.87	-	+	NA	-	-
Posterior urethral valve-1	M	8	109	43.6	47	2.32	-	-	>40	-	+
Posterior urethral valve-2	M	10	147	49.0	40	3.68	-	+	>40	-	+
Posterior urethral valve-3	M	11	5	1.5	107	0.05	+	-	NA	-	-
Hinman syndrome-1	M	8	118	47.2	30	3.93	+	+	>60	-	+
Hinman syndrome-2	M	10	117	39.0	40	2.93	+	-	Incontinent	-	+
Hinman syndrome-3	M	18	303	86.6	10	30.3	+	+	NA	-	+

DO, detrusor overactivity; VUR, vesicouteral reflux; IHC, immunohistochemistry.

A Normal kidney
Normal kidney
B Normal bladder
Normal bladder-1
Normal bladder-2
Normal bladder-3

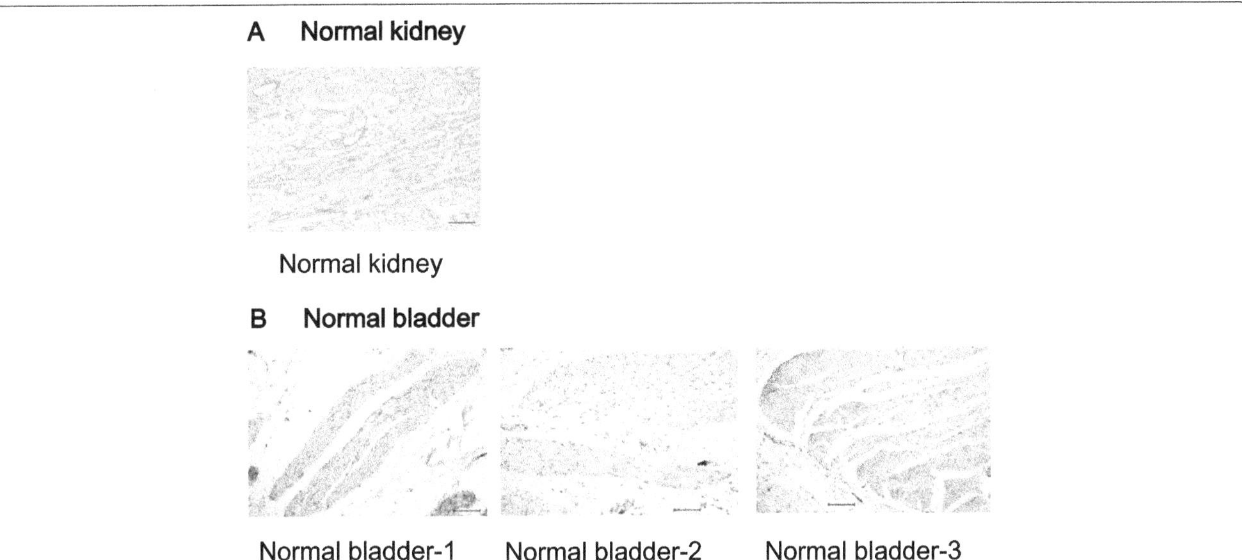

Figure 1 PTH1R immunohistochemical staining of normal kidney tissue and normal control bladder detrusor tissues. (A) Renal tubules were positively stained, in contrast to faint staining in glomeruli. **(B)** Cytoplasm of normal bladder detrusor muscle cells and blood vessels showed positive staining with PTH1R antibody. Scale bar: 100 μm.

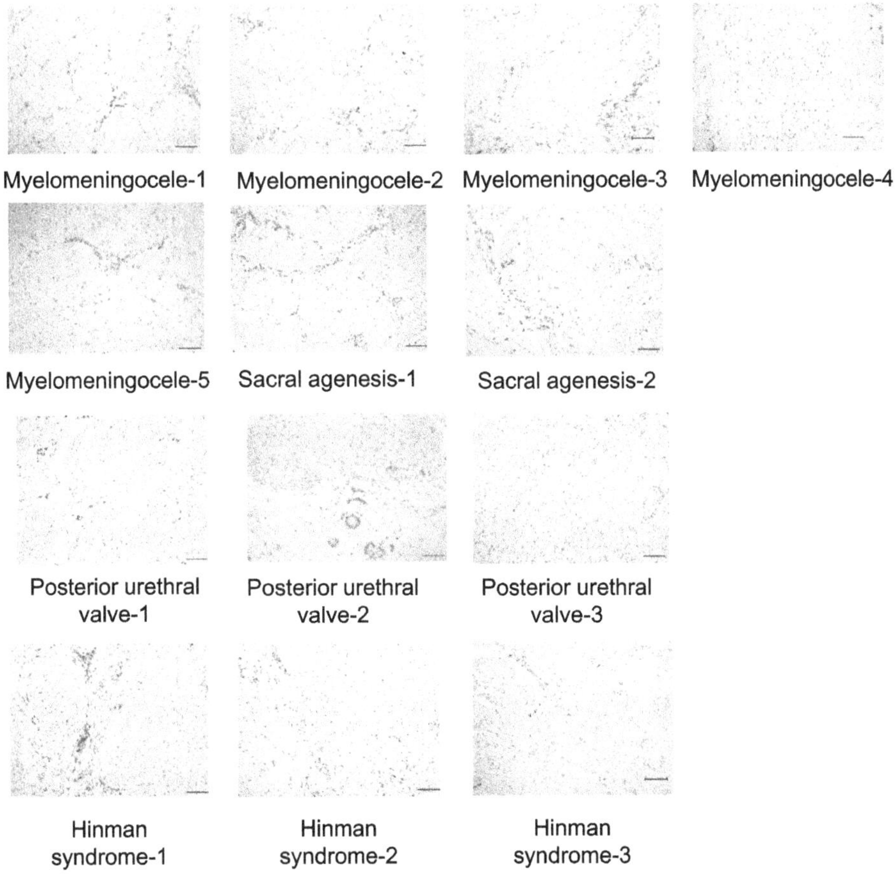

Myelomeningocele-1
Myelomeningocele-2
Myelomeningocele-3
Myelomeningocele-4
Myelomeningocele-5
Sacral agenesis-1
Sacral agenesis-2
Posterior urethral valve-1
Posterior urethral valve-2
Posterior urethral valve-3
Hinman syndrome-1
Hinman syndrome-2
Hinman syndrome-3

Figure 2 PTH1R immunohistochemical staining of diseased bladder detrusor tissues. All diseased bladder detrusor tissues showed negative staining with PTH1R antibody, regardless of the underlying diseases, but positive staining of blood vessels was retained in many specimens. Scale bar: 100 μm.

studies, leaving the physiological relevance of this observation unanswered. In contrast, our recent study in rats showed a potent relaxant effect of PTHrP in suppressing the spontaneous contraction of detrusor strips, and thus increasing bladder compliance in vivo [8]. Our study also demonstrated that PTH1R was expressed primarily in the muscle layer, and not in the urothelial layer. As a logical extension of this previous study, we investigated the expression of PTH1R in the human bladder, and this report supplements and advances the previous study, by investigating the clinical relevance of this axis utilizing human samples.

Detrusor muscle tissues in normal control bladders stained positive for PTH1R, especially in the cytosol. This result seems to contradict the fact that PTH1R is a membrane-anchored G protein-coupled receptor, [14] allowing binding of PTHrP at the membrane surface. However, PTH1R translocation from the plasma membrane into the cytosol after incubation with the PTH1R agonist, PTH (1–34), and positive staining in the cytosol was also seen in other organs such as acinar cells of the prostate gland, cell clusters within the adrenal cortex and cells of the epithelial hair sheath [11].

In sharp contrast, the detrusor muscle in augmented bladders showed negative staining for PTH1R. This lack of staining did not indicate a technical failure, given that blood vessels stained positively in seven out of 13 (53.8%) cases. The negative staining of vessels in the remaining six cases may have been associated with deterioration of the vessels themselves, or technical failure caused by different fixation conditions. If PTH1R is downregulated in these bladders, they may not be able to respond to endogenous PTHrP, which could function as a protective relaxant against excessive distention. Downregulation of PTH1R is thus consistent with low bladder compliance.

In regard of the functional effect in PTHrP-PTH1R axis in the bladder, not only the receptor PTH1R, but expression level of the ligand PTHrP, in normal and diseased bladder is also of a great interest. Perez-Martinez et al. reported about PTHrP immunostaining in rabbit bladder outlet obstruction model [15]. However, we did not succeed in visualizing PTHrP signal in paraffin-embedded human bladder, nor in rat bladder under various fixation conditions. Therefore we did not focus on expression of PTHrP in this study.

Further physiological experiments would have been ideal to confirm these speculations, demonstrating the unresponsiveness of diseased bladder strips to PTHrP peptide. Similarly, it may be of interest whether the difference in expression level of PTH1R may be attributed to altered production, degradation, release, or removal. Unfortunately, it was practically impossible to obtain materials at the separate time of surgery and subsequently perform physiological experiment or obtain enough materials for various biochemical assays. Such mechanistic part should be better studied in experimental model system such as cultured cells and animals, as we did in our previous report, rather than in clinical samples. Therefore it is inevitable limitation of the present study design that it is unidimensional, but supplemented by our previous mechanistic study, it addresses more direct clinical relevance.

Clinical translation of the results of this study may not be straightforward. If downregulation of PTH1R is a feature of low-compliance bladders, it would be difficult to use this axis as a target for treatment. However, it is possible that bladders still positive for PTH1R may retain the ability to relax against excessive distention, while downregulation of PTH1R could be a marker for unresponsiveness to conservative therapy, indicating the need for bladder augmentation. In addition, the PTHrP-PTH1R axis could be a target for treating milder damage in bladders retaining PTH1R expression, including overactive bladder, which affects a far larger percentage of the population than severely diseased bladder. Unfortunately, currently-available PTH1R agonists have systemic side effects that preclude their use for bladder diseases, and bladder-specific derivatives are awaited to allow the clinical translation of the PTHrP-PTH1R axis for treating bladder diseases.

Conclusions

In conclusion, we demonstrated PTH1R expression in the smooth muscle in normal bladders, in contrast to negative expression in muscle from severely diseased bladders. Suppression of the PTHrP-PTH1R axis may therefore be involved in bladder pathophysiology.

Abbreviations

PTH: Parathyroid hormone; PTHrP: Parathyroid hormone-related peptide; PTH1R: Parathyroid hormone/ parathyroid hormone-related peptide receptor 1; PBS: Phosphate-buffered saline.

Competing interests

The authors declare that they have no competing interests.

Authors' contributions

NN and AK participated in the design of the study, evaluated the samples, and performed the analysis. NN drafted the manuscript. YT carried out the immunohistochemical study, and helped to draft the manuscript. RY, YY, MS, and KT provided the clinical samples and clinical data, and YY performed the urodynamic study. HN and MI critically reviewed the manuscript. OO conceived of the study, and participated in its coordination. All authors read and approved the final manuscript.

Acknowledgements

We got financial support from Grant-in-Aid for scientific research from the Japanese Society for Promotion of Science to A.K. (no. 24659719).

Author details

[1]Department of Urology, Kyoto University Graduate School of Medicine, Kyoto, Japan. [2]Department of Cell Physiology, Nagoya City University Graduate School of Medical Sciences, Nagoya, Japan. [3]Department of Urology, Tokyo Women's Medical University, Tokyo, Japan. [4]Department of Urology, Kanagawa Children's Medical Centre, Yokohama, Japan. [5]Department of Urology, Otsu Red Cross Hospital, Otsu, Japan. [6]Department

of Clinical Laboratory Science, Tenri Health Care University, Tenri, Japan.
[7]Department of Urology, Hyogo College of Medicine, Nishinomiya, Japan.

References

1. Ozkan B, Demirkesen O, Durak H, Uygun N, Ismailoglu V, Cetinel B. Which factors predict upper urinary tract deterioration in overactive neurogenic bladder dysfunction? Urology. 2005;66(1):99–104.
2. Stein R, Schroder A, Thuroff JW. Bladder augmentation and urinary diversion in patients with neurogenic bladder: surgical considerations. J Pediatr Urol. 2012;8(2):153–61.
3. Stein R, Schroder A, Thuroff JW. Bladder augmentation and urinary diversion in patients with neurogenic bladder: non-surgical considerations. J Pediatr Urol. 2012;8(2):145–52.
4. Park WH. Management of low complaint bladder in spinal cord injured patients. LUTS. 2010;2(2):61–70.
5. Suva LJ, Winslow GA, Wettenhall RE, Hammonds RG, Moseley JM, Diefenbach-Jagger H, et al. A parathyroid hormone-related protein implicated in malignant hypercalcemia: cloning and expression. Science. 1987;237(4817):893–6.
6. Urena P, Kong XF, Abou-Samra AB, Juppner H, Kronenberg HM, Potts Jr JT, et al. Parathyroid hormone (PTH)/PTH-related peptide receptor messenger ribonucleic acids are widely distributed in rat tissues. Endocrinology. 1993;133(2):617–23.
7. Philbrick WM, Wysolmerski JJ, Galbraith S, Holt E, Orloff JJ, Yang KH, et al. Defining the roles of parathyroid hormone-related protein in normal physiology. Physiol Rev. 1996;76(1):127–73.
8. Nishikawa N, Kanematsu A, Negoro H, Imamura M, Sugino Y, Okinami T, et al. PTHrP is endogenous relaxant for spontaneous smooth muscle contraction in urinary bladder of female rat. Endocrinology. 2013;154 (6):2058–68.
9. Hamano S, Yamanishi T, Igarashi T, Murakami S, Ito H. Evaluation of functional bladder capacity in Japanese children. Int J Urol. 1999;6(5):226–8.
10. Toda Y, Kono K, Abiru H, Kokuryo K, Endo M, Yaegashi H, et al. Application of tyramide signal amplification system to immunohistochemistry: a potent method to localize antigens that are not detectable by ordinary method. Pathol Int. 1999;49(5):479–83.
11. Lupp A, Klenk C, Rocken C, Evert M, Mawrin C, Schulz S. Immunohistochemical identification of the PTHR1 parathyroid hormone receptor in normal and neoplastic human tissues. Eur J Endocrinol. 2010;162(5):979–86.
12. Yamamoto M, Harm SC, Grasser WA, Thiede MA. Parathyroid hormone-related protein in the rat urinary bladder: a smooth muscle relaxant produced locally in response to mechanical stretch. Proc Natl Acad Sci U S A. 1992;89(12):5326–30.
13. Steers WD, Broder SR, Persson K, Bruns DE, Ferguson 2nd JE, Bruns ME, et al. Mechanical stretch increases secretion of parathyroid hormone-related protein by cultured bladder smooth muscle cells. J Urol. 1998;160(3 Pt 1):908–12.
14. Juppner H, Abou-Samra AB, Freeman M, Kong XF, Schipani E, Richards J, et al. A G protein-linked receptor for parathyroid hormone and parathyroid hormone-related peptide. Science. 1991;254(5034):1024–6.
15. Perez-Martinez FC, Juan YS, Lin WY, Guven A, Mannikarottu A, Levin RM. Expression of parathyroid hormone-related protein in the partially obstructed and reversed rabbit bladder. Int Urol Nephrol. 2009;41(3):505–11.

4

Urethral orifice hyaluronic acid injections: a novel animal model of bladder outlet obstruction

Yongquan Wang[1], Zhiyong Xiong[1], Wei Gong[2], Zhansong Zhou[1†] and Gensheng Lu[1*†]

Abstract

Background: We produced a novel model of bladder outlet obstruction (BOO) by periurethral injection of hyaluronic acid and compared the cystometric features, postoperative complications, and histopathological changes of that model with that of traditional open surgery.

Methods: Forty female Sprague-Dawley rats were divided into three groups. Fifteen rats were subcutaneously injected with 0.2 ml hyaluronic acid at 5, 7, and 12 o'clock around the urethral orifice. Another fifteen rats underwent traditional open partial proximal urethral obstruction surgery, and 10 normal rats used as controls. After 4 weeks, filling cystometry, postoperative complications, and histopathological features were evaluated in each group. Three rats were also observed for 12 weeks after hyaluronic acid injection to evaluate the long-term effect.

Results: Hyaluronic acid periurethral injection caused increased maximum cystometric capacity, maximum bladder pressure, micturition interval, and post-void residual urine volume compared with control ($p < 0.01$). The injection group had significantly shorter operative time, less incidence of incision infection and bladder stone formation compared with the surgery group ($p < 0.01$). Hematoxylin and eosin (HE) staining showed suburothelial and interstitial hyperemia edema and smooth muscle hypertrophy in both injection and surgery bladders; these were not observed in the control group. Bladder weight and thickness of smooth muscle in the injection and surgery groups were significantly greater than those in the control group ($p < 0.01$). Urethral epithelial hyperplasia and lamina propria inflammation were observed in the surgery group but not in the injection or control groups. Rats periurethrally injected hyaluronic acid were stable the compound was not fully absorbed in any rat after 12 weeks.

Conclusions: Hyaluronic acid periurethral injection generates a simple, effective, and persistent animal model of BOO with lower complications, compared with traditional surgery.

Keywords: Bladder outlet obstruction, Animal model, Hyaluronic acid

Background

Bladder outlet obstruction (BOO) is a common urological chronic condition in which the urine flow from the urinary bladder through the urethra is impeded. BOO can result from several diseases, including benign prostatic hyperplasia and urethral stricture in adults [1,2]. To better understand the effect of this condition on bladder structure and function, several experimental animal models have been established [3]. Those animal models that recreate BOO are critical to understanding the pathophysiology of many diseases related bladder function, and to evaluating the effects of various pharmacologic therapies.

The most widely used methodological approaches to creating BOO are the partial urethral obstruction (PUO) animal models. In these animal models, a ligature, cuff, or ring is surgically placed around the outlet of the catheterized bladder, so that when the catheter is removed, the bladder experiences increased urethral resistance [4-7]. Although animal models cannot perfectly recapitulate symptoms observed in clinic, evidence indicates that PUO rats have similar storage and micturition symptoms as human BOO patients [8-10].

However, massive trauma caused by open surgery causes some complications such as incision infection and bladder stone formation. It is also difficult to

* Correspondence: lugeng8@hotmail.com
[†]Equal contributors
[1]Center of Urology, Southwest Hospita, Third Militar, Medical University, 400038 Chongqing, China
Full list of author information is available at the end of the article

standardize the firmness of ligation, or exclude foreign material from rings in surgery PUO models. Therefore, establishing a relevant, reproducible, and minimally invasive BOO animal model would be useful.

Bulking agents have previously been injected to treat urinary incontinence in clinic. The injection seeks to increase bladder outlet resistance by oppressing the urethra and thereby reducing urinary leakage in patients with stress urinary incontinence [11]. The establishment of a BOO animal model is possible by a similar principle. Hyaluronic acid is a viscous mucopolysaccharide found in the connective tissue space. It is ideal for BOO model establishment because it is stable and histocompatible. We aimed to establish a novel BOO animal model by hyaluronic acid periurethral injection, and to compare the effects and related complications of this technique with traditional PUO surgery.

Methods

Animal model preparation

All experimental protocols were approved by the Animal Research Ethics Committee of the Third Military Medical University. Forty female Sprague-Dawley rats were studied (weighing 220–260 g, Animal Center of the Third Military Medical University). All animals were anesthetized with sodium pentobarbital (50 mg/kg, i.p.) before procedures. The periurethral injection group (n = 15) underwent PUO by subcutaneous injection of 0.2 ml hyaluronic acid (Restylane, Q-Med, Uppsala,Sweden) at 5, 7, and 12 o'clock around the urethral orifice (Figure 1A). Animals in the surgery group (n = 15) underwent open surgery as previously described [12]. Briefly, a midline abdominal incision was made and the bladder and proximal urethra were dissected from the surrounding tissue. To create intravesical obstruction, a polyethylene tube (1.0 mm outer diameter) was placed beside the proximal urethra and a three-zero silk ligature was tied around the urethra and catheter. Then, the catheter was removed and the abdominal incision was closed (Figure 1B). Another ten normal rats were used as the control group. Four weeks later, mortality rates, complications, filling cystometry, and histopathological studies were evaluated in each group. To evaluate the long-term effect of hyaluronic acid in rats, another three rats were periurethrally injected with hyaluronic acid. The rats were observed for 12 weeks, at which point urethral anatomy was observed to evaluate whether or not hyaluronic acid was still present.

Cystometric study

Four weeks after surgery or injection, cystometric studies were performed on all animals as previously described. Animals were anesthetized as described above, and the bladders were catheterized via an incision at the bladder dome with a 0.6 mm inner diameter catheter. External bladder filling was carried out using an infusion pump (3 M, Saint Paul, MN, USA) at a constant rate of 12 ml/h until micturition was detected. A cystometry catheter was connected to an external pressure transducer (RM-6240B, Chengdu, China) for the measurement of the intravesical pressure. Animals underwent cystometries by irrigation of bladders with normal saline at room temperature and the curves of intravesical pressure and frequency of micturition were recorded. In each animal, approximately 10–12 voiding cycles were recorded and then the mean of the voiding cycles was calculated. The following parameters were evaluated: maximum cystometric capacity (MCC), maximal micturition pressure (Pmax), frequency (micturition interval), post-voiding residual volume (PRV), and detrusor instable contraction (DI). DI was defined as the significant non-voiding detrusor contractions (NVCs) higher than 10 cmH_2O.

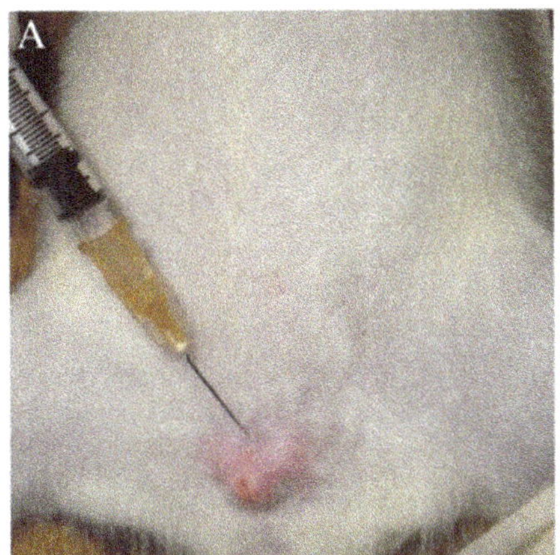

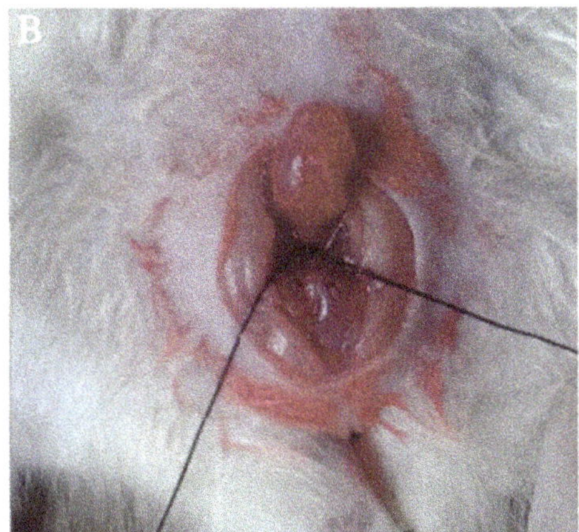

Figure 1 Partial urethral obstruction (PUO) animal model. (A) Hyaluronic acid periurethral injection **(B)** Proximal urethral ligation surgery.

Histopathological study

Four weeks after operation or injection, the animals were sacrificed and the bladders in each group were excised en bloc with the urethra. Bladders were weighed, and the ratio of bladder weight (mg) to body weight (g) was calculated in each surviving animal. Specimens of kidney, ureter, bladder, and urethra from each of the groups were immediately fixed with 10% formalin. After fixation, the tissues were embedded in paraffin, and 5-μm-thick tissue sections were cut. All of the specimens were stained using hematoxylin and eosin (HE) and viewed under a light microscope to evaluate histopathological changes. The thickness of the smooth muscle layer between the serosa and submucosa of the bladder dome were measured and compared among the three groups. All histopathological findings were determined by a pathologist in a blinded fashion.

Statistical analysis

Analysis was performed by SPSS11.0. All data were analyzed for normality of distribution utilizing the Kolmogorov-Smimov test and presented as the mean ± SEM. Data were subjected to t-test. For all statistical tests, $P < 0.05$ was considered significant.

Results

All animals in the injection and control groups survived until the day of evaluation. One of the animals in the surgery group died because of severe incision infection and bladder stones. The average operative time of injection was 3.5 ± 0.3 minutes, which was significantly shorter than that in the surgery group with 15.6 ± 5.4 minutes ($p < 0.01$).

Two animals had incision infections and bladder stone formation (Figure 2) in the surgery group. There were no complications in the injection or control groups (Table 1). All animals with complications were excluded from the cystometric study.

Filling cystometric data showed that both the injection and surgery procedures caused increased MCC, Pmax, frequency, and PRV compared with the control ($p < 0.01$) (Table 2). Both methods of obstruction caused cystometric changes in the bladder consistent with detrusor overactivity, which showed increasing spontaneous activity displayed as non-voiding contractions (NVCs) greater than 10 cmH_2O during the bladder storage period (Figure 3).

Table 1 Post-operative complications in injection, surgery, and control groups

Groups	Mortality	Incision infection	Bladder stone
Injection group N = 15	0	0	0
Surgery group N = 15	1	2	2
Control group N = 10	0	0	0

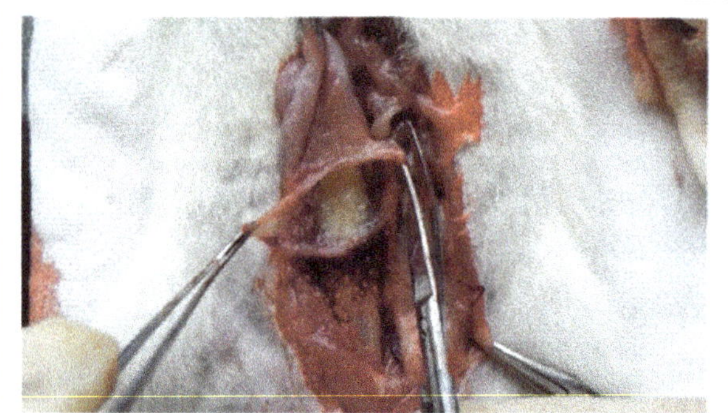

Figure 2 Bladder stone formation in surgery animal after 4 weeks of ligation.

After the animals were sacrificed, gross and microscopic anatomical changes of the organs were examined. There was no significant difference in body weight among the control (209.2 ± 16.2 g), surgery (210.2 ± 14.6 g), and injection (206.1 ± 17.3 g) rats at 4 weeks. However, the bladder weights in the surgery (3.1 ± 0.6 g) and injection (2.6 ± 0.3 g) groups were significantly greater than those in the control group (0.9 ± 0.1 g). The ratio of bladder weight (mg) to body weight (g) was used to evaluate bladder hypertrophy. The ratio increased in both the surgery (14.1 ± 3.7) and injection groups (12.6 ± 1.3) compared with the control group (4.7 ± 0.3, $p < 0.01$). There was a significant increase in the thickness of smooth muscle in the bladders of the injection (805 ± 77 μm) and surgery groups (961 ± 186 μm) compared with the control group (442 ± 39 μm, $p < 0.01$).

HE staining showed that all rats in three groups had normal kidneys and ureters. Examination of the bladder wall revealed an enlarged and hypertrophied bladder in each rat in the surgery and injection groups. Suburothelium inflammatory changes were observed in all surgery rats but not in those rats in the injection group (Figure 4A and B). In the proximal urethra, signs of epithelial proliferation and inflammation were observed around the urethra ligation in all surgery rats (Figure 5B). In some rats (3 of the 12 rats), severe epithelial proliferation caused squamous metaplasia near the ligation in the surgery group (Figure 5E). Unlike the surgery ligation rats, the urethra in the injection rats showed mild smooth muscle hypertrophy without epithelial proliferation and suburothelium inflammation (Figure 5A). Injected hyaluronic acid can be seen as a red dyed zone with a clear boundary, which oppressed the surrounding tissue without any inflammatory signs (Figure 5D). Histological study of the rats in the control group did not reveal any abnormalities (Figures 4C and 5C).

After 12 weeks, three hyaluronic acid injected rats were sacrificed and urethral anatomy was observed. The semitransparent hyaluronic acid gel was still present

Table 2 Filling cystometry results in injection, operation, and control groups

Groups MCC (ml) Micturation interval (s)		Pmax (cmH_2O)		PRV (ml)	NVC#
Injection group N = 15	1.66 ± 0.17*	39.47 ± 3.13*	152.13 ± 20.13*	0.26 ± 0.10*	3.21 ± 0.42*
Surgery group 0.28 ± 0.13* N = 12	1.81 ± 0.59*	42.11 ± 7.99*	165.23 ± 56.30*		2.85 ± 0.67*
Control group N = 10	1.38 ± 0.13	31.28 ± 3.37	256.2 ± 25.55	0	0

Both injection and surgery groups caused typical obstruction characteristics with increasing MCC, Pmax, frequency, and PRV compared with the control group. The data are shown as mean value ± SD.
*$p < 0.05$ compared to control group.
#the frequency of NVC was calculated in every 10 minutes.
MCC, maximum cystometric capacity; Pmax maximum bladder pressure during micturition; PRV, post-void residual urine volume.

around the urethra (Figure 6) in all three rats. The size of the residual hyaluronic acid was the same between the 4 and 12 week rats. Therefore, there was no significant absorption of hyaluronic acid after 12 weeks.

Discussion

The partial bladder neck ligation model is widely used in many studies on BOO, but the procedure is complex and there is a high risk of complications. Operative time and the degree of ligation are difficult to standardize, and severe inflammation around the urethral ligation can often result in excessive obstruction. Further, the fibrous scar in the abdominal skin and muscle, which does not occur in patients with BOO, may affect the accuracy studies using this model [13]. Placing a metal ring loosely around the proximal urethra has been used to create BOO models [7,14]. However, rejection of the foreign material is difficult to avoid.

Using bulking agents to increase bladder outlet resistance has been used in urinary incontinence treatment for some human patients. However, clinical case reports indicate that periurethral polytetrafluoroethylene (Teflon) injection can cause BOO in some patients [15].

Hyaluronic acid is an anionic, nonsulfated glycosaminoglycan that is distributed widely throughout connective, epithelial, and neural tissues. It is popular for filling soft tissue defects such as facial wrinkles or lip augmentation in plastic surgery because it is effective, easy to administer, and safe. Some urologists have attempted to use hyaluronic acid injection to treat vesicoureteral reflux in children [16-18]. Hyaluronic acid is biocompatible and can be exist stably in the body, so it could be used to observe long-term pathophysiological changes in some chronic diseases. Clinical trials indicate that hyaluronic acid can persist up to 6–18 after injection in humans [19]. Therefore, hyaluronic acid appears to be a perfect agent to creating and simulating urinary obstruction. However, no reported

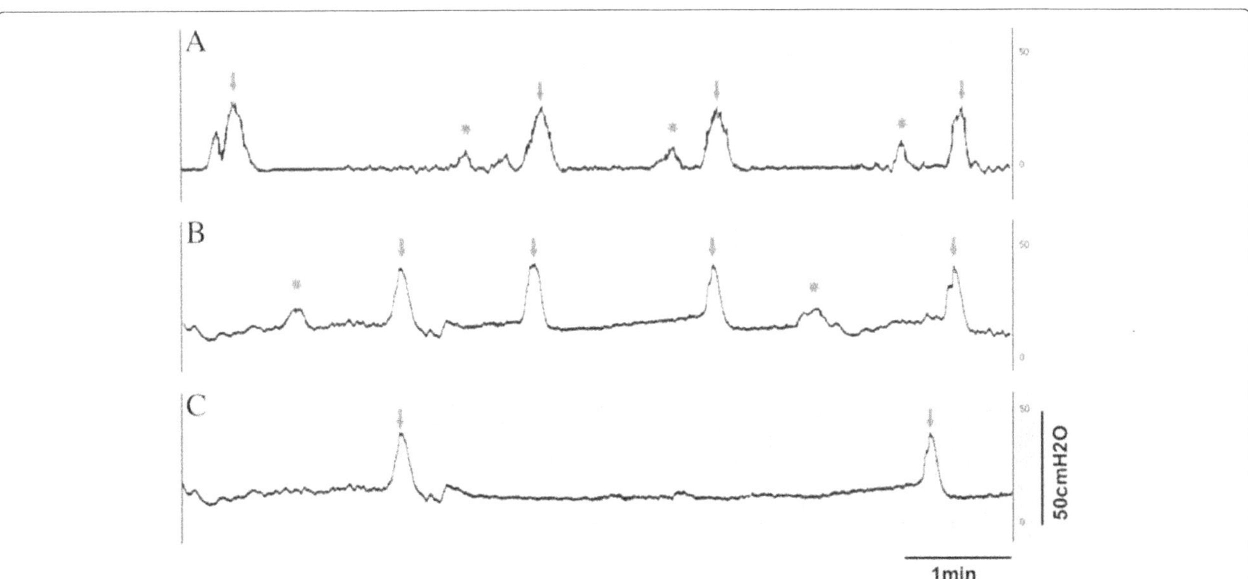

Figure 3 Filling cystometric curves in injection, operation, and control rats. (A) and **(B)** show respective injection and surgery bladders with significant decreases in micturition interval and frequent non-voiding contractions (NVCs) in the storage phase. **(C)** Control bladder displayed micturition frequency and good bladder compliance. *Non-voiding contractions (NVCs); ↓: Micturition.

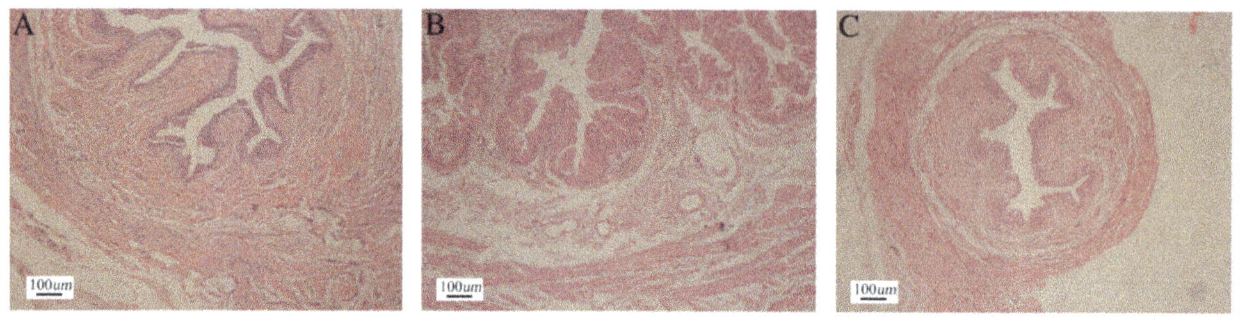

Figure 4 Histological characteristics of injection, operation, and control bladders. There was a significant increase in the thickness of smooth muscle in the bladders of the injection **(A)** and surgery groups **(B)** compared with the control group **(C)**. Suburothelium and interstitial hyperemia edema and smooth muscle hypertrophy were found in both injection and surgery bladders. Severe suburothelium inflammation and hyperemia were observed in the surgery group but not in the injection group.

BOO model has been produced by subcutaneous injection of hyaluronic acid.

In this study, we used hyaluronic acid injection to produce BOO in rats. Using this method, no open surgery or ligation was needed, greatly simplifying the operational process. Therefore, the procedure is safer and more stable compared with traditional surgery. Moreover, the degree of obstruction was easier to control with hyaluronic acid injection. Filling cystometry studies showed that periurethral injection of hyaluronic acid could achieve the same bladder outlet obstructive effects as open surgery. The detrusor overactivity presenting of NVCs appeared in both the injection and surgery bladders. Furthermore, the observed complication rate in the surgery group was higher than that in the injection group. In histological observation, both injection and surgery bladders showed suburothelial and interstitial hyperemia edema and smooth muscle hypertrophy, which are the compensatory responses after urinary tract obstruction. However, significant differences in the bladder and urethra were observed between the surgery and injection groups. In the rats with a urethral ligation, the bladder and urethra showed signs of fibrosis, inflammation, and muscular hypertrophy. The rats with injection

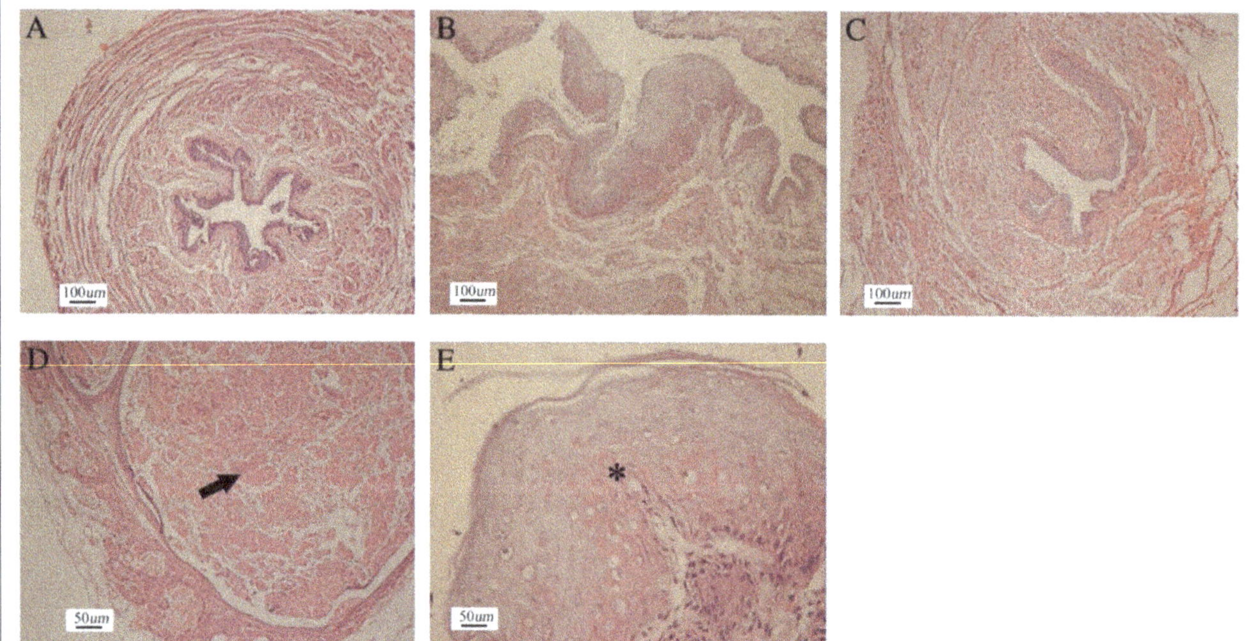

Figure 5 Histological characteristics of injection, operation, and control proximal urethras. The proximal urethra in injection rats showed mild smooth muscle hypertrophy without epithelial proliferation and suburothelium inflammation **(A)** similar to the control **(C)**. Epithelial proliferation and inflammation were seen around the urethra ligation in the surgery group **(B)**. Injected hyaluronic acid is indicated with an arrow **(D)**. Squamous metaplasia because of severe epithelial proliferation and inflammation is indicated with an asterisk in the surgery group **(E)**.

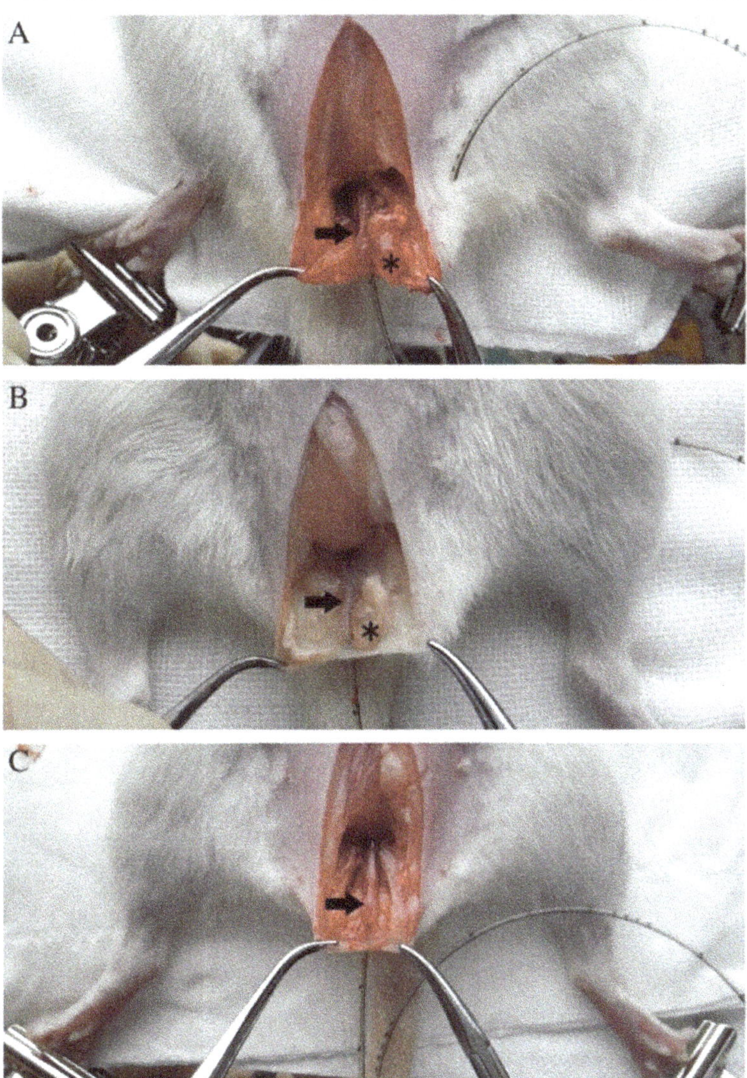

Figure 6 Urethral anatomy after hyaluronic acid injection for 4 and 12 weeks. Injected gel hyaluronic acid stably existed around the urethra. The size of the residual hyaluronic acid was not different from 4 weeks **(A)** to 12 weeks **(B)**. Normal rat urethral anatomy was also performed as control **(C)**. Hyaluronic acid is indicated with an asterisk, and the urethra is indicated with an arrow.

had only mild muscular hypertrophy without epithelial proliferation or lamina propria inflammation. Therefore, the injection of hyaluronic acid seems to cause only some physiological changes in muscular thickening of the bladder wall and increased bladder weight, and minimizes the interference of inflammation. These symptoms more closely mimic those observed of BOO in clinic. To further evaluate the long-term homeostasis of hyaluronic acid, we observed urethral anatomy and found that injected hyaluronic acid was still present after 12 weeks. This suggests that the BOO model is effective for longer examinations. The cystometry data in the injection group had a smaller standard deviation than that in the surgical group, which indicated that the model is more stable and repeatable.

While hyaluronic acid is expensive, the amount necessary for injection in rats is small. Considering that it significantly reduced the amount of animals and time required for study, we believe that it is more cost-effective than the traditional surgery model.

Conclusions

We demonstrated that periurethral injection of hyaluronic acid creates a relatively simple, effective, and persistent animal model of BOO that has fewer complications than that of the traditional surgery model. The model is simple to establish and provides consistent pathophysiological changes of BOO that will be useful for future study.

Abbreviations
BOO: Bladder outlet obstruction; PUO: Partial urethral obstruction; MCC: Maximum cystometric capacity; Pmax: Maximal micturition pressure; PRV: Post-voiding residual volume; DI: Detrusor instable contraction; NVCs: Non-voiding detrusor contractions; HE: Hematoxylin and eosin.

Competing interests
The authors declare that they have no competing interests.

Authors' contributions
WY carried out the animal model design, participated in the cystometric studies, and drafted the manuscript. XY carried out the histopathological studies. GW participated in the cystometric studies and performed the statistical analysis. ZZ participated in the design of the study. LG conceived of the study, participated in its design and coordination, and helped draft the manuscript. All authors read and approved the final manuscript.

Acknowledgments
The study was funded by the Chinese National Natural Sciences Fund (No. 81000288, 81270845).

Author details
[1]Center of Urology, Southwest Hospita, Third Militar, Medical University, 400038 Chongqing, China. [2]Department of Biochemistry and Molecular Biology, College of Basic Medical Sciences, Third Military Medical University, 400038 Chongqing, China.

References
1. Griebling TL. Worldwide prevalence estimates of lower urinary tract symptoms, overactive bladder, urinary incontinence, and bladder outlet obstruction. BJU Int. 2011;108:1138–9.
2. Starkman JS, Duffy 3rd JW, Wolter CE, Kaufman MR, Scarpero HM, Dmochowski RR. The evolution of obstruction induced overactive bladder symptoms following urethrolysis for female bladder outlet obstruction. J Urol. 2008;179:1018–23.
3. McMurray G, Casey JH, Naylor AM. Animal models in urological disease and sexual dysfunction. Br J Pharmacol. 2006;147 Suppl 2:S62–79.
4. Tanaka H, Kakizaki H, Shibata T, Mitsui T, Koyanagi T. Effect of preemptive treatment of capsaicin or resiniferatoxin on the development of pre-micturition contractions after partial urethral obstruction in the rat. J Urol. 2003;170:1022–6.
5. Austin JC, Chacko SK, DiSanto M, Canning DA, Zderic SA. A male murine model of partial bladder outlet obstruction reveals changes in detrusor morphology, contractility and Myosin isoform expression. J Urol. 2004;172(4 Pt 1):1524–8.
6. Gur S, Sikka SC, Chandra S, Koka PS, Agrawal KC, Kadowitz PJ, et al. Alfuzosin attenuates erectile dysfunction in rats with partial bladder outlet obstruction. BJU Int. 2008;102:1651–7.
7. Santis WF, Sullivan MP, Gobet R, Cisek LJ, McGoldrick RJ, Yalla SV, et al. Characterization of ureteral dysfunction in an experimental model of congenital bladder outlet obstruction. J Urol. 2000;163:980–4.
8. Burmeister D, AbouShwareb T, D'Agostino Jr R, Andersson KE, Christ GJ. Impact of partial urethral obstruction on bladder function: time-dependent changes and functional correlates of altered expression of Ca^{2+} signaling regulators. Am J Physiol Renal Physiol. 2012;302:1517–28.
9. Jang H, Han DS, Yuk SM. Changes of neuregulin-1(NRG-1) expression in a rat model of overactive bladder induced by partial urethral obstruction: is NRG-1 a new biomarker of overactive bladder? BMC Urol. 2013;13:54–9.
10. Yuan X, Wu S, Lin T, He D, Li X, Liu S, et al. Role of nitric oxide synthase in bladder pathologic remodeling and dysfunction resulting from partial outlet obstruction. Urology. 2011;77:1001–8.
11. Benshushan A, Brzezinski A, Shoshani O, Rojansky N. Periurethral injection for the treatment of urinary incontinence. Obstet Gynecol Surv. 1998;53:383–8.
12. Kim SO, Oh BS, Chang IY, Song SH, Ahn K, Hwang EC, et al. Distribution of interstitial cells of Cajal and expression of nitric oxide synthase after experimental bladder outlet obstruction in a rat model of bladder overactivity. Neurourol Urodyn. 2011;30:1639–45.
13. Buttyan R, Chen MW, Levin RM. Animal models of bladder outlet obstruction and molecular insights into the basis for the development of bladder dysfunction. Eur Urol. 1997;32 Suppl 1:32–9.
14. O'Connor Jr LT, Vaughan Jr ED, Felsen D. In vivo cystometric evaluation of progressive bladder outlet obstruction in rats. J Urol. 1997;158:631–5.
15. McKinney CD, Gaffey MJ, Gillenwater JY. Bladder outlet obstruction after multiple periurethral polytetrafluoroethylene injections. J Urol. 1995;153:149–51.
16. Mintz BR, Cooper Jr JA. Hybrid hyaluronic acid hydrogel/poly (varepsilon-caprolactone) scaffold provides mechanically favorable platform for cartilage tissue engineering studies. J Biomed Mater Res A. 2014;102:2918–26.
17. Kohn JC, Goh AS, Lin JL, Goldberg RA. Dynamic High-Resolution Ultrasound In Vivo Imaging of Hyaluronic Acid Filler Injection. Dermatol Surg. 2013;39:1630–6.
18. DaJusta D, Gargollo P, Snodgrass W. Dextranomer/hyaluronic acid bladder neck injection for persistent outlet incompetency after sling procedures in children with neurogenic urinary incontinence. J Pediatr Urol. 2013;9:278–82.
19. Beasley KL, Weiss MA, Weiss RA. Hyaluronic acid fillers: a comprehensive review. Facial Plast Surg. 2009;25:86–94.

5

Electrical stimulation of somatic afferent nerves in the foot increases bladder capacity in neurogenic bladder patients after sigmoid cystoplasty

Guoqing Chen[1,2,3], Limin Liao[1,2,3*] and Di Miao[1,2,3]

Abstract

Background: A previous study showed that foot stimulation can delay the bladder filling sensation and increase bladder volume in healthy humans without OAB. The aim of this study was to determine whether or not electrical stimulation of somatic afferent nerves in the foot can increase bladder capacity in neurogenic bladder patients after sigmoid cystoplasty.

Methods: Eleven subjects underwent 30-min foot stimulation using skin surface electrodes connected to a bladder-pelvic stimulator. The electrodes were attached to the bottom of the foot. The subjects completed a 5-day voiding diary, during which time foot stimulation was applied on day 3. The stimulation parameter was a continuous, bi-polar square wave form with a pulse duration of 200 μs and a stimulation frequency of 5 Hz. The stimulation intensity was set by each subject at a maximal level without causing discomfort.

Results: The volume per clean intermittent catheterization (CIC) was 279.4 ± 11.7 ml and 285.4 ± 11.8 ml on the 1st and 2nd days, respectively. On the 3rd day, the average volume per CIC increased to 361.1 ± 18.1 ml after stimulation ($p < 0.05$). The average volume per CIC returned to 295.4 ± 13.4 ml and 275.1 ± 11.5 ml on the 4th and 5th days, respectively.

Conclusions: Foot stimulation can delay the bladder filling sensation and significantly increase bladder capacity in neurogenic bladder patients after sigmoid cystoplasty.

Keywords: Electrical stimulation, Foot, Bladder capacity, Neurogenic bladder, Detrusor overactivity

Background

Augmentation enterocystoplasty (AE) is the reference standard for patients with neurogenic bladder dysfunction (NBD) with the detrimental effects of high-bladder pressure on the upper urinary tract (UUT). The purpose of AE is to create a large-capacity, low-pressure, good-compliance reservoir with a preserved UUT, thus allowing for socially-acceptable continence [1]. Based on our previous research [1], we found that incontinence still occurred and bladder capacity was unsatisfactory within 6 months following sigmoid cystoplasty in some patients because of the weakened function of the sphincter, automatic contraction of the intestinal reservoir, and residual detrusor overactivity (DO) post-operatively. Therefore, we asked these patients to use oral anti-cholinergic agents until the bladder capacity increased and had good compliance.

A previous study showed that foot stimulation using skin surface electrodes inhibits DO and has a long-lasting effect in cats [2], likely as a result of stimulating branches of the tibial nerve in the foot. Recently, Chen [3] reported that foot stimulation can also delay the bladder filling sensation and increase bladder volume in healthy humans without OAB.

In the current study we reported the initial outcome of a clinical study in which we evaluated the effectiveness of electrical stimulation of somatic afferent nerves in the feet of neurogenic bladder patients who emptied the bladder by clean intermittent catheterization (CIC) after sigmoid cystoplasty.

* Correspondence: lmliao@263.net
[1]Department of Urology, China Rehabilitation Research Center, Beijing 100068, China
[2]Department of Urology, Capital Medical University, Beijing, China
Full list of author information is available at the end of the article

Methods

This study was approved by the Ethics Committee of the China Rehabilitation Research Center. All participants signed an informed consent. Foot stimulation was tested in 11 neurogenic bladder patients after sigmoid cystoplasty (7 males, 4 females; mean age, 28.9 ± 3.3 years; age range, 17–46 years) who used CIC to empty the bladder. All the patients were ≥ 1 month post-sigmoid cystoplasty (mean, 4.6 ± 1.2 months; duration, 1–12 months) for neurogenic bladder refractory to conservative treatment. Intra-operatively, a 20–30 cm segment of sigmoid colon was isolated with its vascular pedicle and opened on the anti-mesenteric border to form a patch. The detubulized sigmoid patch was sutured onto the opened bladder. After recovering from surgery, the capacity was increased from 105.6 ± 10.2 ml pre-operatively to 280.5 ± 11.7 ml by urodynamic evaluation. Then the patients were instructed to empty the bladder by CIC for life. Before surgery, all of the patients were diagnosed with incomplete spinal cord damage based on American Spinal Injury Association (ASIA) standards [4] and electrophysiologic assessment.

The subjects were instructed to record CIC volumes during a 5-day period without restriction of daily food and water intake when they returned to the hospital for a follow-up evaluation. The subjects were also instructed to perform CIC when urine leaked or in response to the usual bladder sensations in patients in whom bladder sensations still existed. Foot stimulation was applied for 30 minutes in the morning (9:00–9:30 a.m.) on day 3 with the subject in the sitting position. Two skin surface electrodes (4 × 4 cm) were attached to the plantar surfaces of both feet. A cathodal electrode was placed on the anterior aspect of the foot and an anodal electrode was placed between the inner foot arch and the heel. The two pairs of electrodes were connected to a bladder-pelvic stimulator [Bladder-Pelvic Stimulator (I) developed by Neural Electro-Mechanics Center of Chinese Academy Sciences and Dept. of Urology at China Rehabilitation Research Center, and supported by the China National Technology R&G Program].

The Bladder-Pelvic Stimulator (I) consists of three sub-systems (stimulation circuit, user interface device, and electrode adaptor; Figure 1). The stimulator supports four independent output channels. The stimulator can generate mono- and bi-polar pulse wave with user-defined waveforms and parameters as follows (step sizes are given in parentheses): pulse amplitude 1–50 mA (0.5 mA); pulse frequency 1–100 Hz (1 Hz); pulse width 50–2000 μs (10 μs); pulse train duration 0.1 – 10 s (0.1 s); pulse train interval 0 – 10s (0.1 s); pulse train rising edge 0 – 10s (0.1 s); and pulse train falling edge 0.01 – 10 s (0.1 s). The user interface was developed on the android tablet platform. Clinicians can select and modify stimulation parameters on the tablet. The electrode interface supports multiple types of implantable and surface electrodes, which were not included in this study.

The stimulation applied in this study was a continuous, bipolar square wave form with a pulse duration of 200 μs and a stimulation frequency of 5 Hz. The stimulator was controlled to determine the minimal current needed to induce a toe twitch. The stimulation intensity was then increased to the maximal level, which was comfortable for the subject during the entire 30-min stimulation. The volume per CIC was averaged among subjects during 5 periods, as follows: 1) 48–24 hours before foot stimulation; 2) 24 hours before foot stimulation; 3) up to 24 hours after stimulation; 4) 24–48 hours after stimulation; and 5) 48–72 hours after stimulation.

One-way ANOVA, followed by the Dunnett multiple comparison test, was used to detect statistically significant differences ($p < 0.05$) between voided volumes before and after stimulation.

Results

The baseline characteristics and the stimulation intensities of the patients are shown in Table 1.

The volume per CIC was 279.4 ± 11.7 ml and 285.4 ± 11.8 ml during the 1st and 2nd periods, respectively. During the 3rd period, the average volume per CIC increased to 361.1 ± 18.1 ml after stimulation ($p < 0.05$; Figure 2). The average volume per CIC returned to 295.4 ± 13.4 ml and 275.1 ± 11.5 ml in the 4th and 5th periods, respectively.

The volume per CIC remained increased for 24 h after stimulation in all of the patients. Subjects 4 and 7 had greater bladder capacities 24–48 h after stimulation than before stimulation. Forty-eight hours after stimulation, the volume per CIC returned to pre-stimulation baseline in all patients. Subject 3, who was 1 month post-surgery, felt a desire to void when the capacity was approximately 190 ml, but the bladder filling sensation was delayed and the bladder volume was increased to 246.0 ± 18.3 ml after stimulation.

All subjects tolerated stimulation without discomfort. There were no immediate or long-term adverse events associated with stimulation.

Discussion

In the current study all of the patients underwent sigmoid cystoplasties for 1–12 months (mean, 4.6 ± 1.2 months) because of a neurogenic bladder secondary to incomplete spinal cord injuries, meningoceles, or spina bifida. After recovering from surgery, the patients were asked to empty their bladders by CIC; however, the mean bladder capacity was only 280.5 ± 11.7 ml at early follow-up post-operatively based on urodynamic evaluation, which was unsatisfactory for those subjects who had undergone

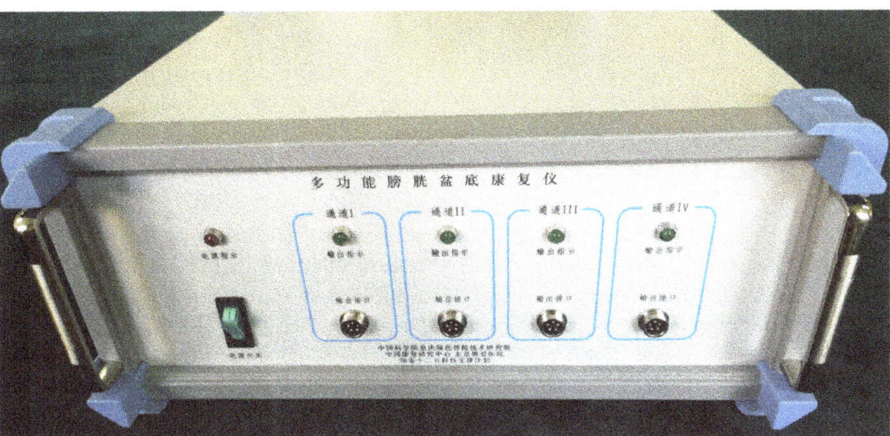

Figure 1 The picture of the Bladder-Pelvic Stimulator (I).

cystoplasty. In our previous research [1], we showed that the most common problem within 6 months post-operatively was incontinence, which might have resulted from the weakened function of the sphincter post-operatively. The presence of an indwelling urethral catheter for a long period could contribute to sphincter weakness because the maximal urethral pressure at rest was significantly decreased during the 6-month follow-up examination compared with the pre-operative pressure. Automatic contraction of the intestinal reservoir could also lead to pressure increase and incontinence. The residual detrusor also may maintain DO post-operatively. New bladder wall edema can result in reduced bladder compliance. The aforementioned four reasons can explain why the bladder capacity of the patients in the current study was not satisfactory at the early follow-up evaluation. The patients continued to use CIC combined with oral anti-cholinergic agents until the bladder capacity became larger 6 months post-operatively. The anti-cholinergic agents have some side effects, e.g., dry mouth, thus the patients cannot take the medications for a long time.

Previous studies in cats showed that transcutaneous electrical stimulation of somatic afferent nerves in the foot inhibits reflex micturition, significantly increases bladder capacity [5], and induces post-stimulation inhibition of

Table 1 The baseline characteristics and the volume per CIC before and after stimulation

Subject-sex-age no.	Neurological pathology	Visiting time (months)	Stimulation intensity (mA)		Mean ± SE Vol/CIC (ml)				
			Left	Right	48 ~ 24 h before	In 24 h before	Up to 24 h after	24 ~ 48 h after	48 ~ 72 h after
1-M-26	Incomplete spinal cord injury	1	15	20	263.3 ± 68.4	266.7 ± 66.7	300.0 ± 57.7	266.7 ± 44.1	270.0 ± 65.1
2-M-43	Incomplete spinal cord injury	3	50	50	310.0 ± 5.8	305.0 ± 9.6	410.0 ± 23.8	290.0 ± 5.8	302.5 ± 13.2
3-M-17	Spina bifida	1	30	30	190.0 ± 4.2	191.7 ± 4.4	246.0 ± 18.3	210.0 ± 7.7	200.0 ± 4.1
4-F-17	Meningocele	1	20	20	291.7 ± 41.7	286.7 ± 21.1	400.0 ± 60.2	358.0 ± 58.9	253.3 ± 36.9
5-M-38	Meningocele	3	15	15	246.7 ± 42.2	260.0 ± 19.2	302.9 ± 21.8	240.0 ± 24.7	258.3 ± 33.5
6-F-17	Meningocele	6	20	15	300.5 ± 33.7	315.0 ± 26.8	385.5 ± 41.2	320.0 ± 38.4	305.8 ± 29.1
7-M-46	Incomplete spinal cord injury	3	22	25	286.0 ± 62.3	300.0 ± 35.8	344.0 ± 50.4	325.0 ± 41.1	253.3 ± 27.7
8-F-24	Meningocele	3	30	27	266.0 ± 15.7	271.4 ± 19.6	364.0 ± 45.8	291.7 ± 14.2	261.7 ± 25.6
9-M-38	Incomplete spinal cord injury	12	50	50	310.0 ± 17.0	328.6 ± 19.6	424.0 ± 31.2	325.0 ± 41.1	320.0 ± 13.7
10-F-22	Spina bifida	6	18	20	276.0 ± 12.9	285.7 ± 12.3	352.0 ± 8.6	281.7 ± 5.4	265.0 ± 5.6
11-M-30	Meningocele	12	25	20	334.0 ± 6.8	328.6 ± 19.6	444.0 ± 11.7	341.7 ± 11.7	336.7 ± 14.1

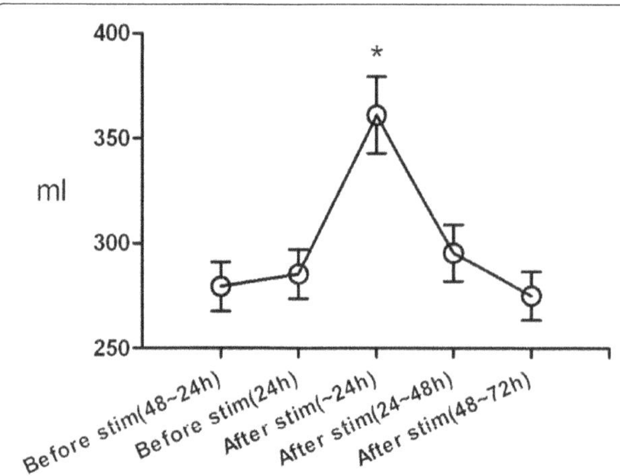

Figure 2 Mean bladder volume per CIC measured in 11 subjects during 48–24 h, 24 h before foot stimulation (Stim), and within 24 h, during 24–48 h and 48–72 h after foot stimulation at 5 Hz frequency, 200 μs pulse width, and 15–50 mA intensity. Asterisks indicate significantly different versus voided volume before stimulation ($p < 0.05$).

reflex bladder activity that persists for 1–2 h [2]. Indeed, the same mechanisms might occur in healthy humans. It has been demonstrated that transcutaneous electrical stimulation of somatic afferent nerves in the foot can delay bladder filling sensations and significantly increase bladder capacity > 50% in healthy humans, and this technology has the potential to be an effective new treatment for patients with DO [3].

In our study, foot stimulation using skin surface electrodes also can delay the bladder filling sensation and significantly increase bladder capacity (Table 1 and Figure 1) in the patients after sigmoid cystoplasty. The volume per CIC was significantly increased compared with baseline, and this effect can last > 1 day.

The mechanism underlying foot stimulation is unknown, but may be mediated by the nerve in the foot [3]. The stimulation electrodes were placed on the skin surface rather than directly on the nerves. Which nerves were activated? The tibial nerve courses from the inner ankle inferiorly to the plantar surface of the foot and branches into the lateral and medial plantar nerves at the location of the electrodes. These nerves further branch into multiple small nerves that course toward the toes. Thus, it is highly likely that foot stimulation activates afferent branches of the tibial nerve in the lateral and medial plantar aspects of the foot.

The spinal segmental distribution of the stimulated somatic afferent pathways is an important factor in the efficacy of this type of neuromodulation [5]; however, inhibition at a supraspinal site cannot be excluded. A previous study in cats showed that the inhibitory effect on bladder activity elicited by electrical stimulation of the nerves from the hind limb muscles was lost after chronic spinal cord transection at the thoracic level, indicating a possible role of the supraspinal mechanisms in somatovesical inhibition [6]. In the current study, all of the patients had incomplete spinal cord damage; therefore we cannot confirm whether or not foot stimulation has the same effects in patients with complete spinal cord damage. The Chen study [3] showed that some subjects voided a larger volume after only 30 minutes of stimulation, indicating that 30 minutes of stimulation might be sufficient to induce an inhibitory effect; thus, foot stimulation was applied for only 30 minutes in the current research.

In the Chen study [3], the average voided volume increased by > 50% or approximately 200 ml, which is more than the increase (approximately 30%) in volume per CIC in the current study. We calculated the mean volume per CIC in 24 hours after stimulation during the 3rd period, which was > 5 hours in the Chen study [3]. It is well known that the stimulation effect will weaken over time. Thus, if we also calculate the average volume per CIC 5 h after stimulation, the result may be close to the volume reported by Chen [3].

Although only a few subjects with neurogenic bladder secondary to incomplete spinal cord injuries, meningoceles, or spina bifida were tested in the study who used CIC to empty the bladder post-sigmoid cystoplasty, our results support proceeding with clinical trials involving foot stimulation in patients with OAB and other types of neurogenic bladder. Currently, CIC combined with an anti-cholinergic medication is the gold standard treatment for NDO; however, many patients are refractory to the medication or have dose-limiting side effects [7]. If foot stimulation can inhibit DO, improve bladder compliance, and increase bladder capacity in patients with neurogenic bladder, foot stimulation can be used to treat the patients instead of anti-cholinergic medications.

This is the first clinical trial in which electrical stimulation of the foot was used to treat patients. We want to determine whether or not this treatment can increase the bladder capacity in patients. Although a positive effect was shown in the current study, there were some flaws and limitations in the study. In the future, we need to conduct a randomized controlled trial to further elucidate and confirm our findings. First, the subjects in the current study all had meningoceles, incomplete spinal cord injuries, or spina bifida who had undergone sigmoid cystoplasties for 1–12 months and they do not represent all types of lower urinary tract disorders, thus we need to continue investigating patients with OAB and other types of neurogenic bladder. Second, we only focused on the changes of volume per CIC; CIC times and the urodynamic data after stimulation require study to verify the effect. Third, additional studies with a larger number of subjects are required to determine the optimal stimulation duration/pattern and further elucidate the post-stimulation effect. Fourth, the neobladder is composed of the residual bladder and sigmoid, still it is not known whether the capacity increased due to residual bladder or the sigmoid from the current data. It is difficult to prove in an augmentation model unless a pre-AE stim response is also recorded; alternatively, a similar study on orthotopic neobladder can also answer the question of whether detubularized bowel can respond to peripheral stimulation. However, no pre-augmentation stim was performed in this study. Though it is verified that neuromodulation is effective for both bladder and bowel dysfunction in previous literature [8], we still need to perform some studies to answer above-mentioned questions in the future. Fifth, all of the patients underwent this procedure at our medical center, but we are designing a portable bladder-pelvic stimulator so that patients can operate it in their own homes.

Conclusions

Electrical stimulation of the foot using skin surface electrodes can delay the bladder filling sensation and significantly increase bladder capacity in neurogenic bladder patients after sigmoid cystoplasty. Thus, foot stimulation will be a promising treatment option if it is shown to be clinically effective in OAB and NDO in the future because it is non-invasive and can be easily managed by patients.

Abbreviations

SNM: Sacral neuromodulation; PNS: Pudendal nerve stimulation; OAB: Overactive bladder; NDO: Neurogenic detrusor overactivity; TNS: Tibial nerve stimulation; DO: detrusor overactivity; CIC: Clean intermittent catheterization; ASIA: American Spinal Injury Association.

Competing interests

The authors declare that they have no competing interests.

Authors' contributions

GC and LL designed and conducted the study. GC and DM performed the electrical stimulation of the foot, and contributed to the statistical analysis and interpretation of the data. GC and LL drafted the manuscript. LL revised the manuscript critically. All authors read and approved the final manuscript.

Authors' information

Guoqing Chen and Limin Liao are co-first authors.

Acknowledgment

This work was supported by the China National Technology R&G Program (2012BAI34B02). All experiments were performed at the clinics of the China Rehabilitation Research Center, Beijing, P. R. China.

Author details

Department of Urology, China Rehabilitation Research Center, Beijing 100068, China. [2]Department of Urology, Capital Medical University, Beijing, China. [3]Center of Neural Injury and Repair, Beijing Institute for Brain Disorders, Beijing, China.

References

1. Zhang F, Liao L. Sigmoidocolocystoplasty with ureteral reimplantation for treatment of neurogenic bladder. Urology. 2012;80:440–5.
2. Chen G, Larson JA, Ogagan PD, Shen B, Wang J, Roppolo JR, et al. Post-stimulation inhibitory effect on reflex bladder activity induced by activation of somatic afferent nerves in the foot. J Urol. 2012;187:338–43.
3. Chen ML, Chermansky CJ, Shen B, Roppolo JR, de Groat WC, Tai C. Electrical stimulation of somatic afferent nerves in the foot increases bladder capacity in healthy human subjects. J Urol. 2014;191:1009–13.
4. Maynard Jr FM, Bracken MB, Creasey G, Ditunno Jr JF, Donovan TB, Garber SL, et al. International Standards for Neurological and Functional Classification of Spinal Cord Injury. American Spinal Injury Association. Spinal Cord. 1997;35:266–74.
5. Tai C, Shen B, Chen M, Wang J, Liu H, Roppolo JR, et al. Suppression of bladder overactivity by activation of somatic afferent nerves in the foot. BJU Int. 2011;107:303–9.
6. McPherson A. The effects of somatic stimuli on the bladder in the cat. J Physiol. 1966;185:185–96.
7. Madersbacher H, Mürtz G, Stöhrer M. Neurogenic detrusor overactivity in adults: a review on efficacy, tolerability and safety of oral antimuscarinics. Spinal Cord. 2013;51:432–41.
8. Fulton M, Peters KM. Neuromodulation for voiding dysfunction and fecal incontinence:a urology perspective. Urol Clin North Am. 2012;39:405–12.

6

Reduced expression of ezrin in urothelial bladder cancer signifies more advanced tumours and an impaired survival: validatory study of two independent patient cohorts

Gustav Andersson[1], Christoffer Wennersten[1], Alexander Gaber[1], Karolina Boman[1], Björn Nodin[1], Mathias Uhlén[2,3], Ulrika Segersten[4], Per-Uno Malmström[4] and Karin Jirström[1*]

Abstract

Background: Reduced membranous expression of the cytoskeleton-associated protein ezrin has previously been demonstrated to correlate with tumour progression and poor prognosis in patients with T1G3 urothelial cell carcinoma of the bladder treated with non-maintenance Bacillus Calmette-Guérin (n = 92), and the associations with adverse clinicopathological factors have been validated in another, unselected, cohort (n = 104). In the present study, we examined the prognostic significance of ezrin expression in urothelial bladder cancer in a total number of 442 tumours from two independent patient cohorts.

Methods: Immunohistochemical expression of ezrin was evaluated in tissue microarrays with tumours from one retrospective cohort of bladder cancer (n = 110; cohort I) and one population-based cohort (n = 342; cohort II). Classification regression tree analysis was applied for selection of prognostic cutoff. Kaplan-Meier analysis, log rank test and Cox regression proportional hazards' modeling were used to evaluate the impact of ezrin on 5-year overall survival (OS), disease-specific survival (DSS) and progression-free survival (PFS).

Results: Ezrin expression could be evaluated in tumours from 100 and 342 cases, respectively. In both cohorts, reduced membranous ezrin expression was significantly associated with more advanced T-stage ($p < 0.001$), high grade tumours ($p < 0.001$), female sex ($p = 0.040$ and $p = 0.013$), and membranous expression of podocalyxin-like protein ($p < 0.001$ and $p = 0.009$). Moreover, reduced ezrin expression was associated with a significantly reduced 5-year OS in both cohorts (HR = 3.09 95% CI 1.71-5.58 and HR = 2.15(1.51-3.06), and with DSS in cohort II (HR = 2.77, 95% CI 1.78-4.31). This association also remained significant in adjusted analysis in Cohort I (HR1.99, 95% CI 1.05-3.77) but not in Cohort II. In pTa and pT1 tumours in cohort II, there was no significant association between ezrin expression and time to progression.

Conclusions: The results from this study validate previous findings of reduced membranous ezrin expression in urothelial bladder cancer being associated with unfavourable clinicopathological characteristics and an impaired survival. The utility of ezrin as a prognostic biomarker in transurethral resection specimens merits further investigation.

Keywords: Ezrin, Urothelial bladder cancer, Prognosis

* Correspondence: karin.jirstrom@med.lu.se
[1]Department of Clinical Sciences, Oncology and Pathology, Lund University, Skåne University Hospital, Lund 221 85, Sweden
Full list of author information is available at the end of the article

Background

In 2008 there were 386 000 estimated new cases of bladder cancer in the world, and approximately 150 000 individuals died from their disease [1]. Bladder cancer is the fourth most common cancer among men in the USA [2].

Standard treatment for non-muscle-invasive carcinoma is transurethral resection of the bladder (TURB), with or without intravesical instillation of bacillus Calmette-Guérin (BCG), to prevent recurrence and progression. In contrast, muscle-invasive carcinoma is treated more aggressively with neoadjuvant chemotherapy and cystectomy [3,4]. However, non-muscle-invasive urothelial carcinoma has a high risk of recurrence and a substantial risk of progression [5], and muscle-invasive carcinoma is associated with a high mortality, despite aggressive treatment [3,6]. Hence, there is a great need for additional biomarkers to predict the risk of recurrence and progression into muscle invasive carcinoma for patients with early stage tumours.

Loss of expression of the membrane-cytoskeletal linking protein ezrin was initially demonstrated to be associated with tumour progression and poor prognosis in patients with T1G3 tumours treated with non-maintenance BCG (n = 92) [7]. In another recent study comprising 104 tumours of different stages and grades, loss of membranous ezrin expression was found to correlate with higher grade and stage, and invasiveness, but the associations with disease progression and survival were not reported [8]. The protein ezrin is closely related to two other membrane associated proteins, radixin and moesin, all three together named ERM proteins. All these proteins are important for regulation of cell adhesion and in the linkage between membrane proteins and the cortical cytoskeleton, thus affecting cell survival, migration and invasion, all factors contributing to tumour progression and development [9-11]. ERM proteins are inactive in the cytoplasm, and activated by binding to the cell membrane [10]. Ezrin is expressed in a variety of cancers [12] and the prognostic value of ezrin expression seems to differ in different cancer forms. In several cancer forms, high expression of ezrin has been associated with more aggressive tumours [13-19], whereas in serous ovarian carcinoma, lost expression of ezrin correlated with a worse prognosis [20], similar to the findings in bladder cancer [7].

The aim of this study was to further evaluate the utility of ezrin as a prognostic biomarker in two independent patient cohorts comprising a total number of 442 cases. Given previous findings of an *in vitro* interaction of ezrin with podocalyxin-like protein (PODXL), an established mediator of metastasis [21], and our recent results demonstrating that membranous PODXL expression is an independent predictor of tumour progression and poor prognosis in urothelial bladder cancer [22], we also examined the correlations between tumour-specific expression of ezrin and PODXL.

Methods

Patients

Cohort I

This cohort is a consecutive cohort of all patients with a first diagnosis of urothelial bladder cancer in the Department of Pathology, Skåne University Hospital, Malmö, from Oct 1st, 2002 until Dec 31st, 2003, for whom archival TURB specimens could be retrieved (n = 110). The cohort includes 80 (72.7%) men and 30 (27.3%) women with a median age of 72.86 (39.25-89.87) years. Information on vital status was obtained from the Swedish Cause of Death Registry up until Dec 31st 2010. Follow-up started at date of diagnosis and ended at death, emigration or Dec 31st 2010, whichever came first. Median follow-up time was 5.92 years (range 0.03-8.21) for the full cohort and 7.71 years (range 7.04-8.21) for patients alive (n = 48) at Dec 31st 2010. Fortyeight patients (43.6%) died within 5 years.

The distribution of T-stage was 48 (43.6%) pTa, 24 (21.8%) pT1, 37 (33.8) pT2 and 1 (0.9%) pT3. Eighteen (16.4%) tumours were Grade I, 34 (30.9%) Grade II and 58 (52.7%) Grade III. The cohort has also been described previously [22]. Permission for this study was obtained from the Ethics Committee at Lund University.

Cohort II

This cohort includes 344 patients from a prospective cohort of patients with newly diagnosed urothelial bladder cancer at Uppsala University Hospital from 1984 up until 2005. TURB specimens have been collected retrospectively and the predominant group of pTa tumours reduced to include 115 cases. Progression-free survival (PFS), overall survival (OS) and disease-specific survival (DSS) were calculated from the date of surgery to date of event or last follow-up. Progression was defined as shift of the tumour into a higher stage. Median time to progression for patients with non-muscle invasive disease was 18.0 months (range 2.0-55.0). Follow-up time for non-recurrent and non-progressing cases were ≥4 and ≥5-years, respectively. The cohort has been described previously [22,23]. Permission for this study was obtained from the Ethics Committee at Uppsala University.

Tissue microarray construction

All tumours were histopathologically re-evaluated and classified according to the WHO grading system of 2004 by a board certified pathologist. Tissue microarrays (TMAs) were constructed as previously described [22,23] using a semi-automated arraying device (TMArrayer, Pathology Devices, Westminister, MD, USA). All tumour samples were represented in duplicate tissue cores (1 mm).

Immunohistochemistry and staining evaluation

For immunohistochemical analysis, 4 μm TMA-sections were automatically pre-treated using the PT Link system and then stained in an Autostainer Plus (DAKO; Glostrup, Copenhagen, Denmark) with a polyclonal, monospecific antibody; HPA021616, Atlas Antibodies AB, diluted 1:1500. The specificity of the antibody has been confirmed by immunofluorescence, Western blotting and protein arrays (www.proteinatlas.org). Ezrin expression was annotated in accordance with previous studies [7], whereby the percentage of cancer cells with membranous protein sub-localization and the intensity of cytoplasmic staining, ranging from 0–3 (negative, weak, moderate, strong), was denoted. When evaluating cytoplasmic staining the dominating intensity for each core was determined. A mean value of the two samples from each tumour was used in the statistical analyses. The staining was evaluated by three independent observers, including one board certified pathologist, who were blinded to clinical and outcome data and every sample was re-evaluated once. Omission of primary antibody was used as a negative control, normal colonic mucosa as positive external control and lymphocytes as an internal positive control. Discrepant cases were re-evaluated once again and discussed in order to reach consensus.

Immunohistochemical expression of PODXL had been performed as previously described, whereby the presence of membranous expression was demonstrated to be prognostic [22].

Statistics

Non-parametric Mann–Whitney U or Kruskal-Wallis tests were applied for analysis of the correlations between membranous ezrin expression and clinicopathological characteristics. Classification and regression tree (CRT) analysis [24] was used to assess optimal prognostic cut-offs for ezrin expression. Receiver operating characteristics (ROC) curve analysis was also applied to verify the CRT-derived cutoffs. Kaplan-Meier analysis and log rank test were used to illustrate differences in 5-year overall survival (OS) and disease-specific survival (DSS) in strata according to high and low ezrin expression. Cox regression proportional hazards modeling was used to estimate the impact of ezrin expression on 5-year OS in both univariable and multivariable analysis, adjusted for age, sex, T-stage and grade. All tests were two sided. P-values <0.05 was considered significant. All statistical analyses were performed using IBM SPSS Statistics version 20.0 (SPSS Inc., Chicago, IL, USA).

Results

Distribution of ezrin expression and its association with clinicopathological characteristics

Following antibody optimisation and staining, ezrin expression could be evaluated in tumours from 100/110 (90.9%) cases in Cohort I and 342/344 (99.4%) cases in Cohort II. Lost cases were either a result of complete tissue loss during IHC preparation or an insufficient quantity of tumour tissue. Sample IHC images are shown in Figure 1 and the distribution of membranous ezrin expression in both cohorts is shown in Figure 2. There was no obvious heterogeneity regarding membranous or cytoplasmic ezrin expression between duplicate cores.

As shown in Table 1, analyses of the relationship between membranous staining and established clinicopathological factors revealed strong, significant associations

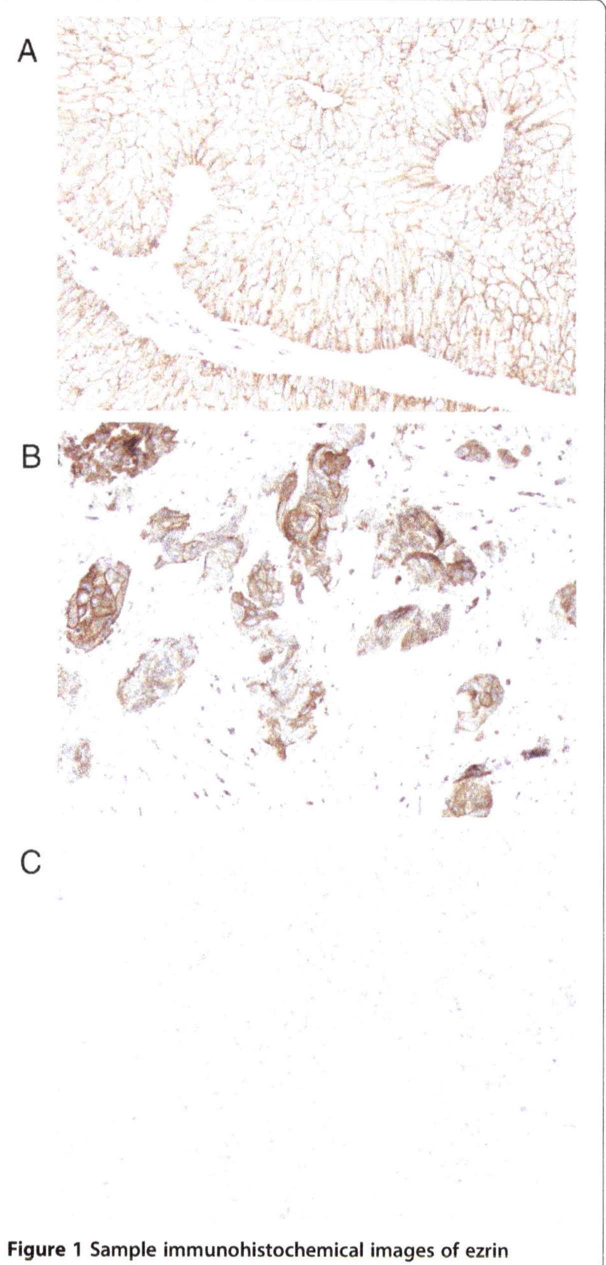

Figure 1 Sample immunohistochemical images of ezrin expression. Images (20x magnification) representing tumours with **(A)** nearly 100%, **(B)** approximately 50% and **(C)** negative ezrin expression.

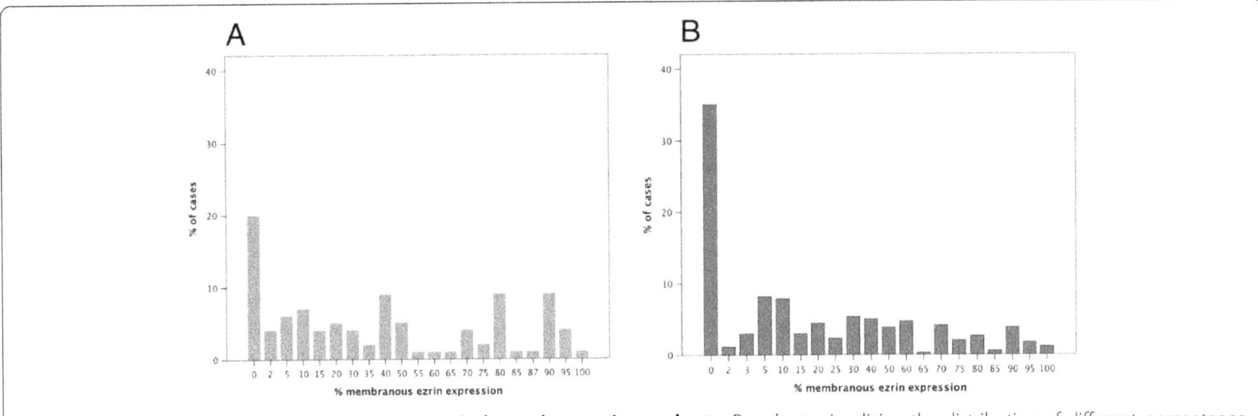

Figure 2 Distribution of ezrin expression in two independent patient cohorts. Bar charts visualizing the distribution of different percentages of ezrin expression in **(A)** cohort I (n = 100) and **(B)** cohort II (n = 342).

between reduced membranous ezrin expression and more advanced T-stage and high grade tumours in both cohorts (p < 0.001 for all). Moreover, there was a significant association between female gender and reduced membranous ezrin expression in both cohorts (p = 0.040 and p = 0.013). No associations were found between membranous ezrin expression and age. Cytoplasmic ezrin expression was not associated with any clinicopathological factors or with membranous ezrin expression (data not shown). In light of the significant associations of ezrin expression with female sex, the distribution of grade and T-stage according to sex was aslo analyzed, whereby it was found that grade did not differ by sex in neither cohort and that the distribution of T-stages was equal in both sexes in cohort I, but not in cohort II, where stage II-IV tumours were more common in women (p = 0.030).

Reduced ezrin expression was also significantly associated with the presence of membranous PODXL expression in both cohorts (p < 0.001 and p = 0.009).

Impact of membranous ezrin expression on survival

CRT analysis determined optimal prognostic cut-offs at 17.5% and 27.5% positive ezrin expression in cohort I and II, respectively, for 5-year OS in cohort I and II (Additional file 1A and 1B). In cohort II, an optimal

Table 1 Associations of membranous ezrin expression with clinicopathological and investigative parameters in two independent patient cohorts of urothelial bladder cancer

Factor	Cohort I (n = 100)			Cohort II (n = 342)		
	n (%)	Ezrin expression median (range)	*p-value*	n (%)	Ezrin expression median (range)	*p-value*
Age						
≤ average	46 (46.9)	30.9 (0.0-100)	0.222	157 (45.9)	10.0 (0.0-100)	0.136
>average	54 (54.0)	35.0 (0.0-95.0)		185 (54.1)	10.0 (0.0-100)	
Gender						
Female	25 (25.9)	10.0 (0.0-90.0)	0.040	82 (24.0)	5.00 (0.0-90.0)	0.013
Male	75 (75.0)	40.0 (0.0-100)		260 (76.0)	10.0 (0.0-100)	
T-stage						
Ta	41 (41.0)	75.0 (0.0-100)	<0.001	115 (33.6)	30.0 (0.0-100)	<0.001
T1	22 (22.0)	25.0 (0.0-95.0)		116 (33.9)	10.0 (0.0-95.0)	
T2-3	37 (37.0)	2.0 (0.0-80.0)		111 (32.5)	0.0 (0.0-60.0)	
Grade						
Low	44 (44.0)	72.5 (0.0-100)	<0.001	82 (24.0)	40.0 (0.0-100)	<0.001
High	56 (56.0)	10.0 (0.0-90.0)		260 (76.0)	5.0 (0.0-95.0)	
PODXL expression						
Negative	78 (78.8)	40.0 (0.0-100)	<0.001	306 (89.7)	10.0 (0.0-100)	0.009
Positive	21 (21.0)	5.00 (0–70.0)		35 (10.2)	(0.0-0.80)	

cutoff for DSS was set at 12.5% (Additional file 1C). The same optimal prognostic cutoffs were obtained by ROC analysis (data not shown).

As demonstrated in Figure 3, loss of ezrin expression was significantly associated with a reduced 5-year OS in cohort I (logrank $p < 0.001$, Figure 3A) and in cohort II (logrank $p < 0.001$, Figure 3B). In cohort II, low ezrin expression was also significantly associated with an impaired DSS (logrank $p < 0.001$, Figure 3C).

The associations between ezrin expression and survival were confirmed in unadjusted Cox regression analysis (Table 2). In adjusted analysis, reduced ezrin expression remained an independent predictor of a significantly reduced 5-year OS in Cohort I (HR = 1.99 (95% CI = 1.05-3.77). In cohort II, however, loss of ezrin expression did not remain prognostic after adjustment for established prognostic factors, neither for 5-year OS nor for DSS (Table 2).

Given the strong association between reduced ezrin expression and the presence of membranous PODXL expression, previously demonstrated to be an independent factor of tumour progression and an impaired survival in the herein investigated cohorts [22], we also compared the prognostic ability of ezrin and PODXL in the multivariable model. This revealed that inclusion of PODXL did not alter the prognostic value of ezrin expression, that was retained in Cohort I but not in Cohort II, neither for 5-year OS nor DSS. Of note, PODXL remained an independent prognostic factor in Cohort II, for both 5-year OS and DSS, but not in cohort I (data not shown).

Since the only previous study on the prognostic value if ezrin expression in bladder cancer was performed on tumours from patients with T1 tumours [7], the prognostic value of ezrin expression in subgroups according to T-stage was also examined. However, ezrin expression was not found to be prognostic in any particular T-stage in neither cohort (data not shown). Furthermore, in contrast to PODXL, reduced ezrin expression was not significantly associated with time to progression in non-muscle invasive (pTa and pT1 or pT1) tumours in cohort II (n = 134 or n = 66, data not shown). Of note, the number of cases that had received BCG treatment was only 17 and 7, respectively, in these two patient categories, hence not allowing for analyses of a potential treatment predictive effect of ezrin. There was no significant association between reduced ezrin expression and a more frequent rate of recurrence (data not shown).

There were no significant associations between cytoplasmic ezrin expression and survival in neither of the analysed cohorts, and a combined score of cytoplasmic and membranous ezrin expression did not add prognostic value (data not shown). Since the percentage of membranous staining was similar between duplicate cores, use of best or worst score did, as expected, not improve the prognostic value of ezrin expression (data not shown).

Discussion

The results from this study demonstrate that loss of membranous ezrin expression in urothelial bladder cancer is strongly associated with a more aggressive tumour phenotype; i.e. higher grade and more advanced tumour stage, and an impaired survival. To our best knowledge, the expression of ezrin in urothelial bladder cancer has only been described in two previous studies; one

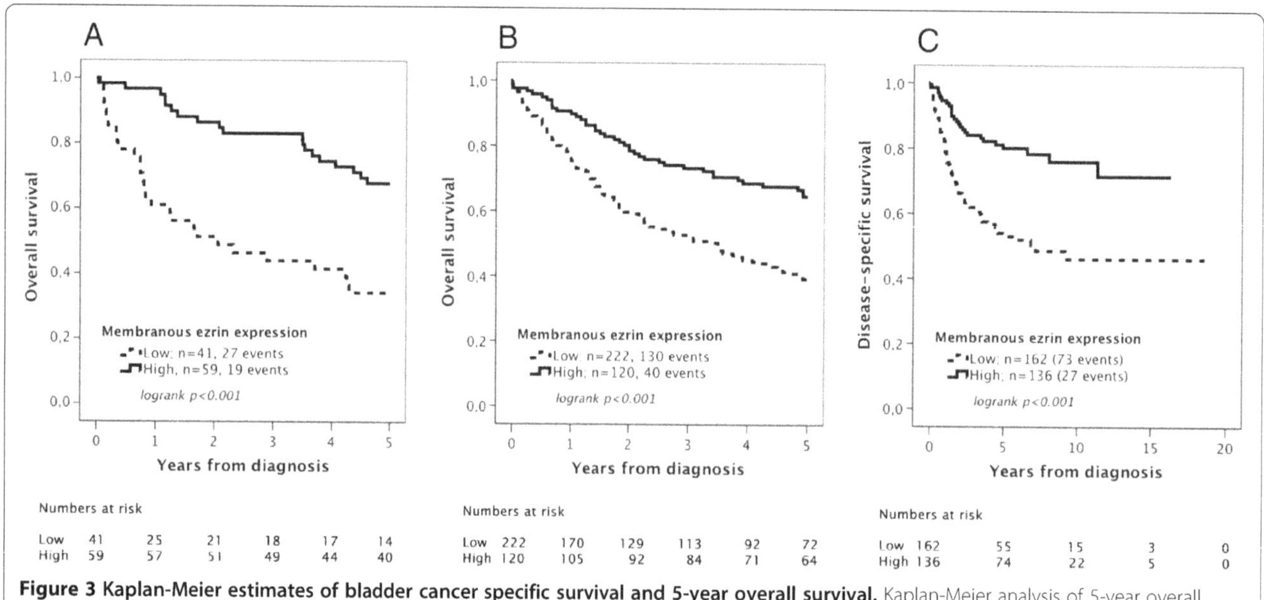

Figure 3 Kaplan-Meier estimates of bladder cancer specific survival and 5-year overall survival. Kaplan-Meier analysis of 5-year overall survival in **(A)** cohort I and **(B)** cohort II, and **(C)** disease-specific survival in cohort II.

Table 2 Relative risks of death from disease and overall death within 5 years according to clinicopathological factors and ezrin expression in two independent patient cohorts

	Cohort I			Cohort II					
	Risk of death within 5 years				Risk of death from disease			Risk of death within 5 years	
		Unadjusted	Adjusted		Unadjusted	Adjusted		Unadjusted	Adjusted
	n (events)	HR (95% CI)	HR (95% CI)	n (events)	HR (95% CI)	HR (95% CI)	n (events)	HR (95% CI)	HR (95% CI)
Age									
Continuous	100(46)	1.05(1.02-1.08)	1.05(1.02-1.08)	300(100)	1.05(1.03-1.07)	1.05(1.02-1.07)	342(170)	1.06(1.05-1.08)	1.07(1.05-1.08)
Gender									
Female	25(11)	1.00	1.00	71(28)	1.00	1.00	82(40)	1.00	1.00
Male	75(35)	0.96(0.49-1.89)	1.12(0.54-2.31)	227(72)	0.79(0.51-1.22)	1.03(0.66-1.61)	260(130)	0.97(0.68-1.38)	1.20(0.83-1.72)
Stage									
Ta	41(7)	1.00	1.00	104(13)	1.00	1.00	115(35)	1,00	1.00
T1	22(15)	5.06(2.06-12.46)	2.20(0.73-6.68)	97(25)	2.20(1.13-4.31)	2.17(1.11-4.25)	116(53)	1.63(1.06-2.50)	1.57(1.02-2.40)
T2-4	37(24)	6.15(2.64-14.31)	2.44(0.73-8.19)	97(62)	8.86(4.86-16.16)	8.70(4.76-15.89)	111(82)	4.34(2.91-6.46)	4.36(2.92-6.52)
Grade									
Low	44(9)	1.00	1.00	75(7)	1.00	1.00	82(20)	1.00	1.00
High	56(37)	4.71(2.27-9.79)	2.94(1.32-6.53)	223(93)	5.75(2.66-12.39)	1.67(0.64-4.35)	260(150)	3.09(1.94-4.93)	1.20(0.67-2.13)
Ezrin expression*									
High	59(19)	1.00	1.00	136(27)	1.00	1.00	120(40)	1.00	1.00
Low	41(27)	3.09(1.71-5.58)	1.99(1.05-3.77)	162(73)	2.77(1.78-4.31)	1.23(0.75-2.02)	222(130)	2.15(1.51-3.06)	1.24(0.84-1.84)

*High and low expression determined by CRT-analysis; cutoff 17.5% for 5-year OS in Cohort I, 27.5% for for 5-year OS in Cohort II and 12.5% for DSS in cohort II.

selected cohort of T1G3 tumours (n = 98) treated with non-maintenance BCG [7], and another unselected cohort (n = 104). In the former study, while correlations of ezrin expression with stage and grade could not be performed, the authors found no associations between ezrin expression and age, sex, substaging, tumour size, focality or the presence of CIS, but that reduced ezrin expression was an independent predictor of progression into muscle-invasive disease and shorter disease- specific survival [7]. In the latter study, loss of ezrin was found to correlate with higher grade and T-stage, and with muscularis propria invasion, but hazard ratios for risk of progression or association with survival were not presented [8].

Thus, the results from our study further validate previous findings of strong significant associations between loss of membranous ezrin expression and more advanced T-stage and high tumour grade in urothelial bladder cancer. Moreover, this study is the first to report the prognostic value of ezrin expression in tumours representing all stages and grades, whereby reduced ezrin expression was found to be associated with a significantly reduced 5-year OS in both examined cohorts, and with a significantly reduced DSS in cohort II. Of note, ezrin expression only retained an independent prognostic value for 5-year OS in the smaller cohort, and neither for 5-year OS nor for DSS in the larger, clinically more well-characterized, cohort. Therefore, further validation of the prognostic value of ezrin expression in additional patient cohorts is warranted. Nevertheless, since tumour stage may be difficult to determine in TURB-specimens, the strong link between loss of ezrin expression and advanced tumour stage found here indicates that assessment of ezrin may be an important surrogate marker for bladder cancer patients at risk of having progressive disease.

In contrast to the findings by Palou et al. [7], we were not able to demonstrate an association between reduced ezrin expression and risk of progression into muscle-invasive disease in pTa-pT1 or pT1-tumours (information only available in cohort II). It should however be pointed out that the number of patients having received BCG-treatment in our study was too small, and since all patients in the study by Palou had received non-maintenance BCG-treatment [7], a potential treatment predictive effect of ezrin cannot be ruled out, and should be taken into consideration in future studies.

The observed significant association between reduced ezrin expression and female sex in both cohorts is noteworthy, not least since the distribution of tumour grades did not differ between sexes in any of the cohorts, and a significant association between female sex and more advanced T-stage could only be found in cohort II. While the risk of bladder cancer is considerably higher in men, there is data indicating an impaired survival from bladder cancer in women [25]. These findings indicate that ezrin may be a relevant investigative biomarker in studies related to the molecular pathological epidemiology of urothelial bladder cancer, in particular studies addressing the influence of sex hormones and reproductive factors on cancer risk and survival.

Despite use of different antibodies for detection of ezrin expression in the two previous studies [7,8] and the present, the results were concordant, which further supports the utility of ezrin as a prognostic and, potentially treatment predictive, biomarker in urothelial bladder cancer. Immunohistochemistry has several advantages compared with other assays, e.g. gene expression analyses, since it is comparatively cheap, can readily be adopted into clinical protocols, and, most importantly, allows for assessment of biomarkers in relation to their subcellular location. In our study, no prognostic value or correlation with clinicopathological factors could be demonstrated for cytoplasmic ezrin expression, which is also in line with previous findings [7,8]. The lack of prognostic value for cytoplasmic ezrin expression is also in agreement with the observation of ERM proteins only being active when bound to the cell membrane and not when located in the cytoplasm [10].

The herein observed inverse association between membranous expression of ezrin and PODXL does not provide evidence of, but may well indicate, a functional link between these proteins in urothelial bladder cancer. This hypothesis is further supported by the previously demonstrated ability of PODXL to form complex with ezrin in breast and prostate cancer cells *in vitro*, thereby inducing phosphorylation of ezrin and changes in its subcellular location, in turn leading to an increased migration and invasion [21]. In light of the apparently contrasting prognostic value and intercorrelation of ezrin and PODXL expression in urothelial bladder cancer, it will be of interest to investigate the existence of a negative functional cooperativity between these proteins in this cancer form.

Of note, although cutoffs selected by CRT-analysis in our study varied somewhat between the cohorts and according to the endpoint, ranging from 12.5% to 27.5% membranous positivity, they still landed closely to the prognostic cutoff determined as the median percentage of ezrin expression at 20% in the study by Palou et al. [7], although all tumours in their study were pT1G3. A different approach was used in the study by Athanasopoulou et al., where four categories of a combined score of percentage and intensity of membranous ezrin immunoreactivity was applied in the statistical analyses [8]. Moreover, in that study, nearly all (103/104) tumours were reported to have positive membranous ezrin expression [8]. Future studies, preferably in the prospective setting, are warranted to determine optimal cutoffs for the potential use of ezrin as a biomarker in clinical practice.

Conclusions

In summary, the results from this study demonstrate that reduced membranous ezrin expression in urothelial bladder cancer is associated with more advanced tumours and a reduced survival. These findings suggest that ezrin may be a useful prognostic biomarker and possibly aid in tailoring the treatment of patients with non-muscle-invasive carcinoma of the bladder. Further studies are warranted in order to confirm the utility of ezrin as a prognostic biomarker in clinical practice.

Abbreviations

TMA: Tissue microarray; CRT: Classification regression tree; DSS: Disease-specific survival; OS: Overall survival; PFS: Progression-free survival; HR: Hazard ratio; CI: Confidence interval.

Competing interests

The authors declare that they have no competing interests.

Authors' contributions

GA and CW evaluated the immunohistochemical stainings, performed the statistical analyses and drafted the manuscript. US, PUM and KB collected clinical data. US and BN constructed the TMAs and BN performed the immunohistochemcal stainings. AG assisted with the statistical analysis and helped draft the manuscript. MU contributed with antibody validation. KJ conceived of the study, evaluated the immunohistochemistry, and helped draft the manuscript. All authors read and approved the final manuscript.

Acknowledgements

This study was supported by grants from the Knut and Alice Wallenberg Foundation, the Swedish Cancer Society, the Gunnar Nilsson Cancer Foundation, Lund University Faculty of Medicine and University Hospital Research Grants.

Author details

Department of Clinical Sciences, Oncology and Pathology, Lund University, Skåne University Hospital, Lund 221 85, Sweden. [2]Science for Life Laboratory, Royal Institute of Technology, Stockholm 171 21, Sweden. [3]School of Biotechnology, AlbaNova University Center, Royal Institute of Technology, Stockholm 106 91, Sweden. [4]Department of Surgical Sciences, Uppsala University, Uppsala 751 85, Sweden.

References

1. Ferlay J, Shin HR, Bray F, Forman D, Mathers C, Parkin DM: **Estimates of worldwide burden of cancer in 2008: GLOBOCAN 2008.** *Int J Cancer* 2010, **127**(12):2893–2917.
2. Jemal A, Siegel R, Xu J, Ward E: **Cancer statistics, 2010.** *CA Cancer J Clin* 2010, **60**(5):277–300.
3. Raghavan D, Shipley WU, Garnick MB, Russell PJ, Richie JP: **Biology and management of bladder cancer.** *N Engl J Med* 1990, **322**(16):1129–1138.
4. Schenkman E, Lamm DL: **Superficial bladder cancer therapy.** *ScientificWorldJournal* 2004, **4**(1):387–399.
5. van der Heijden AG, Witjes JA: **Recurrence, Progression, and Follow-Up in Non-Muscle-Invasive Bladder Cancer.** *Eur Urol Suppl* 2009, **8**(7):556–562.
6. Knowles MA: **Molecular subtypes of bladder cancer: Jekyll and Hyde or chalk and cheese?** *Carcinogenesis* 2006, **27**(3):361–373.

7. Palou J, Algaba F, Vera I, Rodriguez O, Villavicencio H, Sanchez-Carbayo M: **Protein expression patterns of ezrin are predictors of progression in T1G3 bladder tumours treated with nonmaintenance bacillus Calmette-Guerin.** *Eur Urol* 2009, **56**(5):829–836.
8. Athanasopoulou A, Aroukatos P, Nakas D, Repanti M, Papadaki H, Bravou V: **Decreased ezrin and paxillin expression in human urothelial bladder tumors correlate with tumor progression.** *Urol Oncol* 2013, **31**(6):836–842.
9. Mangeat P, Roy C, Martin M: **ERM proteins in cell adhesion and membrane dynamics.** *Trends Cell Biol* 1999, **9**(5):187–192.
10. Bretscher A, Edwards K, Fehon RG: **ERM proteins and merlin: integrators at the cell cortex.** *Nat Rev Mol Cell Biol* 2002, **3**(8):586–599.
11. Curto M, McClatchey AI: **Ezrin…a metastatic detERMinant?** *Cancer Cell* 2004, **5**(2):113–114.
12. Bruce B, Khanna G, Ren L, Landberg G, Jirstrom K, Powell C, Borczuk A, Keller ET, Wojno KJ, Meltzer P, Baird K, McClatchey A, Bretscher A, Hewitt SM, Khanna C: **Expression of the cytoskeleton linker protein ezrin in human cancers.** *Clin Exp Metastasis* 2007, **24**(2):69–78.
13. Li Q, Gao H, Xu H, Wang X, Pan Y, Hao F, Qiu X, Stoecker M, Wang E, Wang E: **Expression of ezrin correlates with malignant phenotype of lung cancer, and in vitro knockdown of ezrin reverses the aggressive biological behavior of lung cancer cells.** *Tumour Biol* 2012, **33**(5):1493–1504.
14. Tan J, Zhang C, Qian J: **Expression and significance of Six1 and Ezrin in cervical cancer tissue.** *Tumour Biol* 2011, **32**(6):1241–1247.
15. Ohtani K, Sakamoto H, Rutherford T, Chen Z, Satoh K, Naftolin F: **Ezrin, a membrane-cytoskeletal linking protein, is involved in the process of invasion of endometrial cancer cells.** *Cancer Lett* 1999, **147**(1–2):31–38.
16. Elliott BE, Meens JA, SenGupta SK, Louvard D, Arpin M: **The membrane cytoskeletal crosslinker ezrin is required for metastasis of breast carcinoma cells.** *Breast Cancer Res* 2005, **7**(3):R365–R373.
17. Weng WH, Ahlen J, Astrom K, Lui WO, Larsson C: **Prognostic impact of immunohistochemical expression of ezrin in highly malignant soft tissue sarcomas.** *Clin Cancer Res* 2005, **11**(17):6198–6204.
18. Jin J, Jin T, Quan M, Piao Y, Lin Z: **Ezrin overexpression predicts the poor prognosis of gastric adenocarcinoma.** *Diagn Pathol* 2012, **7**:135.
19. Kang YK, Hong SW, Lee H, Kim WH: **Prognostic implications of ezrin expression in human hepatocellular carcinoma.** *Mol Carcinog* 2010, **49**(9):798–804.
20. Moilanen J, Lassus H, Leminen A, Vaheri A, Butzow R, Carpen O: **Ezrin immunoreactivity in relation to survival in serous ovarian carcinoma patients.** *Gynecol Oncol* 2003, **90**(2):273–281.
21. Sizemore S, Cicek M, Sizemore N, Ng KP, Casey G: **Podocalyxin increases the aggressive phenotype of breast and prostate cancer cells in vitro through its interaction with ezrin.** *Cancer Res* 2007, **67**(13):6183–6191.
22. Boman K, Larsson AH, Segersten U, Kuteeva E, Johannesson H, Nodin B, Eberhard J, Uhlen M, Malmstrom PU, Jirstrom K: **Membranous expression of podocalyxin-like protein is an independent factor of poor prognosis in urothelial bladder cancer.** *Br J Cancer* 2013, **108**(11):2321–2328.
23. Boman K, Segersten U, Ahlgren G, Eberhard J, Uhlen M, Jirstrom K, Malmstrom PU: **Decreased expression of RNA-binding motif protein 3 correlates with tumour progression and poor prognosis in urothelial bladder cancer.** *BMC Urol* 2013, **13**(1):17.
24. Breiman L: *Classification and regression trees.* New York, N.Y.: Chapman & Hall; 1993.
25. Jung KW, Park S, Shin A, Oh CM, Kong HJ, Jun JK, Won YJ: **Do female cancer patients display better survival rates compared with males? Analysis of the Korean national registry data, 2005–2009.** *PLoS One* 2012, **7**(12):e52457.

7

PET/CT versus conventional CT for detection of lymph node metastases in patients with locally advanced bladder cancer

Firas Aljabery[1,3*], Gunnar Lindblom[2], Susann Skoog[2], Ivan Shabo[3], Hans Olsson[3], Johan Rosell[4] and Staffan Jahnson[1,3]

Abstract

Background: We studied patients treated with radical cystectomy for locally advanced bladder cancer to compare the results of both preoperative positron emission tomography/computed tomography (PET/CT) and conventional CT with the findings of postoperative histopathological evaluation of lymph nodes.

Methods: Patients who had bladder cancer and were candidates for cystectomy underwent preoperative PET/CT using 18-fluorodeoxyglucose (FDG) and conventional CT. The results regarding lymph node involvement were independently evaluated by two experienced radiologists and were subsequently compared with histopathology results, the latter of which were reassessed by an experienced uropathologist (HO).

Results: There were 54 evaluable patients (mean age 68 years, 47 [85 %] males and 7 [15 %] females) with pT and pN status as follows: < pT2-14 (26 %), pT2-10 (18 %), and > pT2-30 (56 %); pN0 37 (69 %) and pN+ 17 (31 %). PET/CT showed positive lymph nodes in 12 patients (22 %), and 7 of those cases were confirmed by histopathology; the corresponding results for conventional CT were 11 (20 %) and 7 patients (13 %), respectively. PET/CT had 41 % sensitivity, 86 % specificity, 58 % PPV, and 76 % NPV, whereas the corresponding figures for conventional CT were 41 %, 89 %, 64 %, and 77 %. Additional analyses of the right and left side of the body or in specified anatomical regions gave similar results.

Conclusions: In this study, PET/CT and conventional CT had similar low sensitivity in detecting and localizing regional lymph node metastasis in bladder cancer.

Background

Accurate clinical staging of localized or regionally advanced urinary bladder cancer remains a challenge. Lymph node (LN) metastasis is correlated with decreased overall survival (OS), and it is plausible that survival in patients with or without such metastasis can be improved by LN dissection [1–5]. Also, patients with LN involvement may be candidates for preoperative chemotherapy if considered for cystectomy [6–10]. Preoperative staging of regional LNs has relied on radiological imaging to identify nodes that meet anatomical criteria. Conventional computed tomography (CT) and magnetic resonance imaging (MRI) are frequently employed as diagnostic tools for staging in evaluation of muscle-invasive bladder cancer. Both these methods use LN size as a criterion for diagnosis and false-negative rates can be as high as 40 % [11–13]. Thus there is a need for a non-invasive imaging modality that can achieve more accurate preoperative staging of bladder cancer.

Positron emission tomography/CT (PET/CT) is an approach in which the capacity to detect specific metabolic tissue changes is combined with simultaneous accurate anatomical depiction. Possible limitations of this combined technique are that the optimal isotope for studying bladder cancer has not yet been determined, and most isotopes have a short half-life and hence require use of an on-site cyclotron or a sophisticated transport modality [14, 15].

* Correspondence: Firas.Abdul-Sattar.Aljabery@regionostergotland.se
[1]Department of Urology, Linköping University Hospital, Linköping, Sweden
[3]Department of Clinical and Experimental Medicine, Faculty of Health Sciences, Linköping University, Linköping, Sweden
Full list of author information is available at the end of the article

Most malignant tumors are characterized by elevated glucose metabolism [16, 17], and therefore increased cell proliferation in tumors can be imaged by PET/CT as increased uptake of 18-fluorodeoxyglucose (FDG). FDG is currently the only isotope approved by the US Food and Drug Administration for use in clinical oncology. FDG has a relatively short half-life (110 min), and it is excreted by the kidneys and accumulated in the urinary tract, which makes it difficult to study the urinary system in detail [18, 19]. Nevertheless, FDG is still the isotope that is most widely used to investigate bladder cancer [14].

In the present study, patients treated by radical cystectomy for locally advanced bladder cancer were investigated to compare the results of preoperative PET/CT and conventional CT with the findings of postoperative histopathological evaluation of LNs.

Methods

Patients

At our hospital, a total of 67 patients with urinary bladder cancer were scheduled for radical cystectomy with pelvic LN dissection between 2010 and 2012. All these patients underwent FDG-PET/CT and conventional CT of the thorax and abdomen as part of pre-cystectomy evaluation. Twelve of the patients did not have a cystectomy for the following reasons: 4 had distant metastasis (M1; positive in both conventional CT and PET/CT); 2 had ASA 4 and high surgical risk; 6 preferred radiation therapy. One of the remaining 55 patients did undergo radical cystectomy but had no LN dissection and was therefore excluded from further analysis. All patients were scheduled for FDG-PET/CT of the thorax and the abdomen 1 to 2 months before cystectomy. However, 6 patients had undergone PET/CT more than 2 months before cystectomy, because the surgery had been delayed to perform necessary investigations to address suspected distant metastases. No patient had preoperative chemotherapy.

The use of PET/CT as an additional mode of investigation of candidates for cystectomy was initiated at our department as a routine procedure in all patients. The method was considered to be safe and well established. We studied herein if additional information could be extracted from PET/CT in this particular setting. No ethical consent was therefore considered to be necessary.

However, we had prior to the start of the investigation an approval from The Regional Ethics Committee (Reference number M42-08). We used oral informed consent from the patients.

Equipment and imaging protocol

The patients scheduled for FDG-PET/CT fasted at least 4 h before injection of the FDG. Blood glucose was monitored immediately before the injection, and a level lower than 8 mmol/L was required to perform the examination. The dose of FDG was 4 MBq/kg body weight. Images were acquired 60 min after the injection, and the patient drank 1 L of fluid or contrast medium during the 60-min interval between injection and imaging. The examination was done using a Siemens Biograph 40 PET/CT scanner with the patient in a dorsal recumbent position with the arms above the head. Full-dose CT with IV contrast was performed first, followed by PET (1.5–mm and 5–mm slices and a resolution of 4.2 mm). CT was performed using a thickness of 1.5 mm and a gap of 1.5 mm at 100 kV while mAS was regulated automatically according to the volume of the patient.

The majority of the patients (88 %) had an indwelling three-way catheter with bladder irrigation for continuous evacuation of the bladder. In patients without such a catheter, a renewed low-dose CT with PET was conducted approximately 30 min after the start of the initial imaging to detect PET-positive foci in the renal pelvis, the ureters, or the bladder after evacuation of all excreted FDG.

Image interpretation

The PET/CT images were evaluated by two radiologists specialized and/or with extensive clinical experience in PET/CT using axial, coronal and sagittal reconstructions. These experts performed the assessments independently and without knowledge of operative or postoperative data. In cases in which the results obtained by the two radiologists were discordant, the investigations were mutually reviewed and discussed to reach consensus. Kappa analysis showed good agreement (Kappa value 0.85) between the PET/CT evaluations conducted by the two radiologists. Conventional CT and PET/CT were evaluated separately. The CT scans were assessed without knowledge of the PET findings. Positive LN findings were recorded for the following anatomical regions used in clinical practice for pelvic LN dissection: obturator fossa, external iliac, internal iliac, and common iliac. All PET images were evaluated by determining the maximum standardized uptake value (SUV), using a SUV-max cut-off of 2.5. LNs were considered to be positive by conventional CT if they had a diameter of ≥ 1 cm, and positive by PET/CT if they exhibited higher levels of activity than the SUV-max cut-off level regardless of their size. No pathological LNs were found in the pelvis outside the surgical templates. Distant metastases were suspected when higher levels of radioactivity were found in other organs, and in such cases evaluation was done to exclude metastasis before surgery.

Surgery

Radical cystectomy was performed with a standardized LN dissection. The upper limit of the LN dissection was at the level of the ureteric crossing of the common iliac vein immediately cranial to confluence of the external and internal iliac veins in 49 (91 %) patients and was extended to the aortic bifurcation in 5 patients. The decision to extend the dissection was made by the surgeon if LN metastases were suspected based on the radiological, clinical, or perioperative data. The dissection extended down to the level of Cooper's ligament, with the genitofemoral nerve as the lateral boundary. Specimens from the following four anatomical regions on both the right and the left side were sent separately for pathological examination: obturator, external iliac, and internal iliac, as well as the common iliac in cases with dissection to the aortic bifurcation. Each LN was sectioned in the middle along the larger axis, and a single 4-μm slice was mounted on a slide and stained with haematoxylin-eosin before analysis.

Histopathological reevaluation

The specimens on the patients' slides from cystectomy and lymph node dissection material were all reevaluated microscopically regarding T-stage, WHO grade, presence of lymphovascular invasion, and LN metastasis. This reassessment was performed by an experienced uropathologist (HO). All positive nodes were completely or almost completely infiltrated by bladder cancer.

Data analysis

Results of PET/CT, conventional CT, and histopathological examination were compared on three levels: first, regarding positive or negative results in general for each patient regardless of node localization; second, according to the four anatomical regions; third, with respect to the side of the body (right or left) of each patient's LN dissection. The third approach was applied because of potential difficulties associated with evaluating an exact anatomical region in both PET and surgery. Using the histopathological examination as gold standard, each PET/CT and conventional CT examination was classified as true positive or false positive, and true negative or false negative. The sensitivity, specificity, positive predictive value (PPV), and negative predictive value (NPV) were calculated.

Results

Of the 54 evaluable patients, 50 (93 %) had urothelial cancer and 4 (7 %) had non-urothelial cancer. Also, 40 (74 %) of the 54 patients had muscle-invasive tumors. The mean time between PET/CT and surgery was 30 (6–133) days. Six patients had undergone PET/CT more than 2 months before cystectomy, because the surgery had been delayed for further investigations due to suspected distant metastasis. In one of these 6 patients, LNs were positive in histopathological examination but negative by both PET/CT and conventional CT; for the remaining 5 patients, all 3 investigations were negative. Thus 54 patients were eligible for evaluation in our study, 47 men and 7 women (mean age 68 years, range 46–85 years). Considering all 54, histopathological examination showed no LN metastasis (N0) in 37 (69 %) but revealed 1 or more positive LNs in 17 (31 %), and 16 (94 %) of those 17 patients had pT3-pT4 disease. FDG uptake was found in 12 patients (22 %), and 7 of those observations were confirmed by pathology. Conventional CT alone showed enlarged LNs in 11 patients (20 %), which was confirmed by pathology in 7 cases. Equivalent findings were obtained by both PET/CT and conventional CT in 43 (80 %) of the 54 patients (Table 1). The following was observed in the remaining 11 patients (20 %): 9 were positive by PET/CT and negative by conventional CT, and only 1 of those findings was confirmed by pathology; 2 were positive by conventional CT and negative by PET/CT, and neither case was confirmed by pathology.

At the first level of analysis, which considered the whole patient, sensitivity was low for both PET/CT and conventional CT (Table 2). At the second level of analysis, we investigated all 1,518 LNs (mean 28 nodes per

Table 1 Patient characteristics

	Pathology findings		
	Positive	Negative	Total
	N	N	N
Gender			
Male	14	33	47
Female	3	4	7
Age			
Mean ≤ 68y	6	22	28
Mean > 68 y	11	15	26
Clinical stage			
cT1	1	8	9
cT2	6	21	10
cT3	10	7	16
cT4	0	1	14
Pathological stage			
pT1	0	14	14
pT2	1	9	10
pT3	7	9	16
pT4	9	5	14
PET/CT			
Positive	7	5	12
Negative	10	32	42
CT findings			
Positive	7	4	11
Negative	10	33	43

Table 2 Different levels of analysis of lymph nodes comparing pathology results and results of conventional CT and PET/CT in 54 patients treated with cystectomy for locally advanced bladder cancer

First level of analysis						
	Patho pos	Patho neg	Sensitivity	Specificity	PPV	NPV
CT pos	7	4	41 %	89 %	64 %	77 %
CT neg -	10	33				
PET pos+	7	5	41 %	86 %	58 %	76 %
PET neg-	10	32				
Second level of analysis						
	Patho pos	Patho neg	Sensitivity	Specificity	PPV	NPV
CT pos	7	10	13 %	97 %	41 %	85 %
CT neg	48	282				
PET pos	14	24	25 %	92 %	37 %	87 %
PET neg	41	268				
Third level of analysis						
	Patho pos	Patho neg	Sensitivity	Specificity	PPV	NPV
CT pos	9	5	31 %	94 %	64 %	79 %
CT neg	20	74				
PET pos	11	14	38 %	82 %	44 %	78 %
PET neg	18	65				

patient) excised from 347 sites in the stipulated anatomical regions, and metastases were confirmed by pathology in 99 LNs (7 % of all LNs) from 55 (16 %) of the 347 sites. FDG-PET/CT was negative in 41 sites with metastases, which was confirmed by pathology, whereas conventional CT was negative in 48 sites with metastases. Also at this level of analysis, sensitivity was low for both PET/CT and conventional CT (Table 2).

Thus there were difficulties in determining the exact location of individual LNs in precise anatomical regions, both during surgery and in radiological evaluation. Accordingly, in the third level of analysis, we considered both the left and the right side of in each patient, which showed low sensitivity for both PET/CT and conventional CT (Table 2).

Discussion

In the present study, we compared FDG-PET/CT and conventional CT regarding the rate of detection of positive LNs as standard investigation of all patients before cystectomy, using histopathological examination of LNs as the gold standard. We found low levels of sensitivity for both FDG-PET/CT and conventional CT, which agrees with the results obtained by Swinnen et al. [20]. However, the levels we observed are lower than those reported by Drieskens et al, Liu et al, and Kibel et al, and Goodfellow et al [21–24], who noted sensitivity rates ranging from 60 to 77 % when using protocols for PET/CT imaging and analyses similar to those employed in our study. There is no obvious explanation for this discrepancy, although most of the mentioned studies were rather small, and hence only a few additional patients with positive PET/CT results might have had a marked impact on the rate of sensitivity.

Another plausible reason for differences in the LN detection rate might be related to the extent of LN dissection. In our series, we used the level of the ureteric crossing of the common iliac vein immediately cranial to confluence of the external and internal iliac veins as the upper limit of dissection in the majority of cases, whereas extended dissection to the aortic bifurcation was used in patients with clinical or radiological suspicion of LN metastases. A similar approach was applied by Kibel et al [22] with 70 % sensitivity. However, Swinnen et al [20] performed dissection to the aortic bifurcation in all patients and despite that observed sensitivity rates comparable to those noted in our series. These findings seem to suggest that the level of LN dissection does not determine the rate of sensitivity of PET/CT. Other investigators have discussed the completeness of LN dissection in terms of the number of extirpated LNs, using cut-offs of 16 and 20 LNs as an indication of a complete dissection [6, 11]. In our patients, a mean of 28 LNs were extirpated, which might represent an acceptable level of completeness in the dissection. Notably, studies of other comparable series have not given any information about the number of LNs removed [21–25].

Optimally, PET/CT should detect a localized pathological LN in order to enable regionally limited LN dissection [16, 20]. However, we found that sensitivity decreased from 41 % on a patient level to 25 % on a regional LN level, and Drieskens et al. [21] have also noted a drop in sensitivity from 60 % to 50 % on the regional level. Even though the indicated lower sensitivity implies that PET/CT is not suitable for exact localization of regional LN metastases, this hybrid imaging technique might nonetheless be useful to achieve improved tumor staging in individual patients, particularly if it is performed in combination with percutaneous biopsies [25]. Furthermore, PET/CT might aid detection of pathological LNs outside the surgical template. Although we did not find any pathological LN outside the surgical template in our small series this might be an advantage of PET/CT to limit LN dissection as suggested by others [16, 20].

Employing novel tracers might also enhance detection of LN metastases. Orevi et al obtained promising PET/CT results using 11C-choline to investigate 18 patients with bladder cancer [26], and Ahlström et al reported 11C-methionine to be superior to FDG in this context [27].

Moreover, 2 recent studies have shown that PET/MRI alone had a greater impact on clinical management compared to PET/CT alone [28, 29]. However we are still awaiting a systematic study PET/MRI in bladder cancer.

PET/CT has a number of limitations, and a potential drawback of our study concerns the difficulty in localizing the exact site of pathological LNs both at surgery and at PET/CT. The resolution of PET is inadequate and needs to be improved to provide better images, although tumor size was not a problem in our study as the image resolution was 4.2 mm and all our positive LNs were massively infiltrated with tumour cells [30]. Other potential weaknesses of our study include aspects related to tumor biology, such as the degree of glucose consumption, which varies considerably and is affected by multiple factors [16]. A major drawback of FDG-PET/CT is urinary elimination of FDG, which can be only partly neutralized by using a bladder washing/rinsing system in combination with diuretic medication and intravenous fluids [18]. It is possible that other isotopes (e.g. 11C-methionine or 11C-choline) can be more useful than FDG as the tracer in PET/CT investigation of bladder cancer [26].

The design of our study also had some limitations. This investigation comprising a small number of patients, and hence no firm conclusions can be drawn from the results. Furthermore, it was our intention to explore the possibility of routine PET/CT for all patients undergoing cystectomy. Considering the substantial number of PET/CT examinations that were negative in our subjects, it might have been more appropriate to study patients who were at greater risk of having positive LNs. Our assessments relied on pathological examination of single sections of LNs, and it is possible that using step-sectioned nodes for comparison would have improved the sensitivity and specificity of PET/CT. Finally, the time from PET/CT to surgery in our study was too long in some cases, which might have influenced the results.

Conclusions

This study showed that, compared to conventional CT, FDG-PET/ CT provided no improvement in detection and localization of regional LN metastases in bladder cancer. Both these imaging approaches showed low sensitivity in detecting LN metastases, and the sensitivity decreased with a more exact degree of LN localization.

Competing interests

The authors declare that they have no competing interests.

Authors' contributions

FJ: Designed the study. Analysis and interpretations of the data. Revising and drafting the manuscript. GL: Participated in designing the study. Carried out the radiological study. SS: Participated in designing the study. Carried out the radiological study. JR: Carried out the statistical analysis. IS: Participated in designing the study. Analysis and interpretations of the data. Revising and drafting the manuscript. HO: Participated in designing the study. Carried out the histopathological analysis. SJ: Designed the study. Analysis and interpretations of the data. Revising and drafting the manuscript. All authors read and approved the final manuscript.

Author details

[1]Department of Urology, Linköping University Hospital, Linköping, Sweden. [2]Department of Radiology, Linköping University Hospital, Linköping, Sweden. [3]Department of Clinical and Experimental Medicine, Faculty of Health Sciences, Linköping University, Linköping, Sweden. [4]Regional Cancer Center Southeast Sweden, County Council of Östergötland, Linköping, Sweden.

References

1. D'Souza AM, Pohar KS, Arif T, Geyer S, Zynger DL. Retrospective analysis of survival in muscle-invasive bladder cancer: impact of pT classification, node status, lymphovascular invasion, and neoadjuvant chemotherapy. Virchows Arch. 2012;461:467.
2. Stephenson AJ, Gong MC, Campbell SC, Fergany AF, Hansel DE. Aggregate lymph node metastasis diameter and survival after radical cystectomy for invasive bladder cancer. Urology. 2010;75:382.
3. Abol-Enein H, El-Baz M, Abd El-Hameed MA, Abdel-Latif M, Ghoneim MA. Lymph node involvement in pyaatients with bladder cancer treated with radical cystectomy: a patho-anatomical study–a single center experience. J Urol. 2004;172:1818.
4. Gakis G, Efstathiou J, Lerner SP, Cookson MS, Keegan KA, Guru KA, et al. ICUD-EAU International Consultation on Bladder Cancer 2012: Radical cystectomy and bladder preservation for muscle-invasive urothelial carcinoma of the bladder. Eur Urol. 2013;63:45.
5. Sanderson KM, Skinner D, Stein JP. The prognostic and staging value of lymph node dissection in the treatment of invasive bladder cancer. Nat Clin Pract Urol. 2006;3:485.
6. Petrelli F, Coinu A, Cabiddu M, Ghilardi M, Vavassori I, Barni S. Correlation of pathologic complete response with survival after neoadjuvant chemotherapy in bladder cancer treated with cystectomy: a meta-analysis. Eur Urol. 2014;65:350.
7. Yuh BE, Ruel N, Wilson TG, Vogelzang N, Pal SK. Pooled analysis of clinical outcomes with neoadjuvant cisplatin and gemcitabine chemotherapy for muscle invasive bladder cancer. J Urol. 2013;189:1682.
8. Sternberg CN, Bellmunt J, Sonpavde G, Siefker-Radtke AO, Stadler WM, Bajorin DF, et al. ICUD-EAU International Consultation on Bladder Cancer 2012: Chemotherapy for urothelial carcinoma-neoadjuvant and adjuvant settings. Eur Urol. 2013;63:58.
9. Culp SH, Dickstein RJ, Grossman HB, Pretzsch SM, Porten S, Daneshmand S, et al. Refining patient selection for neoadjuvant chemotherapy before radical cystectomy. J Urol. 2014;191:40.
10. Weisbach L, Dahlem R, Simone G, Hansen J, Soave A, Engel O, et al. Lymph node dissection during radical cystectomy for bladder cancer treatment: considerations on relevance and extent. Int Urol Nephrol. 2013;45:1561.
11. Paik ML, Scolieri MJ, Brown SL, Spirnak JP, Resnick MI. Limitations of computerized tomography in staging invasive bladder cancer before radical cystectomy. J Urol. 2000;163:1693.
12. Nishimura K, Horii Y, Matsuda T, Okada Y, Takeuchi H, Yoshida O, et al. Clinical application of MRI for urological malignancy. 2: Usefulness of various imaging modalities for local staging of bladder cancer; a comparison between MRI, CT and transurethral ultrasonography. Hinyokika Kiyo. 1988;34:2091.
13. Liedberg F, Bendahl PO, Davidsson T, Gudjonsson S, Holmer M, Månsson W, et al. Preoperative staging of locally advanced bladder cancer before radical cystectomy using 3 tesla magnetic resonance imaging with a standardized protocol. Scand J Urol. 2013;47:108.
14. Nayak B, Dogra PN, Naswa N, Kumar R. Diuretic 18F-FDG PET/CT imaging for detection and locoregional staging of urinary bladder cancer: prospective evaluation of a novel technique. Eur J Nucl Med Mol Imaging. 2013;40:386.
15. Schoder H, Larson SM. Positron emission tomography for prostate, bladder, and renal cancer. Semin Nucl Med. 2004;34:274.
16. Zheng J. Energy metabolism of cancer: Glycolysis versus oxidative phosphorylation (Review). Oncol Lett. 2012;4:1151.
17. Williams RD. Combined metabolic/anatomical imaging in urologic oncology. J Urol. 2006;176:863.

18. Bouchelouche K, Oehr P. Positron emission tomography and positron emission tomography/computerized tomography of urological malignancies: an update review. J Urol. 2008;179:34.
19. Bouchelouche K, Turkbey B, Choyke PL. PET/CT and MRI in Bladder Cancer. J Cancer Sci Ther. 2012;14
20. Swinnen G, Maes A, Pottel H, Vanneste A, Billiet I, Lesage K, et al. FDG-PET/CT for the preoperative lymph node staging of invasive bladder cancer. Eur Urol. 2010;57:641.
21. Drieskens O, Oyen R, Van Poppel H, Vankan Y, Flamen P, Mortelmans L. FDG-PET for preoperative staging of bladder cancer. Eur J Nucl Med Mol Imaging. 2005;32:1412.
22. Kibel AS, Dehdashti F, Katz MD, Klim AP, Grubb RL, Humphrey PA, et al. Prospective study of [18F]fluorodeoxyglucose positron emission tomography/computed tomography for staging of muscle-invasive bladder carcinoma. J Clin Oncol. 2009;27:4314.
23. Liu IJ, Lai YH, Espiritu JI, Segall GM, Srinivas S, Nino-Murcia M, et al. Evaluation of fluorodeoxyglucose positron emission tomography imaging in metastatic transitional cell carcinoma with and without prior chemotherapy. Urol Int. 2006;77:69.
24. Goodfellow H, Viney Z, Hughes P, Rankin S, Rottenberg G, Hughes S, et al. Role of fluorodeoxyglucose positron emission tomography (FDG PET)-computed tomography (CT) in the staging of bladder cancer. BJU Int. 2014;114:389.
25. Mertens LS, Fioole-Bruining A, Vegt E, Vogel WV, van Rhijn BW, Horenblas S. Impact of (18) F-fluorodeoxyglucose (FDG)-positron-emission tomography/computed tomography (PET/CT) on management of patients with carcinoma invading bladder muscle. BJU Int. 2013;112:729.
26. Orevi M, Klein M, Mishani E, Chisin R, Freedman N, Gofrit ON. 11C-acetate PET/CT in bladder urothelial carcinoma: intraindividual comparison with 11C-choline. Clin Nucl Med. 2012;37:67.
27. Ahlstrom H, Malmstrom PU, Letocha H, Andersson J, Långström B, Nilsson S. Positron emission tomography in the diagnosis and staging of urinary bladder cancer. Acta Radiol. 1996;37:180.
28. Partovi S, Robbin MR, Steinbach OC, Kohan A, Rubbert C, Vercher-Conejero JL, et al. Initial experience of MR/PET in a clinical cancer center. J Magn Reson Imaging. 2014;39:768.
29. Catalano OA, Rosen BR, Sahani DV, Hahn PF, Guimaraes AR, Vangel MG, et al. Clinical impact of PET/MR imaging in patients with cancer undergoing same-day PET/CT: initial experience in 134 patients–a hypothesis-generating exploratory study. Radiology. 2013;269:857.
30. Rahmim A, Qi J, Sossi V. Resolution modeling in PET imaging: theory, practice, benefits, and pitfalls. Med Phys. 2013;40:064301.

8

Correlation between psychological stress levels and the severity of overactive bladder symptoms

Henry Lai[1,2*], Vivien Gardner[1], Joel Vetter[1] and Gerald L Andriole[1]

Abstract

Background: The relationship between psychological stress and interstitial cystitis/bladder pain syndrome (IC/BPS) has been well described. Even though there is some overlapping of symptoms between overactive bladder (OAB) and IC/BPS, there have been very few studies that specifically investigated the relationship between psychological stress and urinary symptoms in OAB patients who do not have pelvic pain. Here we examined the relationship between psychological stress levels and the severity of overactive bladder (OAB) symptoms.

Methods: Patients diagnosed with OAB (n=51), IC/BPS (n=27), and age-matched healthy controls (n=30) participated in a case control study that inquired about their psychological stress levels using the perceived stress scale (PSS). PSS reported by the three patient groups were compared. Among OAB patients, their responses on the PSS was correlated to OAB symptoms using the following questionnaires: 1) international consultation on incontinence – urinary incontinence (ICIQ-UI), 2) international consultation on incontinence – overactive bladder (ICIQ-OAB), 3) OAB-q short form, 4) urogenital distress inventory (UDI-6), 5) incontinence impact questionnaire (IIQ-7), 6) urgency severity scale (USS), 7) numeric rating scales of urgency symptom, and 8) frequency symptom. Spearman's correlation tests were performed to examine the relationship between psychological stress levels and the severity of OAB symptoms.

Results: OAB patients reported psychological stress levels that were as high as IC/BPS patients (median 17.0 versus 18.0, p=0.818, Wilcoxon sum rank test), and significantly higher than healthy controls (17.0, versus 7.5, p=0.001). Among OAB patients, there was a positive correlation between perceived stress levels and urinary incontinence symptoms (ICIQ-UI, Spearman's correlation coefficient=0.39, p=0.007), and impacts on quality of life (UDI-6, IIQ-7, OAB-q quality of life subscale; Spearman's correlation coefficient=0.32, 0.31, 0.39, and p=0.028, 0.005, 0.029, respectively). No significant correlation was observed between perceived stress levels and urgency or frequency symptoms (ICIQ-OAB, USS, numeric ratings of urgency and frequency).

Conclusions: OAB patients reported psychological stress levels that were as high as IC/BPS patients, and significantly higher than healthy controls. There was a positive correlation between perceived stress levels and urinary incontinence symptoms, and its impacts on quality of life among OAB patients.

Keywords: Psychological stress, Overactive bladder, Urgency incontinence, Urinary urgency, Interstitial cystitis

Background

The relationship between psychological stress and interstitial cystitis/bladder pain syndrome (IC/BPS) has been well described. Many IC/BPS patients reported that stress exacerbates their bladder symptoms, including urgency [1,2]. There is a positive correlation between psychological stress levels and the severity of urgency and bladder pain symptoms in IC/BPS [3]. This positive correlation becomes progressively stronger in patients with more severe IC/BPS symptoms [3]. Even though there is some overlapping of symptoms between OAB (overactive bladder) and IC/BPS [4], surprisingly there have been very few studies that specifically investigated the relationship between psychological stress and urinary symptoms in OAB patients who do not have pelvic pain.

Knight et al. compared the recent life stress measures between "OAB dry" patients (without urgency incontinence)

* Correspondence: laih@wudosis.wustl.edu
[1]Division of Urologic Surgery, Department of Surgery, Washington University School of Medicine, 4960 Children's Place, Campus Box 8242, St Louis, MO 63110, USA
[2]Department of Anesthesiology, Washington University School of Medicine, 4960 Children's Place, Campus Box 8242, St Louis, MO 63110, USA

and age-matched controls, and found no differences in life stress scores between the two groups [5]. Unfortunately the authors did not recruit "OAB wet" patients with incontinence for comparison. Zhang et al. conducted an epidemiological study to compare the occupational stress levels between female adult Chinese nurses who had OAB-like symptoms versus nurses who did not have OAB-like symptoms [6]. The authors concluded that nurses with OAB-like symptoms had higher occupational stressors and higher psychological strain than nurses without OAB. There are several limitations of that study: (1) the study population were nurses but not a clinical population of OAB patients seeking treatments; (2) the nurses did not have an evaluation or a diagnosis of OAB by a clinician; (3) the OAB-like symptoms reported on the questionnaires may not be bothersome; and (4) the authors used a validated questionnaire that specifically examined occupational stressors but not everyday psychological stressors. Thus, it is difficult to infer the results of the Chinese nurse study to the OAB patients [6].

The objectives of this study were to: (1) compare perceived stress levels in patients with OAB to IC/BPS and controls, and (2) examine the correlation between the level of psychological stress and the severity of OAB symptoms, and its impact on quality of life in patients with OAB.

Methods

Population

Between October 2012 and July 2014, patients diagnosed with OAB or IC/BPS, and healthy controls (age matched to OAB) were recruited into this questionnaire-based study that inquired about their perceived stress levels and OAB symptoms. For OAB, patients must have urinary urgency, with or without urgency incontinence, usually with frequency and nocturia, in the absence of infection or other identifiable causes, in accordance with the 2002 ICS definition of OAB [7]. For IC/BPS, patients must have an unpleasant sensation (pain, pressure, discomfort) perceived to be related to the bladder, associated with lower urinary tract symptoms of more than 6 weeks duration, in the absence of infection or other identifiable causes, consistent with the 2011 AUA IC/BPS Guideline [8]. The clinical assessment followed the published AUA guidelines [8,9]. The majority of OAB patients were undergoing treatments as recommended by the AUA OAB Guideline [9]. OAB patients with concomitant stress incontinence (or mixed incontinence) were also eligible if they reported predominant urgency incontinence by history. Patients with a history of prostate surgery, urinary incontinence surgery, urethral stricture, neurogenic bladder, urinary retention, pelvic radiation, tuberculosis cystitis, cyclophosphamide cystitis, genitourinary cancer, urinary stones, or a documented positive urine culture in the past 6 weeks were excluded. Patients with a positive culture or a post-void residual ≥150 mL (bladder scanner) on the day of visit were excluded.

Age-matched healthy controls were recruited by local advertisement and research database. Controls had no prior diagnosis of OAB or IC/BPS, no significant lower urinary tract symptoms (AUA symptom index < 7), no significant bladder or pelvic pain, and no evidence of infection. Controls were age-matched to the OAB group. All participants signed an informed consent. The Washington University School of Medicine Institutional Review Board approved this study.

Assessment

Perceived stress was measured using the validated 10-item perceived stress scale (PSS) at the time of enrollment to the study [10]. The PSS measures the degree to which situations are perceived as being unpredictable, uncontrollable and overwhelming during the previous month. High scores indicate higher perceived stress.

Participants also completed the following validated questionnaires at the same time to assess their self-reported OAB symptoms and their impact: 1) international consultation on incontinence – urinary incontinence short form (ICIQ-UI) [11], 2) international consultation on incontinence – overactive bladder (ICIQ-OAB) [12], 3) OAB-q short form [13], 4) urogenital distress inventory short form (UDI-6) [14], 5) incontinence impact questionnaire short form (IIQ-7) [14], 6) urgency severity scale (USS) to assess the severity of urgency symptoms [15], 7) numeric rating scale (0 to 10) of the severity of urgency symptom, and 8) numeric rating scale (0 to 10) of the severity of frequency symptom. ICIQ-UI is a 4-item questionnaire that assesses the frequency, amount and interference of urinary incontinence. ICIQ-OAB is a 4-item questionnaire that inquires about daytime frequency, nighttime frequency, urgency, and urgency incontinence. OAB-q contains two sub-scales (symptom bother, quality of life) that assess symptom bother and health-related quality of life of both continent and incontinent OAB patients. UDI-6 and IIQ-7 measures urinary distress and incontinence impact, respectively. USS is a 4-point rating of the degree of urgency sensation (none, mild, moderate, severe). Additional psychosocial factors including childhood traumatic events, anxiety, and depression were assessed using the childhood traumatic event scale and hospital anxiety and depression scale (HADS), respectively [16,17]. Obesity data were not recorded.

Statistical analyses

Wilcoxon rank sum tests were used to compare perceived stress results from OAB, IC/BPS, and controls.

Multivariate linear models were used to compare PSS between the three groups adjusting for age and sex. There were 79 omitted answers out of 5076 possible for the variables of interest (1.6%). Missing data were random and were ignored for the comparisons. $p < 0.05$ was considered significant.

Spearman's correlation analysis was performed to examine the relationship between perceived stress levels and self-reported OAB symptoms. p-values were calculated for the correlation using two-tailed tests using a t approximation testing the null hypothesis of no correlation. $p < 0.05$ was considered significant. All statistical analysis was completed using the open source statistical package R v2.15.1 [18].

Results

Demographics

51 OAB patients, 27 IC/BPS patients, and 30 healthy controls (age matched to OAB) participated in this case control study. The mean age (± SD) of the OAB, IC/BPS and control groups was 53.7 ± 11.9, 44.8 ± 16.6, 54.2 ± 12.3, respectively. There was no age or sex difference between OAB patients and healthy controls (p = 0.984 and 0.14 respectively). OAB patients were significantly older than IC/BPS patients (p = 0.013). OAB patients were also less likely to be females compared to IC/BPS (73% versus 100%, p = 00027, Chi-square test). Their demographics and clinical characteristics were presented in Table 1.

Comparison of perceived stress levels between OAB, IC/BPS and controls

The total scores of the PSS are illustrated in Figure 1 and Table 1. On univariate analysis, OAB patients reported significantly higher psychological stress levels on the PSS compared to age-matched healthy controls (median 17.0, versus 7.5, p = 0.001, Wilcoxon sum rank test). There was no difference in psychological stress levels reported by OAB and IC/BPS patients (median 17.0 versus 18.0, p = 0.818). As expected, IC/BPS patients also reported significantly higher psychological stress levels on the PSS compared to controls (median 18.0 versus 7.5, p = 0.001). Because IC/BPS patients were more likely to be females and older than OAB patients, we incorporated age and sex into our multivariate modeling. On multivariate analysis, PSS remained significant different between OAB and controls (p = 0.001) after adjusting for age and sex.

Table 1 Demographics and clinical characteristics

	OAB	IC/BPS	Controls
No. of participants	51	27	30
Age (mean ± SD)	53.4 ± 11.9	44.8 ± 16.6	54.2 ± 12.3
Sex (% females)	73%	100%	57%
Age of diagnosis of OAB or IC/BPS (mean ± SD)	47.5 ± 15.2	38.8 ± 10.3	NA
% with OAB or IC/BPS symptoms less than one year? (early onset cases)	24%	22%	NA
Comorbidities:			
Hypertension	37%	30%	33%
Diabetes	8%	0%	3%
Stroke, TIA	8%	0%	7%
Angina, MI	0%	0%	0%
Depression	32%	37%	17%
Anxiety	20%	37%	7%
PSS (perceived stress scale, 0–40): Median (1st quartile, 3rd quartile, semi-interquartile range)	17.0 (12.0, 24.0, 6.0)	18.0 (12.5, 21.5, 4.5)	7.5 (5.0, 17.0, 4.75)
OAB symptom scores: (mean ± SD)			
ICIQ-UI (urinary incontinence, 0–21):	12.0 ± 4.9	6.6 ± 5.7	1.4 ± 2.0
UDI-6 (urogenital distress inventory, 0–24):	12.6 ± 5.6	11.0 ± 5.3	0.9 ± 1.4
IIQ-7 (incontinence impact questionnaire, 0–28):	8.8 ± 8.2	4.9 ± 7.0	0.1 ± 0.4
OAB-q quality of life subscale (13–78):	29.7 ± 16.9	25.1 ± 14.9	2.0 ± 3.0
OAB-q symptom bother subscale (6–36):	19.1 ± 6.6	14.2 ± 7.4	2.2 ± 2.8
ICIQ-OAB (overactive bladder, 0–16):	9.3 ± 2.6	7.3 ± 4.1	2.0 ± 1.5
USS (urgency severity scale, 0–3):	2.1 ± 0.7	1.9 ± 0.8	0.5 ± 0.6
Numeric rating scale of **urgency** (0–10):	6.1 ± 2.6	5.9 ± 2.8	0.4 ± 0.6
Numeric rating scale of **frequency** (0–10):	6.4 ± 2.6	6.2 ± 2.3	0.6 ± 0.9

Correlation between perceived stress levels and urinary symptoms among OAB patients

Among OAB patients, high perceived stress levels on the PSS was positively correlated to total scores on ICIQ-UI (Spearman's correlation coefficient $r_s = 0.393$, $p = 0.007$), UDI-6 (Spearman's correlation coefficient = 0.314, $p = 0.028$), IIQ-7 (Spearman's correlation coefficient = 0.393, $p = 0.005$), and quality of life subscale on the OAB-q (Spearman's correlation coefficient = 0.326, $p = 0.029$), see Table 2. No significant correlation between perceived stress levels and the following instruments was observed: ICIQ-OAB, symptom bother subscale on the OAB-q, USS, and the numeric ratings of their urgency or frequency (0 to 10).

When the specific items of the ICIQ-UI questionnaire was examined separately in an exploratory analysis, two of the items ("how often do you leak urine?", "how much urine do you think you leak?") was also positively correlated to perceived stress levels on the PSS (Spearman's correlation coefficient = 0.328, 0.334, and p-value = 0.020, 0.018, respectively).

When the four items of the ICIQ-OAB questionnaire was examined separately in an exploratory analysis ("how many times do you urinate during the day?", "during the night, how many times do you have to wake up to urinate, on average?", "do you have to rush to the bathroom to urinate?", "does urine leak before you can get to the bathroom?), response on the urinary incontinence question (item 4) was positively correlated to perceived stress levels on the PSS (Spearman's correlation coefficient = 0.297, p-value = 0.036). On the other hand, responses on the frequency question (item 1), nocturia question (item 2) and urgency question (item 3) did not show any significant correlation to the PSS (Spearman's correlation coefficient = 0.104, 0.059, 0.238, and p-value = 0.473, 0.689, 0.096, respectively).

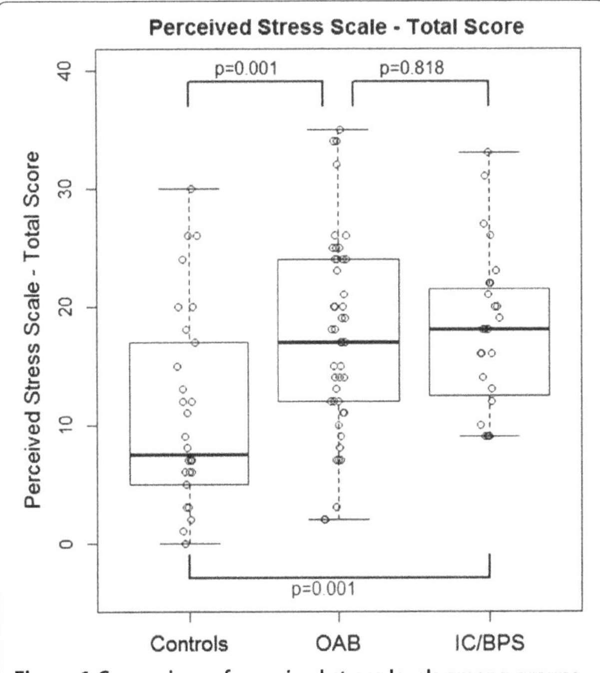

Figure 1 Comparison of perceived stress levels among groups (Wilcoxon rank-sum tests).

Comparison of perceived stress levels between OAB patients with urgency incontinence versus mixed incontinence

OAB patients were recruited if they had urinary urgency, with or without urgency incontinence, in accordance with the 2002 ICS definition of OAB [7]. Patients with concomitant stress incontinence (or mixed incontinence) were also eligible if they reported predominant urgency incontinence by history. Overall, 98% of OAB patients in our cohort reported incontinence symptoms on the ICIQ-UI. Among them, 45% reported urgency incontinence without stress incontinence, and 53% reported mixed incontinence (urgency and stress incontinence) on the ICIQ-UI. There was no difference in PSS between OAB patients with urgency incontinence versus those with mixed incontinence (urgency incontinence PSS = 15.7 ± 1.71, mixed incontinence PSS = 18.8 ± 1.5, $p = 0.17$). Because the percent of OAB patients without any incontinence was too small, we were not able to compare the PSS between OAB patients with incontinence versus OAB patients without incontinence.

Influence of childhood traumatic history, anxiety, and depression on perceived stress levels

Stress levels may be influenced by psychosocial factors such as childhood traumatic events, anxiety and depression. These factors were assessed using the childhood traumatic event scale and the hospital anxiety and depression scale (HADS), respectively [16,17]. OAB patients with a childhood history of sexual trauma or physical trauma reported higher stress levels on the PSS compared to OAB patients without such a history (PSS of 20.6 ± 1.8 versus 15.2 ± 1.4, $p = 0.048$). OAB patients with higher anxiety scores (HADS-A ≥ 8) had higher stress levels than those with lower anxiety scores (HADS-A < 7), PSS of 23.1 ± 1.3 versus 11.9 ± 1.1, $p < 0.0001$. OAB patients with higher depression scores (HADS-D ≥ 8) had higher stress levels than those with lower depression scores (HADS-D < 7), PSS of 22.9 ± 1.2 versus 15.1 ± 1.4, $p = 0.014$.

Discussion

There are two findings in this study: (1) OAB patients reported psychological stress levels that were as high as IC/BPS patients, and significantly higher than healthy controls, (2) among OAB patients, there were significant positive correlation between psychological stress levels perceived by patients and the severity of urinary incontinence

Table 2 Correlation of perceived stress levels and urinary symptoms among OAB patients (Spearman's correlation tests)

	Correlation analysis between PSS total scores and OAB symptoms:	
	Spearman's correlation coefficient (r_s)	p-value
ICIQ-UI (urinary incontinence, 0–21)	0.393	0.007*
UDI-6 (urogenital distress inventory, 0–24)	0.314	0.028*
IIQ-7 (incontinence impact questionnaire, 0–28)	0.393	0.005*
OAB-q quality of life subscale (13–78)	0.326	0.029*
OAB-q symptom bother subscale (6–36)	0.195	0.189
ICIQ-OAB (overactive bladder, 0–16)	0.205	0.158
USS (urgency severity scale, 0–3)	0.127	0.390
Numeric rating scale of **urgency** (0–10)	0.235	0.090
Numeric rating scale of **frequency** (0–10)	0.260	0.068
Specific items on the ICIQ-UI questionnaire:		
ICIQ-UI: "How often do you leak urine?" (0–5)	0.328	0.020*
ICIQ-UI: "How much urine do you think you leak?" (0–6)	0.334	0.018*
ICIQ-UI: "How much does leaking urine interfere with your daily life?" (0–10)	0.270	0.058
Specific items on the ICIQ-OAB questionnaire:		
ICIQ-OAB: "How many times do you urinate during the day" (0–6)	0.104	0.473
ICIQ-OAB: "During the night, how many times do you have to urinate during the night, on average?"	0.052	0.722
ICIQ-OAB: "Do you have to rush to the bathroom to urinate?"	0.238	0.096
ICIQ-OAB: "Does urine leak before you can get to the bathroom?"	0.297	0.036*

*statistical significance, $p < 0.05$.

symptoms (ICIQ-UI), and its impact on quality of life (UDI-6, IIQ-7, OAB-q quality of life subscale).

The clinical implication of our findings is that when treating patients with OAB, a psychological component should be evaluated as possibly contributing to the nature and severity of the lower urinary tract symptoms. Psychological stress might be a potential modifiable risk factor for urgency incontinence. In fact, a recent clinical study suggested that mindfulness-based stress reduction (MBSR) might reduce urgency incontinence episodes [19]. MBSR is a structured, group-based, mind-body intervention with the goal to teach participants stress reduction techniques by a variety of mediation practices, mindful yoga, and discussion of the relation between stress, illness and health. In a non-randomized study that recruited seven women, Baker et al. showed that MBSR reduced urgency incontinence episodes more than it reduced urinary frequency [19].

We have identified a potential link between psychological stress and UI symptoms. Since there were positive correlation between the level of stress and a number of measures (a "dose–response" gradient), this supported the possibility of a causal relationship instead of a pure coincidence. However, the directionality of the relationship cannot be ascertained in this case control study. While it is not surprising that incontinence can increase psychological stress (UI → stress), the reverse may also occur, i.e. high psychological stress may exacerbate existing UI symptoms (stress → UI). The interaction may also be bi-directional (stress ↔ UI). A prospective study is needed to further clarify the causality or directionality of the association between psychological stress and lower urinary symptoms.

The second scenario (stress → UI) is biologically plausible. In animal studies, exposure of female rats to repeated water avoidance stress caused an increase in micturition frequency, reduction of micturition volume, and bladder hypersensitivity [20,21]. Exposure of male rats to rotating stressors had similar effects [22]. Exposure of male rats to repeated social defeat stress had the opposite effect: it caused urinary retention and non-voiding bladder contractions [23]. These stress-induced bladder dysfunctions may be mediated by corticotropin releasing factor (CRF), which functions both as a hormone to regulate the activity of the hypothalamic-pituitary-adrenal (HPA) axis, and as a neurotransmitter in the central nervous system to modulate the function of the pontine micturition center and the descending micturition pathways [23,24]. Currently, it is unknown if there is an alteration in CRF response, HPA axis, or diurnal cortisol levels in patients with OAB. Other factors such as low-grade systemic inflammation or central nervous system changes may be involved [25]. Such changes have been observed in IC/BPS patients [26]. Since there is considerable overlap of urinary symptoms between OAB and IC/BPS (e.g. urgency, frequency) [4,8], these questions deserve further investigation in OAB.

It is not clear why a positive correlation was observed between stress levels and urinary incontinence symptoms, but not with frequency or urgency symptoms. Our results were in agreement with the study by Knight et al. which also found no differences in life stress scores between "OAB dry" patients and controls [5]. Unfortunately the authors did not recruit "OAB wet" patients (with incontinence) for comparison. With IC/BPS, there is a positive correlation between stress levels and the severity of urgency symptom [3]. This correlation becomes progressively stronger in patients with more severe IC/BPS symptoms. In contrast, with OAB we have not observed a correlation between psychological stress levels and the severity of urgency symptom. We did not observe a difference in stress levels between OAB patients with urgency incontinence versus mixed incontinence. However, the sample size might be too small to examine this issue.

The current study has limitations: (1) the case control design did not prove causation or directionality; (2) our cohort did not permit a comparison between "OAB wet" and "OAB dry" patients since 98% of our patients have urgency incontinence (with or without stress incontinence); and (3) the correlation analysis was based on subjective data reported by the patients instead of objective findings (e.g. pad weight, urodynamics). While having objective data might add value to the analysis, they cannot fully replace symptom data or quality of life data, since these patient-reported data reflected patients' own experience of their conditions.

Conclusions

OAB patients reported psychological stress levels that were as high as IC/BPS, and significantly higher than healthy controls. There was a positive correlation between perceived stress levels and urinary incontinence symptoms, and its impacts on quality of life among OAB patients.

Availability of supporting data

Supporting data from the study will be provided to other researchers upon request.

Abbreviations

HADS: Hospital anxiety and depression scale; IC/BPS: Interstitial cystitis/ bladder pain syndrome; ICIQ-OAB: International consultation on incontinence – overactive bladder; ICIQ-UI: International consultation on incontinence – urinary incontinence; IIQ-7: Incontinence impact questionnaire short form; OAB: Overactive bladder; PSS: Perceived stress scale; UDI-6: Urogenital distress inventory short form; USS: Urgency severity scale.

Competing interests

The authors declare that they have no competing interests.

Authors' contributions

HL contributed to the conception, design, analysis and interpretation of the data. In addition, HL also drafted the manuscript, and agreed to be accountable for the accuracy and all other aspects of the work. VG contributed to the design of the study, participant recruitment and acquisition of the data, and revised the manuscript critically. JV contributed to the statistical analysis and interpretation of the data, design and construction of the database, data entry and management, revised the manuscript critically, and agreed to be accountable for the accuracy of the statistical analysis. GA contributed to the design of the study. All authors read and approved the final manuscript.

Acknowledgements

The study is funded by the National Institutes of Health, grant numbers P20-DK-097798 and K08-DK-094964. We would like to thank all the subjects who participated in the study, Aleksandra Klim for recruiting the subjects, and Alethea Paradis for data management.

References

1. Koziol JA, Clark DC, Gittes RF, Tan EM. The natural history of interstitial cystitis: a survey of 374 patients. J Urol. 1993;149:465–9.
2. Lutgendorf SK, Kreder KJ, Rothrock NE, Ratliff TL, Zimmerman B. Stress and symptomatology in patients with interstitial cystitis: a laboratory stress model. J Urol. 2000;164:1265–9.
3. Rothrock NE, Lutgendorf SK, Kreder KJ, Ratliff T, Zimmerman B. Stress and symptoms in patients with interstitial cystitis: a life stress model. Urology. 2001;57:422–7.
4. Lai HH, Vetter J, Jain S, Gereau RW, Andriole GL. The overlap and distinction of self-reported symptoms between interstitial cystitis/bladder pain syndrome and overactive bladder: a questionnaire-based analysis. J Urol. 2014;192(6):1679–85.
5. Knight S, Luft J, Nakagawa S, Katzman WB. Comparisons of pelvic floor muscle performance, anxiety, quality of life and life stress in women with dry overactive bladder compared with asymptomatic women. BJU Int. 2012;109:1685–9.
6. Zhang C, Hai T, Yu L, Liu S, Li Q, Zhang X, et al. Association between occupational stress and risk of overactive bladder and other lower urinary tract symptoms: a cross-sectional study of female nurses in China. Neurourol Urodyn. 2013;32(3):254–60.
7. Abrams P, Cardozo L, Fall M, Griffiths D, Rosier P, Ulmsten U, et al. The standardisation of terminology of lower urinary tract function: report from the Standardisation Sub-committee of the International Continence Society. Am J Obstet Gynecol. 2002;187:116–26.
8. Hanno PM, Burks DA, Clemens JQ, Dmochowski RR, Erickson D, Fitzgerald MP, et al. AUA guideline for the diagnosis and treatment of interstitial cystitis/bladder pain syndrome. J Urol. 2011;185:2162–70.
9. Gormley EA, Lightner DJ, Burgio KL, Chai TC, Clemens JQ, Culkin DJ, et al. Diagnosis and treatment of overactive bladder (non-neurogenic) in adults: AUA/SUFU guideline. J Urol. 2012;188:2455–63.
10. Cohen S, Williamson G. Perceived stress in a probability sample of the United States. In: Spacapan S, Oskamp S, editors. The social psychology of health: Claremont symposium on applied social psychology. Newbury Parl, CA: Sage; 1988.
11. Avery K, Donovan J, Peters TJ, Shaw C, Gotoh M, Abrams P. ICIQ: a brief and robust measure for evaluating the symptoms and impact of urinary incontinence. Neurourol Urodyn. 2004;23:322–30.
12. Jackson S, Donovan J, Brookes S, Eckford S, Swithinbank L, Abrams P. The Bristol Female Lower Urinary Tract Symptoms questionnaire: development and psychometric testing. Br J Urol. 1996;77:805–12.
13. Coyne K, Revicki D, Hunt T, Corey R, Stewart W, Bentkover J, et al. Psychometric validation of an overactive bladder symptom and health-related quality of life questionnaire: the OAB-q. Qual Life Res. 2002;11:563–74.
14. Uebersax JS, Wyman JF, Shumaker SA, McClish DK, Fantl JA. Short forms to assess life quality and symptom distress for urinary incontinence in women: the Incontinence Impact Questionnaire and the Urogenital Distress

Inventory. Continence Program for Women Research Group. Neurourol Urodyn. 1995;14:131–9.
15. Nixon A, Colman S, Sabounjian L, Sandage B, Schwiderski UE, Staskin DR, et al. A validated patient reported measure of urinary urgency severity in overactive bladder for use in clinical trials. J Urol. 2005;174:604–7.
16. Pennebaker JW, Susman JR. Disclosure of traumas and psychosomatic processes. Soc Sci Med. 1988;26:327–32.
17. Snaith RP, Zigmond AS. The hospital anxiety and depression scale. Br Med J (Clin Res Ed). 1986;292:344.
18. R: A language and environment for statistical computation. [http://www.R-project.org/]
19. Baker J, Costa D, Nygaard I. Mindfulness-based stress reduction for treatment of urinary urge incontinence: a pilot study. Female Pelvic Med Reconstr Surg. 2012;18:46–9.
20. Smith AL, Leung J, Kun S, Zhang R, Karagiannides I, Raz S, et al. The effects of acute and chronic psychological stress on bladder function in a rodent model. Urology. 2011;78:967. e961-967.
21. Robbins M, DeBerry J, Ness T. Chronic psychological stress enhances nociceptive processing in the urinary bladder in high-anxiety rats. Physiol Behav. 2007;91:544–50.
22. Merrill L, Malley S, Vizzard MA. Repeated variate stress in male rats induces increased voiding frequency, somatic sensitivity, and urinary bladder nerve growth factor expression. Am J Physiol Regul Integr Comp Physiol. 2013;305:R147–56.
23. Wood SK, Baez MA, Bhatnagar S, Valentino RJ. Social stress-induced bladder dysfunction: potential role of corticotropin-releasing factor. Am J Physiol Regul Integr Comp Physiol. 2009;296:R1671–8.
24. Klausner AP, Steers WD. Corticotropin releasing factor: a mediator of emotional influences on bladder function. J Urol. 2004;172:2570–3.
25. Saini R, Gonzalez RR, Te AE. Chronic pelvic pain syndrome and the overactive bladder: the inflammatory link. Curr Urol Rep. 2008;9:314–9.
26. Lutgendorf SK, Kreder KJ, Rothrock NE, Hoffman A, Kirschbaum C, Sternberg EM, et al. Diurnal cortisol variations and symptoms in patients with interstitial cystitis. J Urol. 2002;167:1338–43.

9

The potential utility of non-invasive imaging to monitor restoration of bladder structure and function following subtotal cystectomy (STC)

David Burmeister[1], Bimjhana Bishwokarma[1], Tamer AbouShwareb[1], John Olson[3], Maja Herco[1], Josh Tan[3], Karl-Erik Andersson[1] and George Christ[1,2*]

Abstract

Background: Restoration of normal bladder volume and function (i.e., bioequivalent bladder) are observed within 8 weeks of performing subtotal cystectomy (STC; removal of ~70 % of the bladder) in 12-week old rats. For analysis of bladder function in rodents, terminal urodynamic approaches are largely utilized. In the current study, we investigated the potential for Computed Tomography (CT) and Magnetic Resonance Imaging (MRI) scans to noninvasively track restoration of structure and function following STC.

Methods: Twelve week old female Fisher F344 rats underwent STC and were scanned via CT and/or MRI 2, 4, 8, and 12 weeks post-STC, followed by urodynamic testing. After euthanasia, bladders were excised for histological processing.

Results: MRI scans demonstrated an initial decline followed by a time-dependent increase to normal bladder wall thickness (BWT) by 8 weeks post-STC. Masson's trichrome staining showed a lack of fibrosis post-STC, and also revealed that the percent of smooth muscle in the bladder wall at 2 and 4 weeks positively correlated with pre-operative baseline BWT. Moreover, increased BWT values before STC was predictive of improved bladder compliance at 2 and 4 weeks post-STC. Cystometric studies indicated that repeated MRI manipulation (i.e. bladder emptying) apparently had a negative impact on bladder capacity and compliance. A "window" of bladder volumes was identified 2 weeks post-STC via CT scanning that were commensurate with normal micturition pressures measured in the same animal 6 weeks later.

Conclusions: Taken together, the data indicate some limitations of "non-invasive" imaging to provide insight into bladder regeneration. Specifically, mechanical manipulation of the bladder during MRI appears to negatively impact the regenerative process *per se*, which highlights the importance of terminal cystometric studies.

Keywords: Subtotal cystectomy, Magnetic resonance imaging, Computed tomography, Regeneration, Urinary bladder

Background

Tissue engineering and regenerative medicine technologies represent a promising approach for development of novel therapeutics for diverse lower urinary tract pathologies [1, 2]. In fact, many different animal models have been employed to evaluate the effectiveness of different cell/scaffold combinations in augmentation of the bladder [3–15]. However, a recent clinical report on bladder augmentation with autologous cell seeded biodegradable scaffolds clearly indicates that current technologies are not yet ready for widespread clinical applications [16]. Such developments speak to the importance of improved understanding of mechanisms of bladder regeneration, repair and remodeling *per se* as an important prerequisite to improved clinical applications of regenerative medicine/tissue engineering technologies to bladder dysfunction and disease.

* Correspondence: gjc8w@virginia.edu
[1]Wake Forest Institute for Regenerative Medicine, 391 Technology Way, Winston-Salem, NC 27101, USA
[2]Departments of Biomedical Engineering and Orthopaedic Surgery, and Laboratory of Regenerative Therapeutics, University of Virginia, 415 Lane Road, Charlottesville, VA 22908, USA
Full list of author information is available at the end of the article

Several studies have suggested that removal of a large part of the bladder without replacement results in some degree of functional bladder regeneration in both rats [17–22] and humans [23–32]. As such, we have focused our recent efforts on developing rodent models and methods that can provide additional insight into the cellular and molecular mechanisms responsible for functional bladder regeneration in mammals. In rodents, however, examining functional regeneration using urodynamic approaches is invasive and limited to evaluation of a single time point [33]. While voiding pattern assays provide an opportunity for longitudinal analysis of bladder function [34, 35], they are also limited in the amount of mechanistic physiological detail they can provide. As such, non-invasive imaging may permit longitudinal analysis of the bladder, providing additional morphological information over time, and potentially leading to novel insights on bladder functional restoration. The goal of this study was to evaluate the potential utility of non-invasive methods for improved understanding of the time course of functional bladder restoration following STC.

Furthermore, if successful, non-invasive imaging could also have great prognostic value in the clinic. Imaging techniques have already been applied to tissue engineering in, for example, cardiac, cartilage and bone regeneration [36–38]. Although a few studies have used Magnetic Resonance Imaging (MRI) and Computerized Tomography (CT) to evaluate the utility of grafts in the bladder, little is known about how changes in the morphology of the bladder relate to bladder function [39–41]. The current study explores the utility of both CT and MRI to inform understanding of bladder function during regrowth/regeneration induced by subtotal cystectomy (STC) in a well-characterized rodent model. The results of this study demonstrate a potential for non- invasive imaging as a prognostic indicator for the functional success or failure of bladder regeneration.

Methods

Animals

Twenty-eight 12-week old (170–200 g) female Fisher F344 rats underwent subtotal cystectomy (STC), and the experimental design is shown in Fig. 1. All animals underwent MRI scanning pre-operatively, with cohorts of animals also scanned at 2, 4, 8, and 12 weeks post-STC. For cystometric studies, 5 animals were designated for analysis at 2, 4, and 12 weeks, while 10 were designated for analysis at 8 weeks. Of these 10 animals at 8 weeks post-STC, half (n = 5) were utilized for CT scanning in addition to MRI. MRI procedures were completed the day before CT scanning and catheter implantation. Additionally, retrospective analysis was performed on previously published data from animals of the same strain, age, and gender [21]. All methods were approved by the Animal Care and Use Committee, Wake Forest University.

Trigone-sparing cystectomies

Animals underwent trigone-sparing STC as previously described [21, 22, 42]. Briefly, two stay sutures were made on either side of the bladder, just above the uretero-vesical junction, using 6–0 polyglycolic acid. The dome portion of the bladder was excised and the remaining portion of the bladder was then sutured continuously using one of the original stay sutures. Animals were allowed to recover and given food and water *ad libitum*.

Magnetic resonance imaging (MRI)

All MRI experiments were performed in a 7 T horizontal bore magnet (Bruker Biospin, Billerica, MA) equipped with an actively shielded gradient insert. RF signal transmission and reception was performed with a 50 mm I.D. quadrature Litzcage RF coil (Doty Scientific, Columbia, SC) tuned and matched with each rat to 300.2 MHz. Rats were anesthetized with oxygen (2 L/min) and isoflurane (2 %) and the bladder was manually expressed. The animal was then placed in the RF coil in the prone position with the bladder centered in the RF coil. Anesthesia was maintained during the scan via nose cone which provided oxygen (1 L/min) and isoflurane (1.5 %). Body temperature was kept constant by thermostatically controlled warm air (SA Instruments, Stoney Brook, NY). A three plane localizer scan was acquired using a Rapid Acquisition with Relaxation Enhancement (RARE) spin echo pulse sequence with an echo train of 8 echos to ensure that the bladder of each rat was centered in both the RF coil and the magnet. A 3D FLASH pulse sequence allowed for the acquisition of 8 slices, each 250 microns thick. The low slice thickness reduced partial volume effects, thus allowing for better detection of the inner and outer surfaces of the bladder wall. The coronal 3D FLASH slab was positioned using the tri plane localizers as scout images so that the slices in the center of the slab were perpendicular to the surface of the bladder wall. Scanning parameters were as follows: TR = 50 ms, TE = 6 ms, flip angle = 15 degrees, FOV = 3 cm, matrix = 256x256, giving an in-plane resolution of 117um, NEX = 8. Acquisition was also respiratory gated to avoid breathing motion artifacts. Analysis of bladder wall thickness was performed using TeraRecon 3D visualization and image analysis software using the linear measurement tool. This was performed in triplicate, on five different locations of the bladder wall, denoted "base" to "dome".

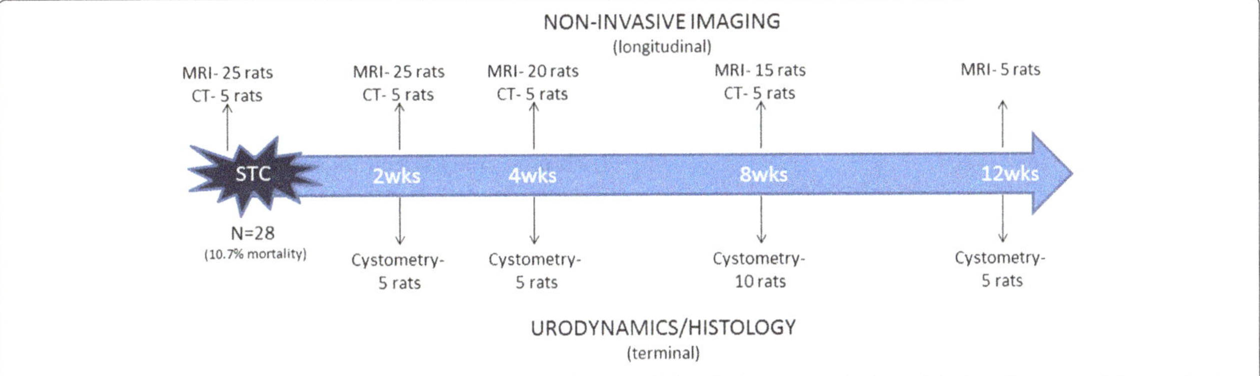

Fig. 1 Schematic showing experimental design. Of the 28 rats undergoing STC, 3 died post-operatively, and the baseline scans of those animals were omitted. All rats underwent MRI at every timepoint, while 5 of those rats had CT scans performed at every timepoint until 8 weeks. 5 rats were used for terminal urodynamic studies at 2, 4, and 12 weeks. 10 rats had urodynamic testing at 8 weeks, including the 5 rats that received CT scans. STC- subtotal cystectomy

CT imaging

The day after MRI testing, CT Scans of the animals were taken with a Siemens MicroCATII @ 70 kV, 500 μA (BIN Factor of 4, 200° rotation, 500 steps, 73 micron cuts), and the scans were centered on the bladder. Contrast medium (288 mg/ml Iothalamate Meglumine, diluted 1:3) was applied via transurethral catheterization and injected until bladder was full. All images were reconstructed using COBRA EXXIM version 4.9.52, and converted to DICOM images with Amira version 3.1. Analysis was done after transfer of images to TeraRecon Aquarius Workstation. Briefly, the entire image except the bladder was removed using the erase function. A bladder template was optimized with the following parameters: Window Width (WW) of 1116, Window Level (WL) of 657, and 11 % opacity. Finally, the volume measurement tool was used for quantification of bladder volume.

Cystometric analysis

Bladder catheters were implanted and cystometric studies were performed 3 days after catheter implantation in conscious, freely moving rats as previously described [21, 42, 43]. Briefly, the indwelling catheter was connected to a pressure transducer and infusion pump. The pressure transducer was connected to an ETH 400 (CD Sciences, Dover, New Hampshire) amplifier and read with a MacLab/8e (Analog Digital Instruments, New South Wales, Australia) acquisition board. Equipment was calibrated in cmH_20 before each experiment. Room temperature saline was infused at a rate of 10 mL/h. Voided fluid was diverted into a collection tube attached to a force displacement transducer. The following cystometric parameters were investigated: basal pressure (BP, lowest pressure between voids), maximum pressure (MP, the highest pressure during micturition), threshold pressure (TP, pressure which initiates a voiding contraction), bladder capacity (B_{cap}, residual volume plus amount of saline infused), micturition volume (MV, amount of expelled urine), residual volume (RV, B_{cap} – MV), and bladder compliance ($B_{com} = B_{cap}/(TP\text{-}BP)$).

Histology

An additional subset of bladders were preserved for histological analysis of smooth muscle content ($n = 4/$ timepoint). Bladders distal to the UVJ were fixed in 10 % buffered formalin overnight, processed, embedded in paraffin and then cut into 7 μM axial slices. Slides were cleared in xylene and rehydrated to water. Masson's trichrome stain (Newcomer Supply Catalog #9176A) was performed on at least 2 different areas of the bladder (i.e. a section closest to the base or UVJ/original plane of excision, and a section taken towards the dome or more distally). Four high magnification images were taken in each section, and image analysis was performed with ImagePro software 6.3 (Media Cybernetics, Bethesda, MD). The color selection tool was used to determine quantity of red (muscle) and blue (collagen) pixels, and the percentage of muscle corresponds to the number of red pixels/total number of selected pixels.

Statistical analysis

Non-invasive image reconstruction was performed with TeraRecon AquariusNET software version 4.4.5.49 (TeraRecon, Inc., San Mateo, CA). Statistical evaluations and regression analysis were performed using GraphPad Prism software. (GraphPad software Inc.) One-way ANOVAs with Neumann-Keuls post testing were performed on bladder wall thickness, cystometric parameters, and Trichrome analysis. Additionally, t-tests were performed on cystometric parameters obtained at 8 weeks in order to determine the effect of MRI. A two-way ANOVA was used to determine any regional variations in bladder wall thickness. P values less that 0.05 were considered significant. All results are expressed as the mean ± SEM.

Results

Subtotal cystectomy

Of the 28 rats that underwent STC, three animals died within three days after surgery due to urine leakage into the peritoneum (10.7 % mortality rate).

MRI scanning

An example of a sagittal bladder slice and associated measurements are shown in Fig. 2a, with demonstration of measurements in Fig. 2b. Analyzable scans were attained in 24/25, 22/25. 18/20, 14/15, and 4/5 possible scans at the 0, 2, 4, 8, and 12 week time points, respectively. Analysis of sagittal slices of MRI scans revealed an initial decrease in bladder wall thickness (BWT) after STC, which normalized to control values by 8 weeks post-STC (Fig. 2c). Values for BWT were 402.1 ± 18.82 microns, 269.6 ± 12.21 microns, 315.3 ± 17.55 microns, 384.7 ± 19.11 microns, and 399.8 ± 25.12 microns at the 0, 2, 4, 8, and 12 week time points, respectively. Analysis of BWT variations from the bladder base to the bladder dome revealed no significant differences between any of the time points studied (8 weeks shown in Fig. 1d).

Trichrome analysis and regression

A representative trichrome image is shown in Fig. 3 and analysis revealed no changes in percent smooth muscle values at any time after STC, which were 66.16 ± 1.41, 64.14 ± 3.35, 65.46 ± 2.09, 59.10 ± 1.67, and 63.48 ± 1.35 % at 0,2,4,8, and 12 weeks post-STC, respectively. However, the percent smooth muscle in the bladder wall at the 8 and 12-week time points was positively correlated with MRI-determined bladder wall thickness at those same time points.

Cystometric analysis

All cystometric parameters are displayed in Fig. 4. Bladder capacity was higher at 8 weeks compared to every

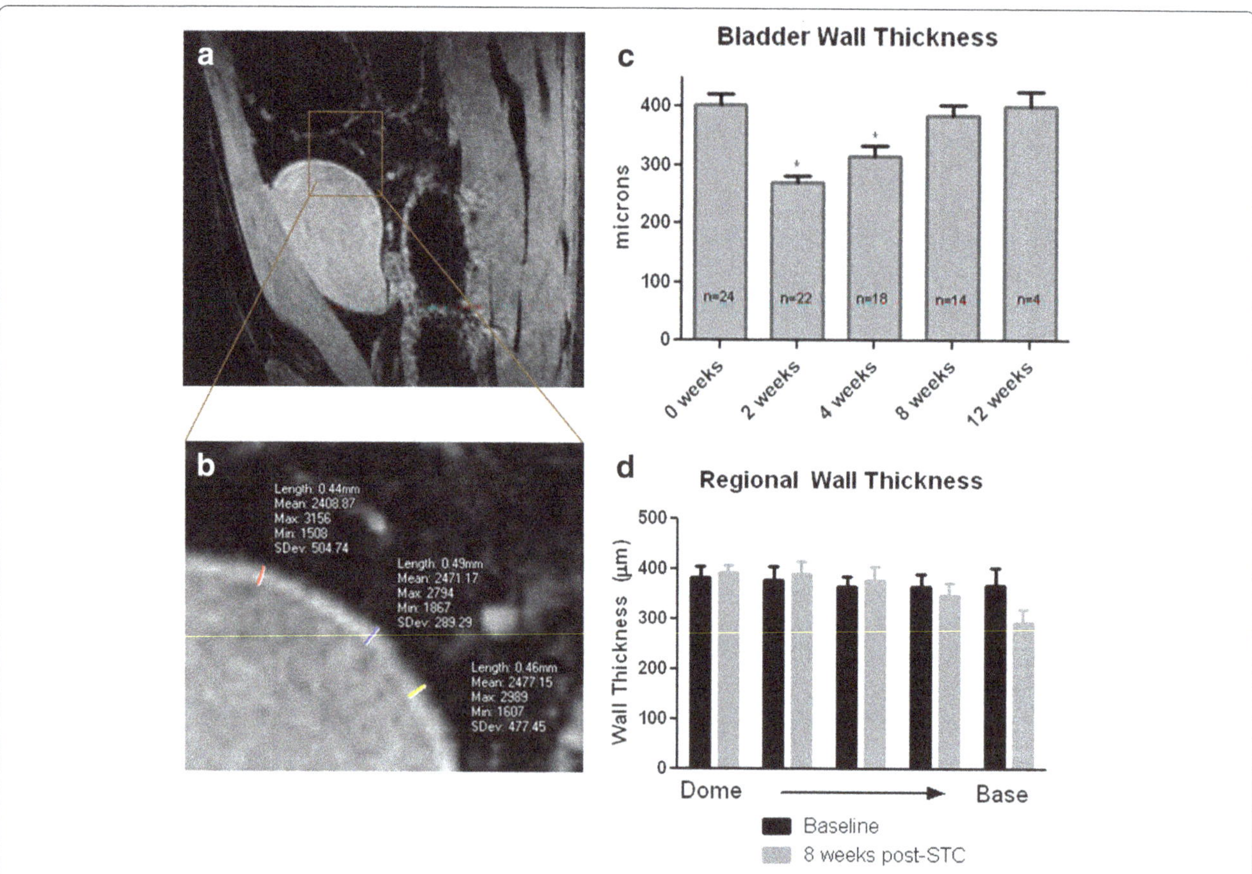

Fig. 2 Bladder wall thickness normalizes thickness 8 weeks after STC. **a** Example of a sagittal view of a control (pre-STC) bladder visualized by magnetic resonance imaging (MRI), magnified in **b**. **c** 1 Way ANOVA analysis of quantified bladder wall thickness using MRI scans reveals that the bladder wall is thinner than pre-STC values 2 and 4 weeks post-STC ($P < 0.01$). The number of observations at each timepoint represent the number of successful scans at each timepoint, as instances of gating artifact did lead to some unsuccessful scans. The ratio of unsuccessful scans to total number of possible scans was 1/25, 3/25, 2/20, 1/15, and 1/5 at 0, 2, 4, 8, and 12 weeks, respectively. **d** Analysis of regional wall thickness shows no differences from control ($n = 24$) and 8 weeks post-STC ($n = 14$)

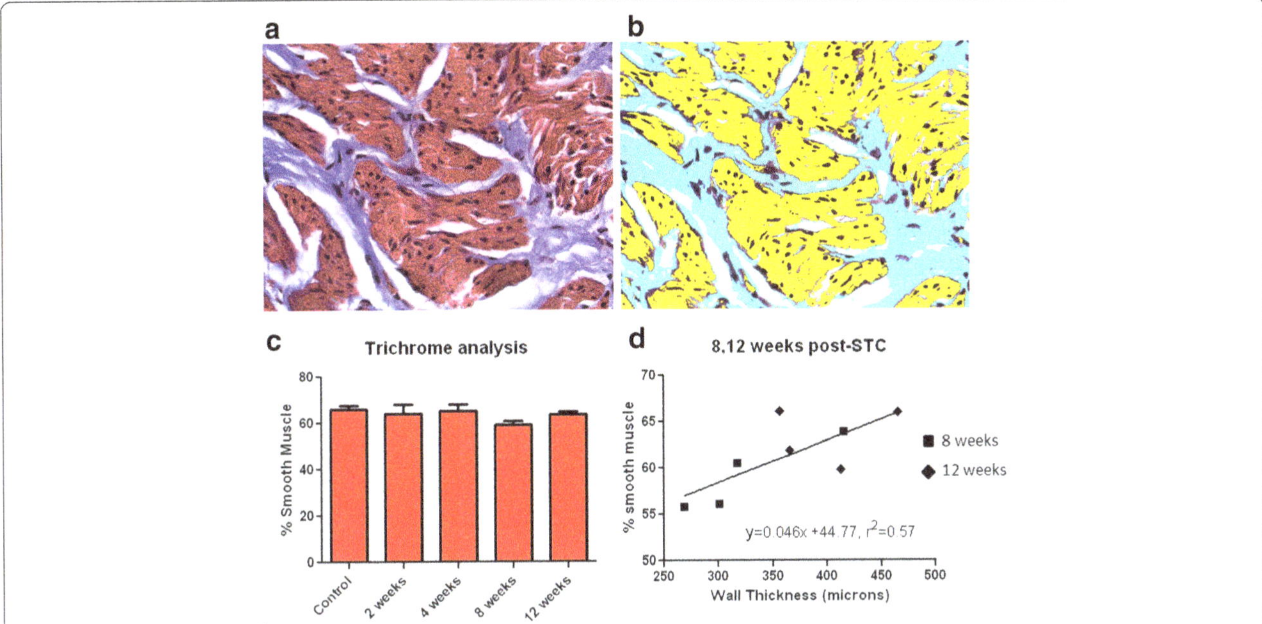

Fig. 3 Quantification of smooth muscle to collagen ratios using semi-quantitation of Masson's trichrome staining. **a** Representative image of excised STC bladder used for quantification by choosing pixel intensity **b. c** Analysis shows no differences accross time, however linear regression **d** reveals that the amount of smooth muscle is correlated with bladder wall thickness determined via MRI ($P < 0.05$)

other time point post-STC. Consistent with previous studies, the average measured bladder capacity increased until the 8-week time point, however in contrast to those studies, bladder capacity declined afterwards. Upon closer inspection, there was significant variation in bladder capacity at the 8-week time point (the only time point at which CT was also performed). Subdivision of the animals at the 8-week time point into those animals that received both CT and MRI vs. those that received MRI alone revealed statistically significant increases in bladder capacity, micturition volume and bladder compliance in CT-scanned animals when compared to

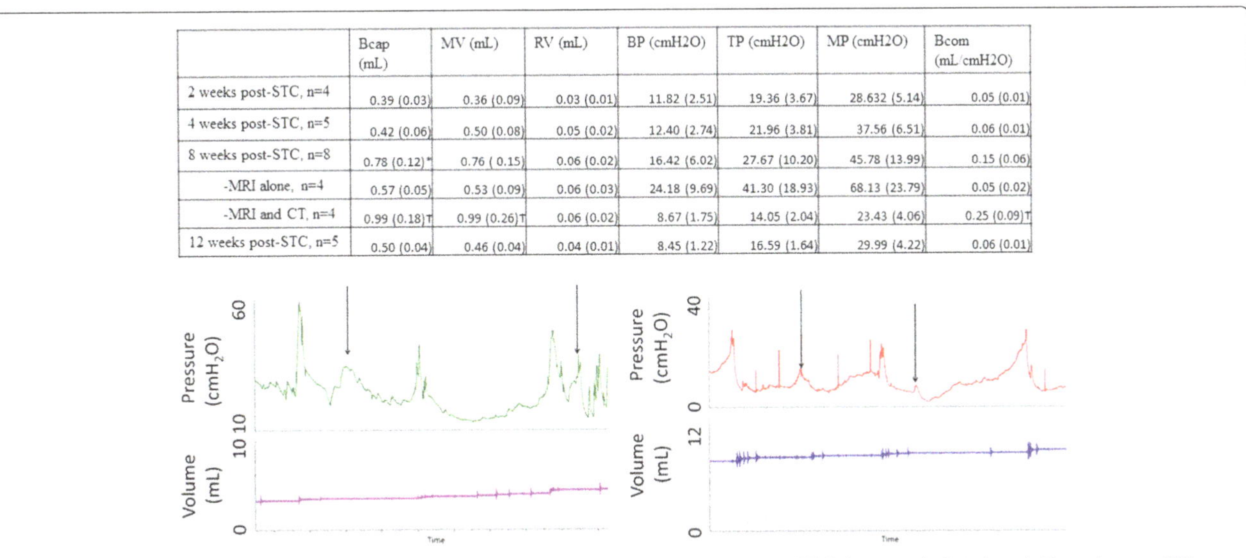

	Bcap (mL)	MV (mL)	RV (mL)	BP (cmH2O)	TP (cmH2O)	MP (cmH2O)	Bcom (mL/cmH2O)
2 weeks post-STC, n=4	0.39 (0.03)	0.36 (0.09)	0.03 (0.01)	11.82 (2.51)	19.36 (3.67)	28.632 (5.14)	0.05 (0.01)
4 weeks post-STC, n=5	0.42 (0.06)	0.50 (0.08)	0.05 (0.02)	12.40 (2.74)	21.96 (3.81)	37.56 (6.51)	0.06 (0.01)
8 weeks post-STC, n=8	0.78 (0.12)*	0.76 (0.15)	0.06 (0.02)	16.42 (6.02)	27.67 (10.20)	45.78 (13.99)	0.15 (0.06)
-MRI alone, n=4	0.57 (0.05)	0.53 (0.09)	0.06 (0.03)	24.18 (9.69)	41.30 (18.93)	68.13 (23.79)	0.05 (0.02)
-MRI and CT, n=4	0.99 (0.18)ϯ	0.99 (0.26)ϯ	0.06 (0.02)	8.67 (1.75)	14.05 (2.04)	23.43 (4.06)	0.25 (0.09)ϯ
12 weeks post-STC, n=5	0.50 (0.04)	0.46 (0.04)	0.04 (0.01)	8.45 (1.22)	16.59 (1.64)	29.99 (4.22)	0.06 (0.01)

Fig. 4 Urodynamic parameters as determined by in vivo cystometry. Top table shows mean (SEM) for animals 2, 4, 8, and 12 weeks post-STC. *- Bladder capacity was higher 8 weeks post-STC compared with all other timepoints ($P < 0.05$). Cystometric parameters at 8 weeks post-STC are further broken down into animals that were imaged via CT, and those that only underwent MRI scanning. ϯ- Bcap, MV, and Bcom are significantly different between animals with MRI alone ($P < 0.05$). Bcap- Bladder Capacity, MV- Micturition Volume, RV- Residual Volume, BP- Basal Pressure, TP- Threshold Pressure, MP- Maximal Pressure. Bcom- Bladder Compliance. Lower panels show representative cystometrograms from animals at 8 weeks subjected to MRI alone revealing abnormal readings in the form of non-voiding contractions (arrows)

animals that had MRI alone. Importantly, bladders still emptied completely in all animals as evidenced by low residual volume.

Linear regression of urodynamic parameters and MRI Scans

Linear regression analysis revealed that BWT, as determined via MRI (see Fig. 5), correlated with some cystometric parameters early post-STC (i.e., 2 and 4 weeks). Specifically, BWT at the time of sacrifice was negatively correlated with bladder capacity at that same time point (Fig. 5a). Additionally, pre-operative (baseline) BWT values were positively correlated with the bladder compliance and percent smooth muscle seen at 2 and 4 weeks post-STC ($P = 0.049$, and 0.016, respectively).

CT scanning

A previous report documented that the anterior bladder circumference measured via CT scans positively correlated with maximum pressures generated by the bladder post-STC [21]. Here, we conducted a retrospective analysis to further examine CT-determined bladder volume with other cystometric parameters from the same animal. Retrospective analysis revealed a negative correlation between total bladder volumes measured by CT scans 2 weeks post-STC and the maximum pressures generated *in vivo* 8 weeks post-STC (Fig. 6). A bladder volume of less than 0.2 mls at 2 weeks post-STC was associated with high pressures and detrusor overactivity at 8 weeks (i.e., the appearance of non-voiding contractions). Conversely, a bladder with a large volume at 2 weeks (>0.8 mls) resulted in significantly diminished pressure generation during micturition at 8 weeks post-STC. Bladders in which volumes ranged between 0.2 and 0.6 mls 2 weeks post-STC estimated by CT imaging were subsequently observed to have normal urodynamic profiles at 8 weeks post-STC.

Discussion

The present study investigated the utility of Magnetic Resonance Imaging (MRI) and Computerized Tomography (CT), in conjunction with traditional measures, to provide longitudinal mechanistic insight into restoration of bladder structure and function. MRI can be challenging in rodent models because of the small size of organs/tissues (rat bladder). We were able to overcome difficulties by using a 7 Tesla magnet coupled with respiratory gating, although a few instances of motion artifact prevented acquisition of analyzable images (8/90 possible scans). We noted that bladder wall thickness (BWT) drastically decreased immediately after STC, but returned to normal pre-operative values by 8 weeks post-STC (Fig. 2). Although absolute values of BWT reported here with MRI (≈400 μm) are lower than our previous report based on histological evaluation (≈550 μm), it is still within the normal range reported for BWT [21, 44]. Discrepancies between tissue thickness via MRI and histology have been shown previously in, for example, the retina [45, 46]. Although

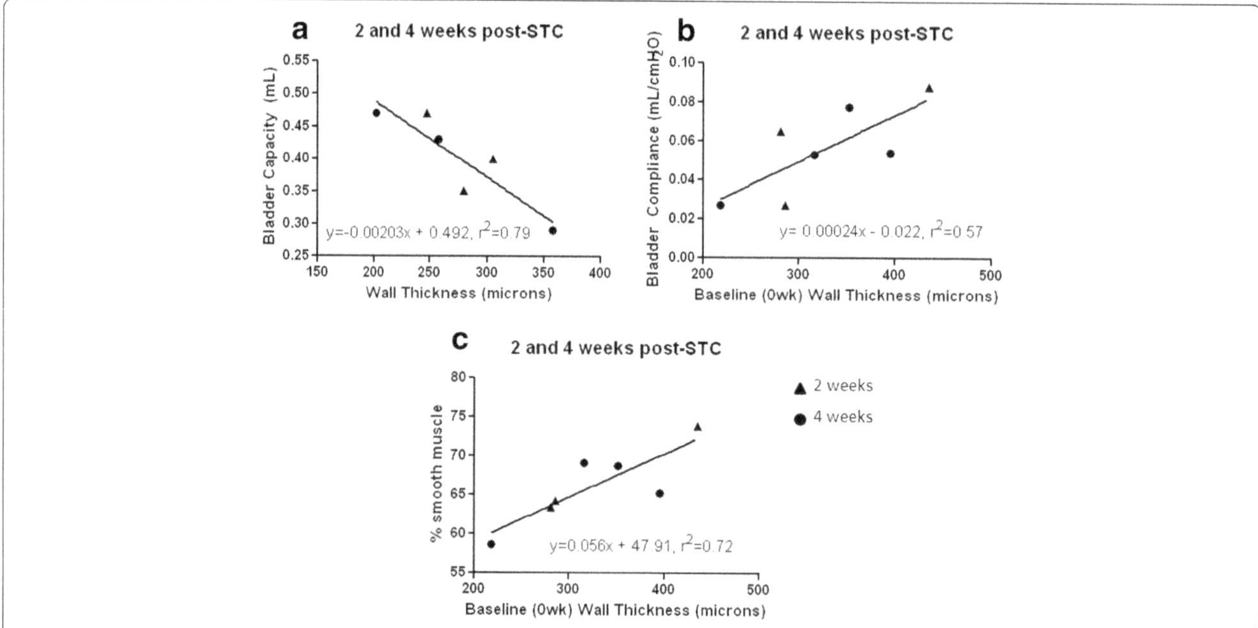

Fig. 5 Linear regression analysis of cystometric parameters with MRI-determined bladder wall thickness. **a** At early timepoints (i.e., 2,4 weeks) after STC, the bladder capacity is negatively correlated with bladder wall thickness at that same timepoint. The pre-operative thickness of the bladder wall (baseline) is positively correlated with bladder compliance (**b**) and smooth muscle content (**c**) seen at early time points post-STC. ($P < 0.05$)

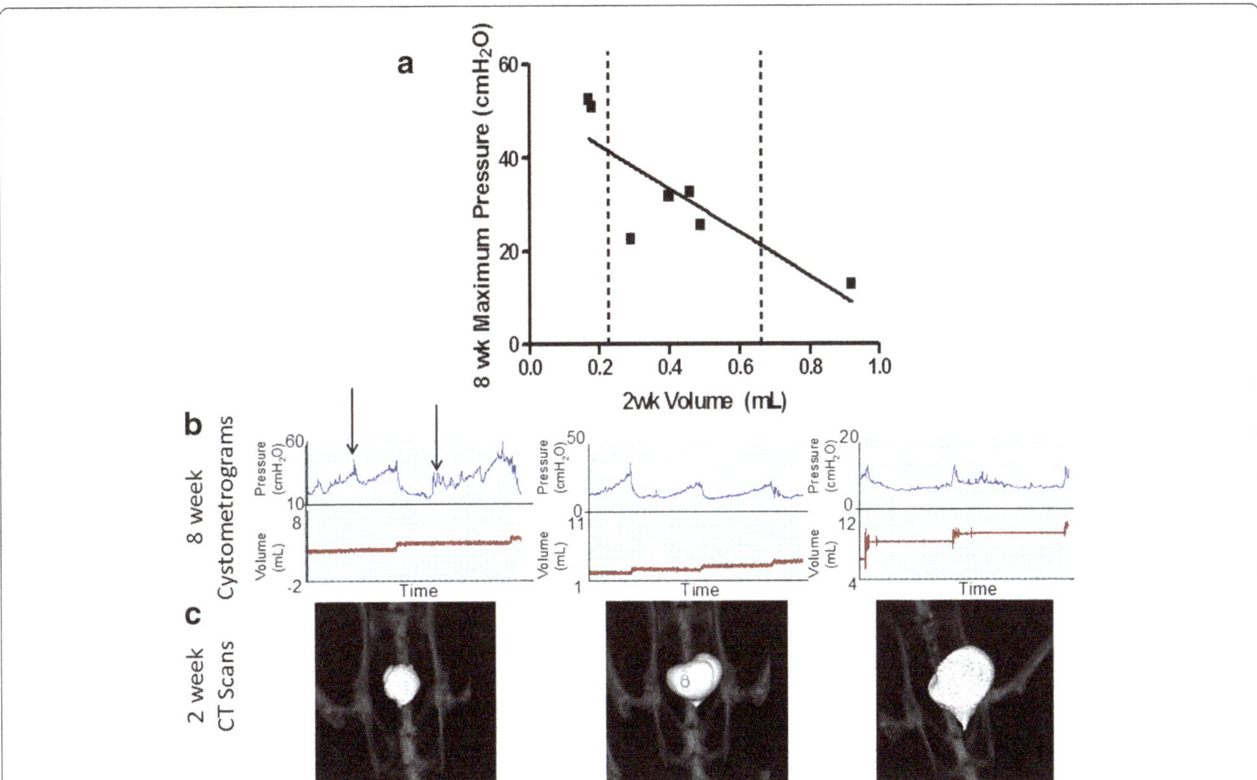

Fig. 6 Retrospective regression analysis of animals subjected to STC reveals a predictive value for CT Scanning. This graph represents 2 week CT and 8 week cystometric data from 4 animals in this study, along with 3 animals from a previous study (Burmeister et al., 2010). **a** X-axis represents bladder volume 2 weeks post-STC as determined by CT Scanning, and Y-axis represents maximum pressure (MP) generated by bladders 8 weeks post-STC as determined by *in vivo* urodynamic studies in the SAME ANIMAL. **b** Representative cystometrograms at 8 weeks and (**c**) CT scans at 2 weeks of 3 individual animals. This analysis displays that animals with minimal bladder growth seen upon CT scanning 2 weeks post-STC (left of the dashed lines) display bladder overactivity (arrows show non-voiding contractions), while the animal with a large bladder volume 2 weeks post-STC (right of the dashed lines) generates low maximum pressures (i.e. ~13 cmH_2O). Normal bladder function was seen in animals with intermediate bladder volumes determined by CT 2 weeks post-STC. $y = -46.65x + 52.12$, $r = 0.82$, $P = 0.02$

statistically thinner at 2–4 weeks after STC, the bladder did not display any significant fibrosis at any time point, as illustrated by the percent smooth muscle in the bladder wall displayed in Fig. 3c.

Urodynamic studies revealed increased bladder capacities 8 weeks post-STC similar to our prior report [21]; however this was not maintained 12 weeks post-STC (Fig. 4). Significant variability in cystometric parameters 8 weeks post-STC prompted subdivision of the animals based on whether they had an MRI only or MRI plus CT on the day following MRI. Manual bladder emptying during MRI apparently had an adverse impact on the regeneration process leading to instances of non-voiding contractions, abnormal basal pressures, and small bladder capacities (Fig. 4). At all time points, animals assessed via MRI showed diminished recovery of normal bladder volumes. Conversely, animals in which MRI scanning/bladder emptying was followed by bladder filling during CT scanning showed complete restoration of bladder volume and improved bladder compliance. While the precise mechanism(s) responsible for this observation remain unclear, it is interesting to speculate that it may be related to untoward mechanical manipulation of the bladder emptying during critical periods of bladder regrowth and regeneration. Consistent with this supposition is recent data in a murine model of STC (Christ et al., unpublished observations) that indicates that MRI without bladder emptying results in normal recovery of bladder volume. Despite diminished recovery of bladder volume in this study, residual volume never increased in any animal, and there was no decrease in bladder wall thickness (Fig. 2) or smooth muscle percentage in the bladder wall (Fig. 3).

A limitation of the current study involves technical difficulties in standardizing the state of the bladder during imaging (i.e. how full/empty the bladder is during scanning). Ideally, the bladder would be filled to a standard pressure during scans to atone for dynamic BWT due to filling. However, these MRI scans lasted approximately one hour, and starting from empty presumably minimizes the effect on BWT due to physiological filling. Similarly, CT scanning requires filling the bladder with contrast medium, and clamping of the catheter to prevent emptying. It is logistically difficult to ensure a consistent pressure during these scans, resulting in comparison of thoroughly and comparably full bladders. Regardless, there is reasonable consistency in these procedures as reflected in small variability shown in MRI and CT parameters. While we acknowledge these technical limitations, as noted above, the BWT measurements derived from MRI were still a reasonable approximation of prior reports using more standard measures [21, 44].

Given these considerations, MRI studies still yielded potentially interesting relationships between BWT and bladder capacity and compliance (Fig. 5). Specifically, during the first month of bladder regeneration, BWT was negatively correlated with bladder capacity, perhaps due to non-optimal cellular proliferation/organization in the regenerating bladder wall at early time points. We also found that baseline BWT (i.e., pre-STC) was positively correlated with both bladder compliance and the percent of smooth muscle found in the bladder during the first month post-STC. These correlations point to an overall improved outcome of bladder regeneration in animals that have a thicker bladder wall pre-STC, and earlier recovery of BWT post-STC. While these metrics, as well as their putative mechanism(s) require further investigation, they may provide valuable insight into important correlates of successful regenerative responses in the bladder.

A previous report documented that bladder volumes estimated by CT imaging accurately tracked bladder capacity measured via cystometry [21]. Here we report a retrospective analysis of those results, illustrating a significant correlation observed between CT-determined bladder volumes 2 weeks post-STC and maximal pressure determined cystometrically in the same animal 8 weeks post-STC. This suggests that there may be a normal volume range for bladder re-growth during the first two weeks post-STC, such that bladder volumes outside this range may result in abnormal bladder function (Fig. 6b). Specifically in the 2 weeks post-STC, a small increase in bladder capacity (<0.2 mls) results in bladder overactivity (i.e. high pressure and non-voiding contractions), while a large amount of bladder growth (>0.8) results in a substantial deficiency for pressure generation *in vivo*. If further validated as an index for the eventual success of bladder regeneration, the use of CT scans at early time points during bladder regrowth may provide a critical opportunity for intervention(s) to correct an otherwise failed therapeutic recovery.

Conclusions

To summarize, we have demonstrated that although non-invasive imaging may be a useful tool for obtaining mechanistic insight into bladder regeneration during the first 3 months post-STC, these methods alone are not yet ready to replace well-established functional analyses (i.e. cystometry), as well as more descriptive measures of bladder voiding patterns [35, 36]. Specifically, the impact of mechanical emptying of the bladder during critical stages of regeneration using these modalities must be carefully monitored to ensure that their utilization does not affect the remodeling response being measured. Further investigation will hopefully identify appropriate boundary conditions such that both CT and MRI can be more effectively used and provide important noninvasive mechanistic insight into functional bladder regeneration. While current urodynamic approaches (i.e. cystometry and voiding pattern analysis) must still be employed, non-invasive imaging may eventually allow researchers to follow important aspects of the morphogenesis/bladder regeneration longitudinally. Ultimately, this approach could identify noninvasive metrics early on in the regenerative process where one might be able to not only predict the extent and outcome of regeneration/re-growth, but also develop effective interventions for therapeutic restoration of bladder re-growth/regeneration.

Abbreviations

STC: Subtotal Cystectomy; BWT: Bladder Wall Thickness; MRI: Magnetic Resonance Imaging; CT: Computed Tomography.

Competing interests

The authors declare that they have no competing interests.

Authors' contributions

DB organized the study design, performed statistical analysis and drafted the manuscript. BB participated in cystometric and histological studies. TA participated in design of the study and animal surgeries. JO performed all MRI procedure troubleshooting. MH analyzed all MRI images and participated in cystometric studies. JT helped design and interpret CT and MRI studies. KEA was involved in conception, design, coordination of the study and helped draft the manuscript. GJC was involved in conception, design, coordination of the study and helped draft the manuscript. All authors have read and approved the final manuscript.

Acknowledgements

The authors would like to thank the Center for Biomolecular Imaging at Wake Forest University, including Kerry Link, Debra Fuller, and Sandy Kaminsky for their support and technical assistance with this manuscript. This work was supported by NIH USPHS (grant no. R21DK081832).

Author details

[1]Wake Forest Institute for Regenerative Medicine, 391 Technology Way, Winston-Salem, NC 27101, USA. [2]Departments of Biomedical Engineering and Orthopaedic Surgery, and Laboratory of Regenerative Therapeutics, University of Virginia, 415 Lane Road, Charlottesville, VA 22908, USA. [3]Wake Forest Department of Biomolecular Imaging, Medical Center Blvd, Winston-Salem, NC 27157, USA.

References

1. Atala A. Tissue engineering of human bladder. Br Med Bull. 2011;97:81–104.
2. Atala A, Bauer SB, Soker S, Yoo JJ, Retik AB. Tissue-engineered autologous bladders for patients needing cystoplasty. Lancet. 2006;367(9518):1241–6.

3. Obara T, Matsuura S, Narita S, Satoh S, Tsuchiya N, Habuchi T. Bladder acellular matrix grafting regenerates urinary bladder in the spinal cord injury rat. Urology. 2006;68(4):892–7.
4. Oberpenning F, Meng J, Yoo JJ, Atala A. De novo reconstitution of a functional mammalian urinary bladder by tissue engineering. Nat Biotechnol. 1999;17(2):149–55.
5. Roth CC, Mondalek FG, Kibar Y, Ashley RA, Bell CH, Califano JA, et al. Bladder regeneration in a canine model using hyaluronic acid-poly(lactic-co-glycolic-acid) nanoparticle modified porcine small intestinal submucosa. BJU Int. 2011;108(1):148–55.
6. Sharma AK, Bury MI, Marks AJ, Fuller NJ, Meisner JW, Tapaskar N, et al. A nonhuman primate model for urinary bladder regeneration using autologous sources of bone marrow-derived mesenchymal stem cells. Stem Cells. 2011;29(2):241–50.
7. Urakami S, Shiina H, Enokida H, Kawamoto K, Kikuno N, Fandel T, et al. Functional improvement in spinal cord injury-induced neurogenic bladder by bladder augmentation using bladder acellular matrix graft in the rat. World J Urol. 2007;25(2):207–13.
8. Yoo JJ, Meng J, Oberpenning F, Atala A. Bladder augmentation using allogenic bladder submucosa seeded with cells. Urology. 1998;51(2):221–5.
9. Chung SY, Krivorov NP, Rausei V, Thomas L, Frantzen M, Landsittel D, et al. Bladder reconstitution with bone marrow derived stem cells seeded on small intestinal submucosa improves morphological and molecular composition. J Urol. 2005;174(1):353–9.
10. Drewa T, Joachimiak R, Kaznica A, Sarafian V, Pokrywczynska M. Hair stem cells for bladder regeneration in rats: preliminary results. Transplant Proc. 2009;41(10):4345–51.
11. Engelhardt EM, Micol LA, Houis S, Wurm FM, Hilborn J, Hubbell JA, et al. A collagen-poly(lactic acid-co-varepsilon-caprolactone) hybrid scaffold for bladder tissue regeneration. Biomaterials. 2011;32(16):3969–76.
12. Jack GS, Zhang R, Lee M, Xu Y, Wu BM, Rodriguez LV. Urinary bladder smooth muscle engineered from adipose stem cells and a three dimensional synthetic composite. Biomaterials. 2009;30(19):3259–70.
13. Sharma AK, Hota PV, Matoka DJ, Fuller NJ, Jandali D, Thaker H, et al. Urinary bladder smooth muscle regeneration utilizing bone marrow derived mesenchymal stem cell seeded elastomeric poly(1,8-octanediol-co-citrate) based thin films. Biomaterials. 2010;31(24):6207–17.
14. Zhang Y, Lin HK, Frimberger D, Epstein RB, Kropp BP. Growth of bone marrow stromal cells on small intestinal submucosa: an alternative cell source for tissue engineered bladder. BJU Int. 2005;96(7):1120–5.
15. Zhu WD, Xu YM, Feng C, Fu Q, Song LJ, Cui L. Bladder reconstruction with adipose-derived stem cell-seeded bladder acellular matrix grafts improve morphology composition. World J Urol. 2010;28(4):493–8.
16. Joseph DB, Borer JG, De Filippo RE, Hodges SJ, McLorie GA. Autologous Cell Seeded Biodegradable Scaffold for Augmentation Cystoplasty: Phase II Study in Children and Adolescents with Spina Bifida. J Urol. 2014;191(5):1389–95.
17. Frederiksen H, Arner A, Malmquist U, Scott RS, Uvelius B. Nerve induced responses and force-velocity relations of regenerated detrusor muscle after subtotal cystectomy in the rat. Neurourol Urodyn. 2004;23(2):159–65.
18. Liang DS, Goss RJ. Regeneration of the bladder after subtotal cystectomy in rats. J Urol. 1963;89:427–30.
19. Piechota HJ, Gleason CA, Dahms SE, Dahiya R, Nunes LS, Lue TF, et al. Bladder acellular matrix graft: in vivo functional properties of the regenerated rat bladder. Urol Res. 1999;27(3):206–13.
20. Saito M, Yoshikawa Y, Ohmura M, Yokoi K, Kondo A. Functional restoration of rat bladder after subtotal cystectomy: in vivo cystometry and in vitro study of whole bladder. Urol Res. 1996;24(3):171–5.
21. Burmeister D, Aboushwareb T, Tan J, Link K, Andersson KE, Christ G. Early stages of in situ bladder regeneration in a rodent model. Tissue Eng Part A. 2010;16(8):2541–51.
22. Peyton CC, Burmeister D, Petersen B, Andersson KE, Christ G. Characterization of the early proliferative response of the rodent bladder to subtotal cystectomy: a unique model of mammalian organ regeneration. PLoS One. 2012;7(10):e47414.
23. Baker R, Maxted WC, Dipasquale N. Regeneration of Transitional Epithelium of the Human Bladder after Total Surgical Excision for Recurrent, Multiple Bladder Cancer: Apparent Tumor Inhibition. J Urol. 1965;93:593–7.
24. Baker R, Tehan T, Kelly T. Regeneration of urinary bladder after subtotal resection for carcinoma. Am Surg. 1959;25(5):348–52.
25. Bohne AW, Urwiller KL. Experience with urinary bladder regeneration. J Urol. 1957;77(5):725–32.
26. Folsom AI, O'Brien HA, Caldwell GT. Subtotal Cystectomy in the treatment of Hunner Ulcer. J Urol. 1940;44:650.
27. Liang DS. Bladder regeneration following subtotal cystectomy. J Urol. 1962;88:503–5.
28. McCallum DC. Gangrene of the bladder with subsequent regrowth. J Urol. 1965;94(6):669–70.
29. Portilla Sanchez R, Blanco FL, Santamarina A, Casals Roa J, Mata J, Kaufman A. Vesical regeneration in the human after total cystectomy and implantation of a plastic mould. Br J Urol. 1958;30(2):180–8.
30. Richardson EJ. Bladder regeneration case report and review of the literature. Minn Med. 1952;35(6):547–9.
31. Sisk IR, Neu VF. Regeneration of the Bladder. Trans Am Assn GU Surg. 1939;32:197.
32. Tucci P, Haralambidis G. Regeneration of the Bladder: Review of Literature and Case Report. J Urol. 1963;90:193–9.
33. Andersson KE, Soler R, Fullhase C. Rodent models for urodynamic investigation. Neurourol Urodyn. 2011;30(5):636–46.
34. Bjorling DE, Wang Z, Vezina CM, Ricke WA, Keil KP, Yu W, et al. Evaluation of voiding assays in mice: impact of genetic strains and sex. Am J Physiol Renal Physiol. 2015;308(12):F1369–78.
35. Hodges SJ, Zhou G, Deng FM, Aboushwareb T, Turner C, Andersson KE, et al. Voiding pattern analysis as a surrogate for cystometric evaluation in uroplakin II knockout mice. J Urol. 2008;179(5):2046–51.
36. Lau JF, Anderson SA, Adler E, Frank JA. Imaging approaches for the study of cell-based cardiac therapies. Nat Rev Cardiol. 2010;7(2):97–105.
37. Saldanha KJ, Doan RP, Ainslie KM, Desai TA, Majumdar S. Micrometer-sized iron oxide particle labeling of mesenchymal stem cells for magnetic resonance imaging-based monitoring of cartilage tissue engineering. Magn Reson Imaging. 2011;29(1):40–9.
38. Young S, Kretlow JD, Nguyen C, Bashoura AG, Baggett LS, Jansen JA, et al. Microcomputed tomography characterization of neovascularization in bone tissue engineering applications. Tissue Eng Part B Rev. 2008;14(3):295–306.
39. Cheng HL, Wallis C, Shou Z, Farhat WA. Quantifying angiogenesis in VEGF-enhanced tissue-engineered bladder constructs by dynamic contrast-enhanced MRI using contrast agents of different molecular weights. J Magn Reson Imaging. 2007;25(1):137–45.
40. Newport JP, Dusseault BN, Butler C, Pais VM, Jr. Gadolinium-enhanced computed tomography cystogram to diagnose bladder augment rupture in patients with iodine sensitivity. Urology. 2008; 71(5):984 e989-911.
41. Ramalingam M, Senthil K, Murugesan A, Pai MG. Laparoscopic undiversion in a child with sacral agenesis into augmentation cystoplasty. JSLS. 2013;17(3):450–3.
42. Burmeister DM, AbouShwareb T, Bergman CR, Andersson KE, Christ GJ. Age-related alterations in regeneration of the urinary bladder after subtotal cystectomy. Am J Pathol. 2013;183(5):1585–95.
43. Burmeister D, AbouShwareb T, D'Agostino Jr R, Andersson KE, Christ GJ. Impact of partial urethral obstruction on bladder function: time-dependent changes and functional correlates of altered expression of Ca(2)(+) signaling regulators. Am J Physiol Ren Physiol. 2012;302(12):F1517–28.
44. Auge C, Chene G, Dubourdeau M, Desoubzdanne D, Corman B, Palea S, et al. Relevance of the cyclophosphamide-induced cystitis model for pharmacological studies targeting inflammation and pain of the bladder. Eur J Pharmacol. 2013;707(1–3):32–40.
45. Chen J, Chiang CW, Zhang H, Song SK. Cell swelling contributes to thickening of low-dose N-methyl-D-aspartate-induced retinal edema. Invest Ophthalmol Vis Sci. 2012;53(6):2777–85.
46. Li G, De La Garza B, Shih YY, Muir ER, Duong TQ. Layer-specific blood-flow MRI of retinitis pigmentosa in RCS rats. Exp Eye Res. 2012;101:90–6.

Neoadjuvant chemotherapy for primary adenocarcinomas of the urinary bladder

Bin Yu[1,2†], Jin Zhou[3†], Hongzhou Cai[1†], Ting Xu[1], Zicheng Xu[1,2], Qing Zou[1*] and Min Gu[2*]

Abstract

Background: Adenocarcinoma of the urinary bladder is a rare malignancy. Radical surgery is suggested as the best available treatment for early-stage disease, but there is currently no consensus on standard chemotherapy regimen for advanced stage. We assessed the feasibility and effect of neoadjuvant chemotherapy with gemcitabine and cisplatin (GC) plus S-1 for patients with locally advanced primary adenocarcinomas of the urinary bladder.

Methods: Six patients with locally advanced urachal or non-urachal (n = 3, each) primary adenocarcinoma of the bladder were treated from October 2010 to October 2013 at a single center. All the patients were treated with 3 cycles (21d, each) of GC plus S-1 (gemcitabine, 1000 mg/m^2, days 1 and 8; cisplatin, 70 mg/m^2, day 2; and S-1, 50 mg bid, day 1-14). After neoadjuvant chemotherapy, patients with urachal cancer were treated with *en bloc* radical cystectomy and umbilectomy; the remaining 3 patients were treated with cystectomy.

Results: All patients successfully completed the neoadjuvant chemotherapy without serious side effects. Two patients were assessed as complete response, 2 as partial response, 1 as stable disease and 1 as progressive disease.

Conclusions: Despite the limitations of a small study population, the GC plus S-1 regimen for locally advanced primary adenocarcinoma of the urinary bladder was effective, and facilitated the success of surgery to a certain extent. Short follow-up time was also a limitation of our study. More studies are needed to evaluate the results.

Keywords: Neoadjuvant chemotherapy, Primary adenocarcinomas of bladder, Survival

Background

Primary adenocarcinomas of the bladder account for less than 2% of primary bladder cancers, and are rarely encountered [1,2]. Primary adenocarcinomas of the urinary bladder can be subdivided into urachal and non-urachal adenocarcinoma. Radical surgery is considered the best available treatment, but the 5-year survival rates (11%-61%) have not been satisfactory [3]. Patients with urachal adenocarcinoma often present with higher stage disease because the disease arises out-side of the bladder and causes fewer symptoms before its invasion of surrounding organs. For patients with locally advanced primary adenocarcinomas of the bladder, neoadjuvant chemotherapy can be a good option: it helps downstage the cancer before radical surgery, eradicates potential micrometastases, and may avoid local and distant failure [4,5]. However, primary adenocarcinomas of the urinary bladder are so rare that experience of chemotherapy is limited [6]. The National Comprehensive Cancer Network (NCCN; version 2.2014) suggests that chemotherapy with methotrexate, vinblastine, doxorubicin, and cisplatin (MVAC) is not effective for primary adenocarcinomas of the urinary bladder, and according to some reports a 5-fluorouracil (5-FU)-based regimen should be tried [6,7]. Furthermore, gemcitabine plus cisplatin (GC) has proved viable as first-line chemotherapy for urothelial (transitional) cell carcinoma with overall survival comparable to that of MVAC but with fewer side effects [8]. Herein, we report our experience in treating 6 cases of

* Correspondence: 343463975@qq.com; caihong12006@gmail.com
†Equal contributors
[1]Department of Urologic Surgery, Affiliated Cancer Hospital of Jiangsu Province of Nanjing Medical University, Nanjing, China
[2]Department of Urology, First Affiliated Hospital of Nanjing Medical University, Nanjing, China
Full list of author information is available at the end of the article

locally advanced primary adenocarcinomas of the bladder, 3 urachal and 3 non-urachal.

Methods

This prospective observational study was approved by the Institutional Review Board of Nanjing Medical University, Nanjing, China. Each patient provided written informed consent before treatment. Six patients with pathologically diagnosed locally advanced primary adenocarcinoma of the bladder were treated between October 2010 and October 2013 at Affiliated Cancer Hospital of Jiangsu Province of Nanjing Medical University. The patients' demographics and clinical data were collected. All the pathology gained through biopsy via cystoscopy was confirmed as adenocarcinoma before chemotherapy. Computed tomography of cranial, chest and abdomen was done to exclude the metastatic adenocarcinoma. All patients were confirmed primary adenocarcinoma of the bladder at a locally advanced stage, with clinical stage $\geq T_2$, without distant metastasis, and with or without lymph node metastasis. All the patients were treated with GC plus S-1 chemotherapy for 3 cycles, 21 d/cycle: gemcitabine, 1000 mg/m^2, days 1 and 8; cisplatin, 70 mg/m^2, day 2; and S-1, 50 mg bid, days 1-14. The adenocarcinomas were classified as as urachal or non-urachal prior to surgery. Tumors were considered urachal if the tumor was located at the dome of the bladder rather than the anterior bladder wall, with the most critical features being the presence of a sharp demarcation between the tumor and the surface epithelium, and the exclusion of a primary adenocarcinoma elsewhere. Patients with urachal bladder cancer were treated with *en bloc* radical cystectomy and umbilectomy. Non-urachal patients were treated with cystectomy after neoadjuvant chemotherapy. The response of the target lesions to treatment was evaluated by computed tomography scan, in accordance with the Response Evaluation Criteria In Solid Tumors (RECIST 1.1) guidelines: complete response (disappearance of target lesion); partial response (≥30% decrease in the sum of the longest diameter of the target lesion, from baseline); stable disease (between a partial response and progressive disease); and progressive disease (≥20% increase in the sum of the longest diameter of the target lesion, from nadir) [9]. The patients were followed, beginning at diagnosis.

Results

Six patients were enrolled in this study: 5 men and 1 woman, aged 49 to 79 years (mean 62.5 y; Table 1). Hematuria and lower abdominal pain were the most frequently reported symptoms at presentation. Specifically, 4 patients presented with hematuria and 3 with lower abdominal pain (1 patient with both symptoms). One, 3, and 2 patients were in stages T_2, T_3, and T_4, respectively. One month after the 3 cycles of neoadjuvant chemotherapy, 2, 2, 1, and 1 patient were evaluated as complete response, partial remission, stable disease, and progressive disease, respectively. No patient stopped chemotherapy because of side effects. Three patients were judged to have non-urachal adenocarcinoma. Two of these received *en bloc* radical cystectomy and umbilectomy. One patient refused surgery. The 3 patients with non-urachal adenocarcinoma were treated by cystectomy. After surgery, pathology confirmed pure primary adenocarcinoma in 5 patients.

Four patients experienced grade 2 myelosuppression. Three patients had transient elevated serum creatinine (averaging 1.5-fold normal). Three patients had nausea, vomiting, and loss of appetite. All the patients recovered from the side effects after completion of chemotherapy.

Discussion

Adenocarcinoma of the urinary bladder is a rare malignancy with a poor prognosis. Patient survival is similar to that of muscle-invasive urothelial carcinoma [10]. Unlike other cancers, there is currently no consensus regarding a standard chemotherapy regime for adenocarcinoma of the urinary bladder. In the present study, we used GC plus S-1 for neoadjuvant chemotherapy. Johnson et al. [11] reported that adenocarcinomas of the urinary bladder have a clinical behavior similar to that of urothelial (transitional) cell carcinoma of the bladder, and GC as first-line chemotherapy for urothelial cell carcinoma has fewer side effects and similar overall survival compared with MVAC. 5-FU is widely used in the treatment of adenocarcinomas (such as

Table 1 Case summaries of 6 patients with primary adenocarcinomas of the urinary bladder

Patient	Age	Gender	Symptom	Tumor	Stage	Response[a]	PFS, mo[b]	Survival, mo
1	71	Male	Pain	Non-urachal	T3b	Complete	3	7
2	68	Male	Hematuria	Non-urachal	T2b	Partial	>18	18[c]
3	79	Female	Hematuria	Non-urachal	T4b	Stable disease	6	12
4	67	Male	Pain	Urachal	T3b	Complete	>20	20[c]
5	51	Male	Hematuria	Urachal	T3b	Partial	>10	10[c]
6	49	Male	Pain and hematuria	Urachal	T4a	Progressive disease	>6	6[c]

[a]After neoadjuvant chemotherapy; [b]progression-free survival; [c]still alive.

stomach cancer), and Logothetis et al. [6] reported using 5-FU to treat urachal cancers, but continuous 5-FU infusion has recently been replaced by S-1, to avoid some of the inconveniences and adverse effects of 5-FU [12,13]. S-1 is a novel oral Xuoropyrimidine derivative that consists of tegafur, 5-chloro-2, 4-dihydropyrimidine (CDHP), and potassium oxonate.

All the 6 patients of the present study received GC plus S-1 for 3 cycles, and no patient failed to complete the cycles because of side effects. The most severe side effect was grade 2 myelosuppression such as leucopenia and thrombocytopenia. This was resolved within 2 to7 days after symptomatic treatment with granulopoietin. More severe side effects can be treated by blood transfusion. No patient suffered renal function impairment because of chemotherapy. Three patients experienced transient elevated serum creatinine (averaging 1.5-fold normal). However, this also returned to normal after the end of treatment. Thus, the safety of this chemotherapy regime was acceptable.

In the present study, we applied GC plus S-1. Two patients had a partial response, and 2, 1, and 1 patient had complete response, stable disease, and progressive disease, respectively. In contrast, a study conducted by the MD Anderson Cancer Center (MDACC) used combinations of 5-FU and cisplatin and reported a 33% response rate [7]. Thus, our results are encouraging. Several factors may contribute to the difference in response rate. Firstly, the composition of patients is different. The patients in MDACC report are pure with urachal cancers, while in our study, NU adenocarcinoma patients are included. Secondly, the differences in the predominant ethnicities of the study populations (Houston, TX cf. Nanjing, China) may have influenced the response rate to chemotherapy. Many studies report that genetic polymorphisms exist in different races, especially in drug-metabolizing enzymes, drug targets, and drug receptors [14,15]. These genetic polymorphisms may have contribution to the response rate. Compared with western populations, the patients in China have more attention from their family. Better food and family care may encourage the nutrients and psychological healthy of patients. More importantly, adenocarcinomas of the urinary bladder are rare and all studies are limited in the small cases. The choice of chemotherapy regimens has been based largely on case reports and single institution experiences and the statistical power is limited.

After 3 cycles of neoadjuvant chemotherapy, 5 patients received surgery. The surgeries were straightforward and uneventful. Considering neoadjuvant chemotherapy may lead to increased edema and adhesion of the bladder to the surrounding tissue, increasing the difficulty of the operation. However, no unusual bleeding or postoperative infection was observed in our cases. Patient 1 rejected surgery because he had no medical insurance and could not bear any further financial burden. This patient had complete response after 3 cycles of chemotherapy, but after 3 months, the tumor recurred.

The majority of relevant studies have indicated that tumor stage is a highly significant predictor of outcome [16,17]. The shorter follow-up time, small case number, and the heterogeneity of patient 1 (who refused surgery and even other treatments) handicapped our analysis in this study. However, our results are enough to warrant further clinical studies with a larger number of patients with primary adenocarcinomas of the urinary bladder, to evaluate the efficacy of GC plus S-1 combination chemotherapy for neoadjuvant chemotherapy, and even for adjuvant chemotherapy.

Despite the limitations, the preliminary results of this study show that chemotherapy with GC plus S-1 for primary adenocarcinomas of the urinary bladder is effective. For patients at a locally advanced stage, this regimen effectively downstaged the tumor and may eradicate potential micrometastases, without increasing the difficulty of surgery.

Conclusions

Chemotherapy with the GC plus S-1 regimen for patients with primary adenocarcinomas of the urinary bladder is effective. To a certain extent, neoadjuvant chemotherapy facilitates surgery of patients at the locally advanced stage. Our treatments should be investigated in a randomized controlled trial to confirm these outcomes.

Competing interests

The authors declare that they have no competing interests.

Authors' contributions

QZ and MG contributed substantially to the conception and design. BY and HC helped to acquire the data and draft the manuscript. QZ, TX and ZX performed statistical analyses. JZ contributed to language editing. All authors read and approved the final manuscript.

Acknowledgments

We are grateful to Professor Changjun Yin (First Affiliated Hospital of Nanjing Medical University), and are thankful for the funding support (ZQ 201302) we received from the Affiliated Cancer Hospital of Jiangsu Province of Nanjing Medical University, Nanjing, China.

Author details

[1]Department of Urologic Surgery, Affiliated Cancer Hospital of Jiangsu Province of Nanjing Medical University, Nanjing, China. [2]Department of Urology, First Affiliated Hospital of Nanjing Medical University, Nanjing, China. [3]Department of Hospital Infection Control, Affiliated Cancer Hospital of Jiangsu Province of Nanjing Medical University, Nanjing, China.

References

1. Jemal A, Bray F, Center MM, Ferlay J, Ward E, Forman D. Global cancer statistics. CA Cancer J Clin. 2011;61(2):69–90.
2. Abol-Enein H, Kava BR, Carmack AJ. Nonurothelial cancer of the bladder. Urology. 2007;69(1 Suppl):93–104.
3. Dahm P, Gschwend JE. Malignant non-urothelial neoplasms of the urinary bladder: a review. Eur Urol. 2003;44(6):672–81.

4. Calabro F, Sternberg CN. Neoadjuvant and adjuvant chemotherapy in muscle-invasive bladder cancer. Eur Urol. 2009;55(2):348–58.
5. Clark PE. Neoadjuvant versus adjuvant chemotherapy for muscle-invasive bladder cancer. Expert Rev Anticancer Ther. 2009;9(6):821–30.
6. Logothetis CJ, Samuels ML, Ogden S. Chemotherapy for adenocarcinomas of bladder and urachal origin: 5-fluorouracil, doxorubicin, and mitomycin-C. Urology. 1985;26(3):252–5.
7. Siefker-Radtke AO, Gee J, Shen Y, Wen S, Daliani D, Millikan RE, et al. Multimodality management of urachal carcinoma: the M. D. Anderson Cancer Center experience. J Urol. 2003;169(4):1295–8.
8. von der Maase H, Hansen SW, Roberts JT, Dogliotti L, Oliver T, Moore MJ, et al. Gemcitabine and cisplatin versus methotrexate, vinblastine, doxorubicin, and cisplatin in advanced or metastatic bladder cancer: results of a large, randomized, multinational, multicenter, phase III study. J Clin Oncol. 2000;18(17):3068–77.
9. Sohaib A. RECIST rules. Cancer Imaging. 2012;12:345–6.
10. Ploeg M, Aben KK, de Hulsbergen-van Kaa CA, Schoenberg MP, Witjes JA, Kiemeney LA. Clinical epidemiology of nonurothelial bladder cancer: analysis of the Netherlands Cancer Registry. J Urol. 2010;183(3):915–20.
11. Johnson DE, Hogan JM, Ayala AG. Primary adenocarcinoma of the urinary bladder. South Med J. 1972;65(5):527–30.
12. Cunningham D, Starling N, Rao S, Iveson T, Nicolson M, Coxon F, et al. Capecitabine and oxaliplatin for advanced esophagogastric cancer. N Engl J Med. 2008;358(1):36–46.
13. Kang YK, Kang WK, Shin DB, Chen J, Xiong J, Wang J, et al. Capecitabine/cisplatin versus 5-fluorouracil/cisplatin as first-line therapy in patients with advanced gastric cancer: a randomised phase III noninferiority trial. Ann Oncol. 2009;20(4):666–73.
14. Barter ZE, Tucker GT, Rowland-Yeo K. Differences in cytochrome p450-mediated pharmacokinetics between chinese and caucasian populations predicted by mechanistic physiologically based pharmacokinetic modelling. Clin Pharmacokinet. 2013;52(12):1085–100.
15. Chiurillo MA. Genomic biomarkers related to drug response in Venezuelan populations. Drug Metabol Drug Interact. 2014; doi:10.1515/dmdi-2014-0019.
16. Zhang H, Jiang H, Wu Z, Fang Z, Fan J, Ding Q. Primary adenocarcinoma of the urinary bladder: a single site analysis of 21 cases. Int Urol Nephrol. 2013;45(1):107–11.
17. Siefker-Radtke A. Urachal carcinoma: surgical and chemotherapeutic options. Expert Rev Anticancer Ther. 2006;6(12):1715–21.

Treatment efficacy and tolerability of intravesical Bacillus Calmette-Guerin (BCG) - RIVM strain: induction and maintenance protocol in high grade and recurrent low grade non-muscle invasive bladder cancer (NMIBC)

Naim B Farah[1*], Rami Ghanem[2] and Mahmoud Amr[3]

Abstract

Background: BCG-RIVM strain was used in many treatment protocols for non-muscle invasive bladder cancer only as induction courses. Cho et al. *(Anticancer Res 2012)* compared BCG-RIVM induction and 'standard' maintenance *(Lamm et al., J Urol. 2000)* to mitomycin C. They found no statistically significant differences regarding disease recurrence and progression. The purpose of our study was to determine the efficacy & tolerability of this specific BCG RIVM strain, using six-weekly, induction course and single monthly instillations as maintenance for one year, in high risk recurrent, multifocal low grade and multifocal high grade pTa/pT1, CIS transitional cell carcinoma of bladder.

Methods: From 2003 - 2012, BCG-naive patients treated with intravesical BCG-RIVM for high-risk multifocal NMIBC were identified. Transurethral resection of bladder tumor (TURBT) and re-staging TURBT within six weeks, was done for accurate staging and complete elimination of disease. A six-weekly induction course, started 2-3 weeks after the last TURBT, followed by monthly maintenance protocol for one year. Recurrence, progression, cystectomy free survivals, cancer specific and over-all survival were determined.

Results: Sixty evaluable patients - median age 63, median follow-up 3.98 years. Forty-two patients (70%) completed BCG-RIVM treatment as planned. BCG termination was necessary in 18 patients (30%). Recurrence occurred in 16 patients (26.7%) at a median follow-up of 24.2 months while progression occurred in five patients (8.3%) at a median follow-up of 33 months. Recurrence-free survival and progression-free survival rates were 73% and 92% respectively. Cystectomy was performed in seven patients (12%) with a cystectomy-free survival of 88%. There were no cancer specific deaths. Two patients died of other causes (3.3%). The overall survival rate was 97%.

Conclusions: Our study is the first to show the clinical efficacy and tolerability of BCG-RIVM strain in the management of high risk NMIBC when given in a schedule of six-weekly induction with monthly maintenance for one year. Our maintenance protocol, achieved equivalent recurrence-free, progression-free, disease specific survival and overall survival to the reported literature and the more intense three-years South West Oncology Group (SWOG) protocol.

Keywords: Bladder cancer, BCG-RIVM, Intravesical, Maintenance

* Correspondence: dr.nbfarah@hotmail.com
[1]From the department of surgery, section of Uro-oncology, King Hussein Cancer Center, Amman, Jordan
Full list of author information is available at the end of the article

Background

Bacille Calmette-Guerin for urothelial carcinoma has been the most successful use of immunotherapy to date and represents the standard of care for urothelial CIS and superficial bladder tumors [1]. Although BCG has been in use for over 35 years, the optimal dose and instillation schedule remains unclear. Nevertheless several meta-analyses showed the overall superiority of intravesical BCG with some form of maintenance therapy over chemotherapy in terms of recurrence-free and progression-free survival rates [2-5]. The two Dutch trials [6,7] that failed to show superiority of RIVM or Tice BCG over mitomycin C, could be explained by a sub-optimal BCG schedule, recruitment of high percentage of low risk patients, the type of BCG strain used or short follow-up. Other trials [8] that showed no advantage of maintenance BCG over induction course alone, may also be related to the BCG maintenance schedule, which may have t been sub-optimal for immunological boosting [9].

One of the major obstacles to a meaningful comparisons between different trials has been the adoption of variable maintenance schedules and BCG doses. Lamm et al. [10] advocated the use of an intense protocol of maintenance that he described as, "the current gold standard", which consisted of intravesical BCG - standard dose - every week for 3 weeks given at 3, 6, 12, 18, 24, 30 and 36 months from initiation of induction therapy; however, only 16% of patients completed the treatment protocol as planned.

When designing a maintenance protocol, two main factors should be considered: efficacy and compliance. Both of these factors depend on: BCG strain, dose volume, duration of treatment, total number and frequency of instillations [11].

Several different BCG strains are currently available for intravesical instillation [3,4,12]. These strains show differences in its phenotype, antigenicity and immune reactivity which may influence their antitumor activity, toxicity and clinical efficacy [13]. Despite BCG strain differences, very few studies were conducted to compare their efficacy, optimal dose and toxicity in the clinical setting.

Although BCG-RIVM is the third most commonly used BCG strain world-wide after Tice and Connaught [14], for unclear reasons, it is one of the less frequently used BCG strains in the reported clinical trials.

Since no clinical assumptions can be made regarding the individual BCG strain, unless efficacy and tolerability is proven in the clinical setting [5], we reviewed our experience in the use of this specific BCG -RIVM strain, with an induction course of one instillation every week for 6 weeks and a single monthly instillation as maintenance for one year, to determine its tolerability and efficacy in preventing recurrence, progression and cancer specific death and to determine the cystectomy-free survival and over-all survival.

Methods

From January 2003 to December 2012 all patients who were treated with intravesical BCG-RIVM therapy at our institution were reviewed. All patients had histologically proven transitional cell carcinoma (TCC) of the urinary bladder pTa/pT1 with or without concomitant carcinoma in situ (CIS) or primary carcinoma in situ (2002 TNM classification of urinary bladder cancer and 2004 WHO grading system). Only two patients had Lymphovascular invasion. According to our institution's clinical practice guidelines, intravesical BCG-RIVM therapy was offered to all patients who were BCG naive, had high grade (TCC) Ta/T1 and CIS and to patients with low grade TCC but who were considered at high risk of recurrence and/or progression (multifocal and recurrent TCC). Complete transurethral resection of the bladder tumor (TURBT) and re-staging TURBT within six weeks prior to starting intravesical BCG therapy was done to all patients (including pT1 and pTa) to eliminate any residual tumor and confirm the stage of the disease. All patients had basic blood tests & computed tomography (CT) scan for chest, abdomen and pelvis and restaging CT scans & bone scan prior to radical cystectomy.

Ethical approval

The study was approved by the King Hussein Cancer Center Institutional Review Board (No. 12 KHCC 70).

Patients consent

Written informed consent to intravesical BCG therapy was obtained from all patients in this study. The consent was obligatory and a standard requirement in accordance with King Hussein Cancer Center Clinical Practice Guidelines.

BCG protocol and treatment schedule

Intravesical BCG therapy was started 2 - 3 weeks after the restaging TURBT. The BCG strain used was: Seed RIVM (derived from seed 1173 -P2, 2 x 10 [8] -3 x 10 [9] viable units). Marketing authorization Holder and Manufacturer: Medac, Gesellschaft fur, klinischeSpezialpraparatembH, FehlandtstraBe 3, D-20354 Hamburg, Germany. BCG-RIVM strain was the only strain available at our institution. The choice was made on the basis of a competitive price, the commitment by the manufacturing company to ensure a steady supply of the medicine and on the presumption (at the time) that all commercially available BCG strains were equally effective.

The BCG-medac powder was re-suspended with 50 ml of 0.9% normal and introduced into the bladder via a 12 French urethral catheter.

Patients were instructed to hold on the medicine in the bladder for two hours and to lie on their back, right side, left side and face-down for 30 minutes each before voiding. They were also instructed to refrain from oral fluid intake four hours prior to and two hours after each treatment session. Induction course consisted of one instillations every week for 6 consecutive weeks, while maintenance course consisted of one instillations every month for one year in patients with no evidence of disease after the re-staging TURBT. Full BCG dose was used for both induction and maintenance therapy.

Cystoscopy schedule

Cystoscopy +/- TURBT was done every three monthly for the first two years, then every six monthly for the next two years, then annually thereafter. If recurrence occurs then the clock for cystoscopy is re-set at every three months.

Definitions of BCG responses

BCG resistance: defined as persistent disease at three months following induction course. *BCG refractory*: failure to achieve disease-free state at six months because of persistent or rapidly recurring disease. *BCG relapse*: recurrence of disease *after* six months of disease-free state. *BCG intolerance*: when patient discontinue treatment because of severe lower urinary tract side effects; (If this occurs during the induction course then it would not be considered BCG failure as treatment was not actually given). *BCG failure*: persistence of high grade disease at six months (or at three months if the initial tumor was pT1G3), any worsening of disease parameters (higher grade, stage, number of recurrences or appearance of CIS) or detection of pT2 disease during follow-up [15].

Progression was defined in this study as any worsening of disease parameters including change of pTa low grade to high grade or to pT1 or detection of pT2 disease during follow-up.

Salvage therapy

Cystectomy was offered to patients who progressed, developed worsening disease parameters, were BCG resistant or BCG refractory. However for patients who declined cystectomy, intravesical therapy with MMC was offered. MMC treatment protocol was 40 mg in 40 ml of 0.9% normal saline one instillation every week for six weeks then one instillation every month for six months and a single instillation after every TURBT.

Statistical method

Patients' characteristics such as age group, gender, histology and others were presented in terms of counts and percentages as shown in the tables and figures of this study. Treatment outcome (recurrence and progression) was compared among the treatment groups using Log rank test. Survival and event-free survival were presented by Kaplan-Meier curves showing their three/five year rates and standard error. Hazard ratios (HR) and their corresponding 95% confidence intervals (CI) were calculated to compare the risk between the different categories of each factor. All analyses were performed using: SAS version 9.1 (SAS Institute Inc, Cary, NC).

Results

Sixty evaluable patients with a median age of 63 years (range 37 - 81; mean 61.7 years) were available. Median follow up was 3.98 years (range 8.28 - 93.6 months, mean 4.1 years). According to histological grade the study population of this cohort, consisted of two groups; **group 1:** 37 patients (61.7%) of **'high risk' low grade**, recurrent and multifocal TCC and **group 2:** 23 patients (38.3%) of **high grade** multifocal TCC. In 55 out of 60 patients (92%) the tumors were papillary, while primary CIS or concomitant CIS and papillary were present in 5 out of 60 (8%). A great emphasis in this study was placed on complete elimination of disease by re-staging TURBT prior to start of intravesical BCG therapy, close endoscopic surveillance and early counseling for radical cystectomy at the earliest sign of BCG failure.

Forty two out of 60 patients (70%) completed the intravesical BCG treatment protocol as planned, while BCG termination was necessary in 18 out of 60 patients (30%). The mean, median and minimum number of BCG instillations were 15.7, 18 and 3 respectively. In 16 patients, the terminations were related to sever lower urinary tract symptoms. BCG intolerance occurred in 11 of 18 patients (61.1%); BCG refractory state occurred in 3 of 18 patients (16.7%) and BCG resistance and sepsis in 2 of 18 patients each (11.1%). Complete demographic data are presented in (Table 1). The two patients who developed BCG sepsis, defined as: systemic BCG infection with persistent high grade fever and positive blood cultures for BCG; they required anti-tubercular therapy and further intravesical BCG was discontinued.

Forty four out of 60 patients (73.3%) remained free of recurrence during the entire follow up period while 16 out of 60 patients (26.7%) had recurrences at different time; five patients in the first year, 10 patients at 1 - 5 years and only one patient had a recurrence after five years. Median time to recurrence was 24.2 months (range 3.12 - 78). Recurrences occurred with equal frequency in the low grade and high grade groups, at 27% (10 of 37 patients) and 26% (6 of 23 patients) respectively (Figure 1). For low grade group, the recurrence-free survival rates at three and five years were 74% and 69% respectively, while the values for the high grade group were 69.9% for both periods. There was no statistical difference between the two groups ($p = 0.88$). When all grades where combined the three and five year recurrence-free survival rates were **72.5%** (95% CI: 57.67 - 82.98, SE: +/- 6.4) and **68.9%** (95% CI: 52.9 - 80.5, SE: +/- 7.05) respectively. Analysis of Kaplan-Meier curves for the recurrence-free survival of

Table 1 Demographic data of study patients

Total number of patients = 60				N (Percent %)
Gender	Female			10(16.7%)
	Male			50(83.3%)
Smoking	Ex-smoker			33(55.0%)
	Non-smoker			9(15.0%)
	Smoker			18(30.0%)
No. of tumors	2-7			57(95.0%)
	>8			3(5.0%)
Stage	Primary CIS			2(3.3%)
	T1			24(40.0%)
	Ta			34(56.7%)
Grade	High grade			23(38.3%)
	Low grade			37(61.7%)
Histology	Papillary			55(91.7%)
	Concomitant CIS and papillary			3(5.0%)
	Primary CIS			2(3.3%)
BCG	BCG Complete			42(70%)
	BCG Termination			18(30%)
	BCG Termination reasons	BCG Refractory		3(16.7%)
		BCG intolerance		11(61.1%)
		BCG resistance		2(11.1%)
		BCG sepis		2(11.1%)
	Median	Maximum	Minimum	Mean
Age (Years)	63	81	37	61.7
Cigarette pack-year	60	150	10	55.4
No. of BCG installation	18	18	3	15.7
Follow up time (Years)	3.98	7.8	8.28 months	4.1

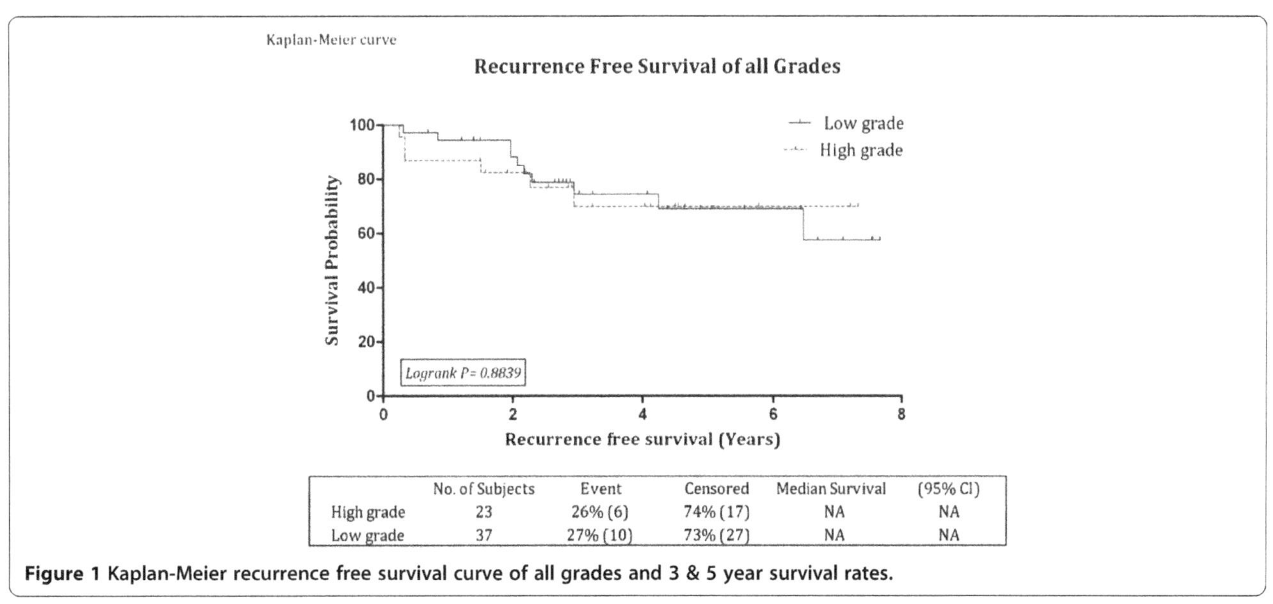

	No. of Subjects	Event	Censored	Median Survival	(95% CI)
High grade	23	26% (6)	74% (17)	NA	NA
Low grade	37	27% (10)	73% (27)	NA	NA

Figure 1 Kaplan-Meier recurrence free survival curve of all grades and 3 & 5 year survival rates.

the whole cohort (Figure 2) and for the two study groups separately (Figure 1) showed that most recurrences (in 14 patients) occurred within the first three years, while recurrence occurred in one patient each at the 4th and 6th year.

Progression occurred in five patients (8%) between one and four years after the start of BCG therapy. Median time to progression was 33 months (range 13.9 - 43.2). Three patients progressed from pTa/pT1 low grade to pT1G3 and only two patients progressed from T1G3 to pT2 disease; interestingly, both of these patients had Lymphovascular invasion at their initial histology. For the low grade group, the progression-free survival rates at three and five years were 96.9% and 92.4% respectively, while the values for the high grade group, were 88.7% and 78.8% respectively (Figure 3). There was no statistical difference between the two groups (P = 0.19). The three and five years progression-free survival rates for all grades combined were **93.9%** (95% CI: 82.4 - 98, SE: +/- 3.4) and **87.9%** (95% CI: 72.8 - 94.9, SE: +/- 5.2) respectively. Analysis of Kaplan-Meier curves for progression-free survival for both groups combined (Figure 4) and for the two groups separately (Figure 3) showed that all progressions occurred within the first 4 years. Although the five year progression-free survival rate of low grade and high grade groups were 92.4% and 78.8% respectively, with a hazard ratio of 3.07 (Figure 3), it did not reach statistical significance. However the number of progressions were too few for definitive conclusion - two out of 37 patients (5%) in the low grade group and three out of 23 patients (13%) in the high grade group.

During follow up, patients who developed progression, BCG resistance, BCG refractory or BCG relapse were counseled and offered radical cystectomy. In this cohort radical cystectomy and bilateral pelvic lymphadenectomy - standard template - was performed in seven patients (12%), all within the first three years. The mean and median lymph node yield was 16 (range 8 - 29). Lymph nodes were negative in all patients. The final histology of the radical cystectomy specimens were as follows:- 2 patients: pT2 N0, 2 patients: CIS N0, 2 patients: pT0 N0 *(T1 G3 tumors were resected prior to the radical cystectomy)* and one patient: pTa G3 N0. The cystectomy-free survival rate was 88% (Figure 5). All cystectomy patients are currently alive; six patients without evidence of disease but one patient, during follow-up, developed retroperitoneal lymph node metastasis and was treated with systemic chemotherapy. One patient who progressed to pT2 disease (at 30 months of follow up) had radiologic evidence of pulmonary nodules, pelvic and retroperitoneal lymphadenopathy suggestive of metastasis; he was treated with systemic chemotherapy and is still alive at last follow-up with stable disease. Of the 12 patients who had recurrences but declined cystectomy at first sign of BCG resistance or refractory state, six patients were treated with intravesical MMC according to the above described protocol and six patients were kept on surveillance cystoscopy as they refused any form of intravesical therapy. Further recurrences occurred in eight of the 12 patients, of which one patient had radical cystectomy, two patients continued on MMC and five patients were kept on surveillance cystoscopy (Table 2).

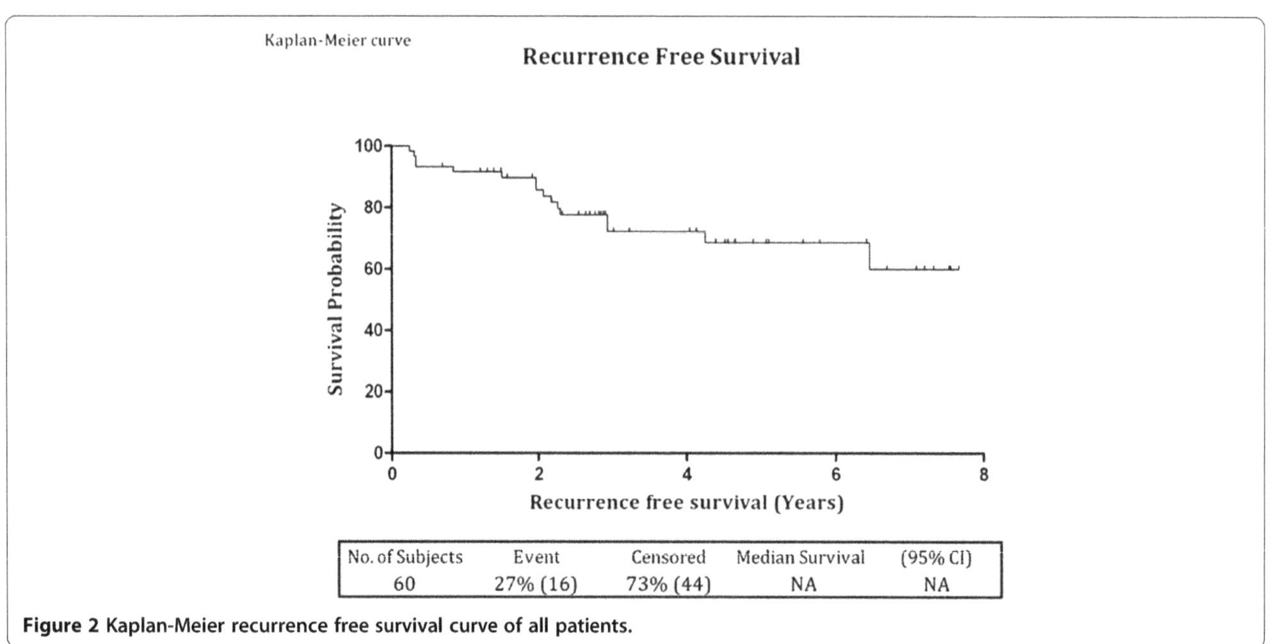

No. of Subjects	Event	Censored	Median Survival	(95% CI)
60	27% (16)	73% (44)	NA	NA

Figure 2 Kaplan-Meier recurrence free survival curve of all patients.

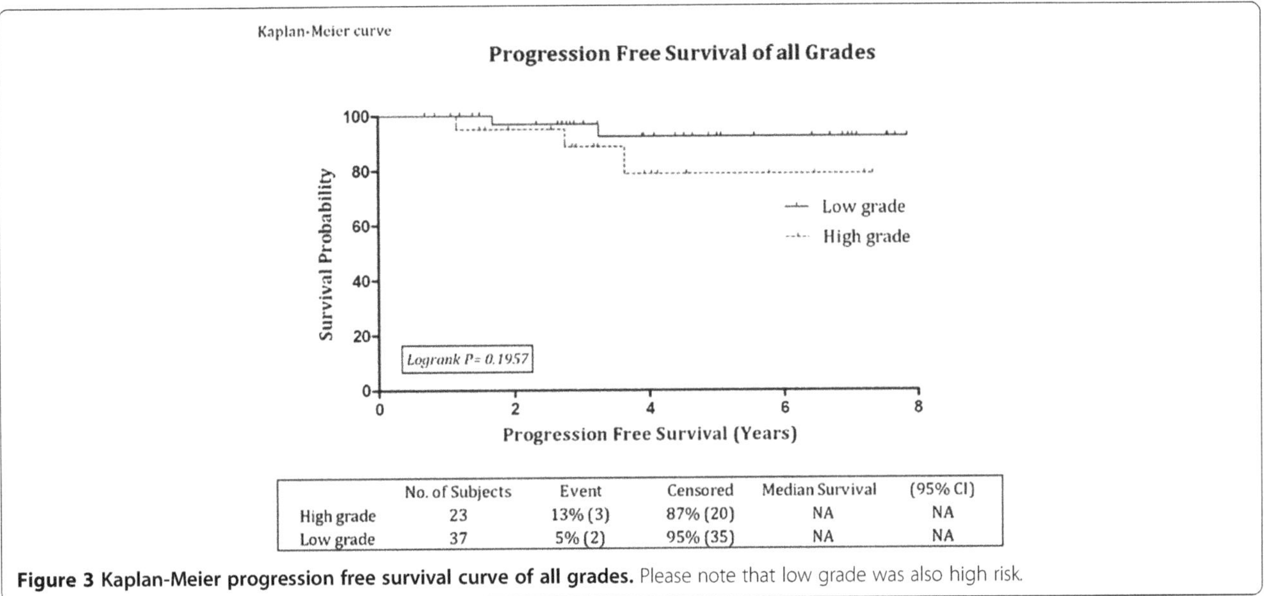

	No. of Subjects	Event	Censored	Median Survival	(95% CI)
High grade	23	13% (3)	87% (20)	NA	NA
Low grade	37	5% (2)	95% (35)	NA	NA

Figure 3 Kaplan-Meier progression free survival curve of all grades. Please note that low grade was also high risk.

There were no cancer specific deaths at a mean follow up of 4.1 years and the overall survival was 97% (Figure 6).

Current status

At last follow up, 58 patients (96.7%) were alive. Two patients died (3.3%), one patient from myocardial infarction while the other patient died from bacterial sepsis secondary to perforated neobladder. The perforation occurred 11 months after the radical cystectomy with no evidence of recurrent disease; both of these deaths occurred around the 4th year of follow up. There were no cancer specific deaths in this cohort (Figure 1). The three and five year overall survival rates were estimated at **100%** (95% CI: NA and SE: NA) and **92.7%** (95% CI: 73.7 - 98.2, SE: +/- 4.98) respectively.

Discussion

Several studies have established the superiority of intravesical BCG with maintenance over chemotherapy in intermediate and high-risk NMIBC with regard to long-term tumor recurrence, progression and mortality [9,10,16].

However, Malmstrom et al. [4] reported on an individual data meta-analysis of nine trials with 2820 patients, comparing long-term outcome of intravesical MMC versus BCG in NMIBC. All The trials included in that meta-analysis had some sort of maintenance MMC. The authors

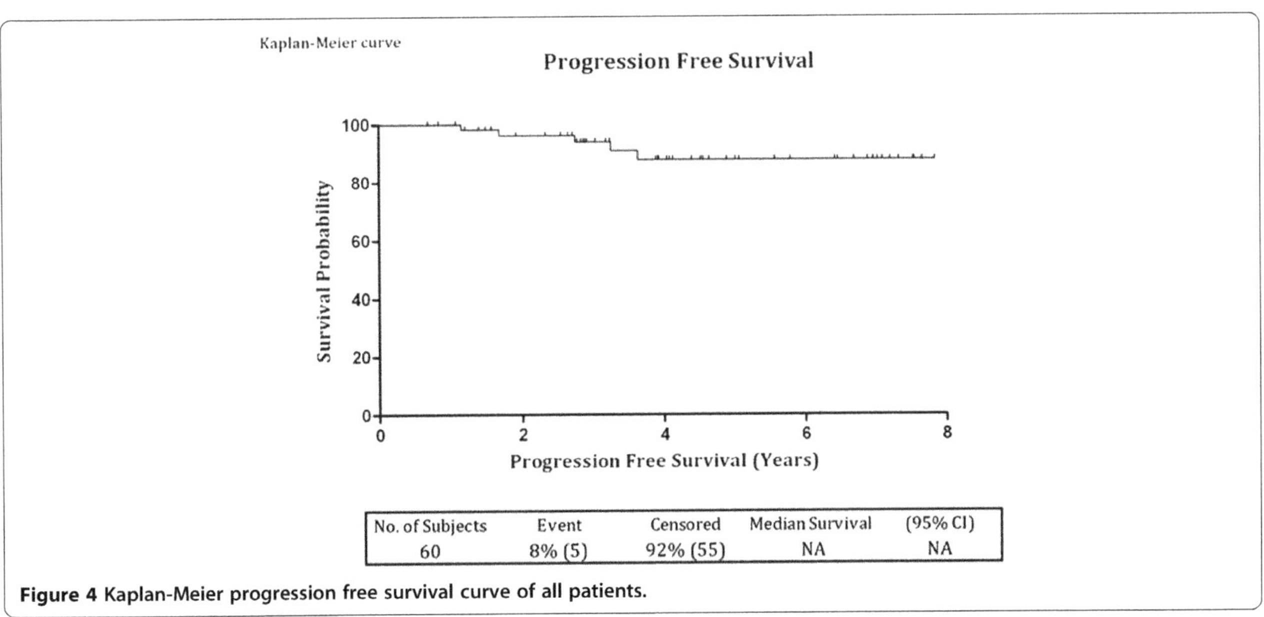

No. of Subjects	Event	Censored	Median Survival	(95% CI)
60	8% (5)	92% (55)	NA	NA

Figure 4 Kaplan-Meier progression free survival curve of all patients.

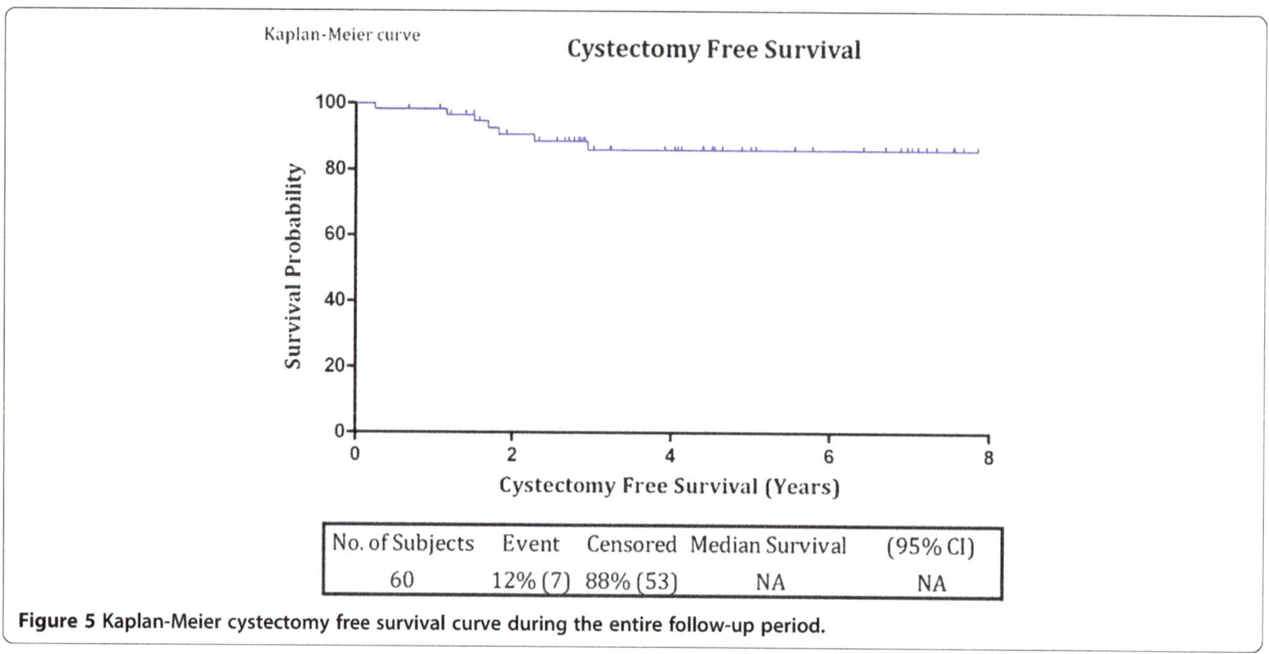

Figure 5 Kaplan-Meier cystectomy free survival curve during the entire follow-up period.

Table 2 Summary of follow-up results

Total number of patients			**60**
Disease recurrence	No		44(73.3%)
	Yes		16(26.7%)
	Histology of recurrence	T1-High grade	4(25.0%)
		Ta-High grade	2(12.5%)
		Ta-Low grade	10(62.5%)
	Salvage therapy	Cystectomy	4(25.0%)
		Mitomycine C	6(37.5%)
		Surveillance cystoscopy & TURBT	6(37.5%)
Further recurrence	No		52(86.7%)
	Yes		8(13.3%)
	Histology further recurrence	T1-Low grade	1(12.5%)
		Ta-Low grade	7(87.5%)
	Further Salvage therapy	Cystectomy	1(12.5%)
		Mitomycine C	2(25%)
		Surveillance cystoscopy & TURBT	5(62.5%)
Disease progression	No		55(91.7%)
	Yes		5(8.3%)
	Histology of progression	T1-High grade	3(60.0%)
		T2	2(40.0%)
	Further Salvage therapy	Cystectomy	2(40.0%)
		Surveillance cystoscopy & TURBT	2(40.0%)
		Systemic chemotherapy	1(20.0%)
Outcome	Alive		58(96.7%)
	Death from other cause (one, myocardial infarction and one, sepsis secondary to perforated neobladder)		2(3.3%)

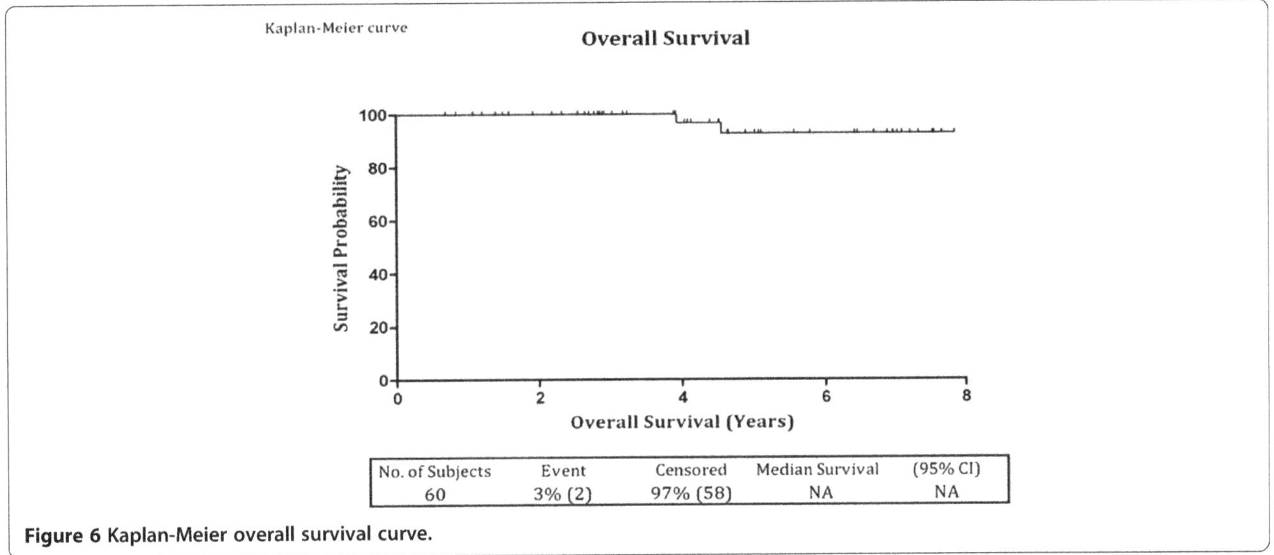

Figure 6 Kaplan-Meier overall survival curve.

found that, for prophylaxis of recurrence, maintenance BCG was needed to be more effective than MMC. Prior intravesical chemotherapy was not a confounder, and did not bias the results in favor of BCG. However there were no statistically significant differences regarding progression, overall survival and cancer specific survival between the two treatments.

Although a majority consensus suggests that BCG with maintenance is superior to MMC in recurrence free survival, the debate is likely to continue, regarding progression and cancer specific survival, unless researchers address in their studies, the type of the BCG strain used among other variables.

The emphasis on the use of BCG with maintenance in the treatment of NMIBC was further highlighted by Saint et al. [2] who reported on a meta-analysis of 24 trials with some form of BCG maintenance involving 1685 patients. They found that, at a mean follow-up of 41 months the average recurrence free survival rate was 70%, the average progression rate was 8% and the disease-free specific survival rate was 91%. Our results are in concordance with the above meta-analyses and others (Table 3). The three and five year recurrence-free survival rates in our study were, 72.5% and 68.9% respectively, and the progression-free survival rates for the same periods were, 93.9% and 87.9% respectively. However, it is important to note that our cohort are *high grade and low grade with 'high risk'* for recurrence and progression because of the recurrent and multifocal nature of the disease (Table 1); thus accounting for a similar biological behavior in terms of recurrence and progression rates for the two treatment groups.

In our study only two patients progressed to muscle invasive disease during the follow-up period. One patient underwent immediate Radical cystectomy, while in the other patient, re-staging studies showed pulmonary nodules and retroperitoneal lymphadenopathy suggestive of metastatic disease and was treated with chemotherapy. Both of these patients had Lymphovascular invasion at the initial histology suggestive of a bad prognosis.

However, Cho et al. [17] reported in their series, the presence of Lymphovascular invasion in 29 out of the 107 patients (27%), but made no reference to this finding in the analysis of the results. In fact European Association of Urology Guidelines makes no reference to Lymphovascular invasion in the management of NMIBC.

Table 3 Results of studies that used different BCG strains and maintenance protocols

Author	No. of patients	Follow-up months (median)	Recurrence %	Progression %	Disease specific survival	BCG strain	Maintenance protocol
Lamm 2000 [9]	192	98	40	24	*83*	Connaught	3 weekly at 3, 6, 12, 18, 24, 30, 36
Peyromaure 2003 [26]	57	53	42	23	88	Pasteur	3 weekly at 3, 6, 12, 18, 24, 30, 36
Pansadoro 2003 [27]	86	91	35	14	94	Pasteur	Every 2 weeks × 6, every month × 6, every 3 months × 6
Yoo 2012 [18]	92	43	35.6	20	85.3	Tice	Monthly for 12 months
Present series	60	47.8	26.7	8.3	100	RIVM	Monthly for 12 months

Yoo et al. [18] reported on 92 patients treated with a monthly maintenance protocol (BCG-Tice strain) for one year, and showed similar median recurrence-free (RSF) and survival rates to that of the SWOG protocol (BCG-Connaught strain) [9]. In the SWOG study, the median RFS was 76.8 months with 83% 5-year survival rate, and for Yoo et al. [18] study the corresponding figures were 87 months and 85.3%. Our study also achieve similar results with a protocol of monthly maintenance (BCG-RIVM) for one year. In our series the overall survival was 97% with no cancer specific deaths and an even lower progression rates (8.2%), compared to SWOG [9]and Yoo series [18] which were (24%) and (20%) respectively. This difference could be related to the different BCG-RIVM strain in our study, racial (Jordanian population) or to our protocol which included a mandatory re-staging TURBT prior to BCG therapy.

Cho et al. [17] compared the efficacy of BCG-RIVM and MMC in 107 Korean patients with pT1G3 bladder cancer. The BCG arm consisted of 53 patients, of which 26 were treated with only 6-weekly induction course, and 27 patients treated with similar induction course plus three once-weekly maintenance at 3, 6, 12 and 18 months; while The MMC arm consisted of 54 patients, of which 29 were treated only with (30 mg) weekly instillations for 6 weeks, and 25 patients with similar 6-weekly instillations plus monthly instillation for one year. The authors then combined the data of both groups in each treatment arm for analysis. They found that the 2-year recurrence-free rate for BCG and MMC to be 45.7% and 52.1% respectively, while progression occurred in 9.4% and 7.4% of patients respectively. The authors concluded that there was no statistically significant difference between the two treatment arms in terms of recurrence and progression rates. The authors did not report the compliance rate in the BCG maintenance group. In our view, the results should be interpreted with caution, since half of the patients in each of the treatment arms were treated with induction courses only, which is now considered sub-optimal therapy [19] and would have undoubtedly, diluted the results. A more meaningful analysis would have been, a comparison between the two maintenance groups.

The fact that, so many treatment protocols existed in just as many trials confirms that the ideal protocol is still unknown. The mechanism of action of intravesical BCG is incompletely characterized. However BCG-induced anti-tumor activity, depends on both, local and systemic immunological responses [20]. After initiating intravesical BCG instillation, immune stimulation generally peaks at 6 weeks. However with subsequent instillations (as in maintenance therapy) the immune stimulation peaks at 3 weeks, and is suppressed at weeks 4, 5, and 6 [9,11]. This would explain the negative results of maintenance protocols that used repeated six-weekly instillations. However, whether the ideal 'immune stimulation schedule' is, every month, every 3 months or otherwise, remains to be determined for the individual patient and for the specific BCG strain in the clinical setting. Thus, the 'gold standard' for BCG maintenance schedule is yet to be determined.

BCG intolerance and the development of complications are important factors in further determining the ideal maintenance protocol. BCG tolerance appears to be relate to dose, BCG strain, frequency and total number of instillations. Badalament et al. [21] reported a 36% compliance - Pasteur strain - on a schedule of one instillation every month for 24 months, and in Palou et al. series [22] this value was 33.8% (Connaught strain) on a schedule of 6 instillation every 6 months for 2 years. However, in Akaza et al. series [8] the compliance was 65.5% using 1/2 dose of BCG Tokio strain at one instillation every month for 1 year.

In our study, 70% of patients completed the 'once monthly maintenance' protocol while in Yoo et al. [18] study (BCG Tice strain) using a similar protocol, 100% of patients completed the treatment as planned. Cho et al. [17] al also reported a 100% patient's compliance using BCG-RIVM, on a maintenance protocol based on SWOG recommendation but for only 18 months. Clearly, such variable results, reported from different geographical locations may also have a racial explanation among others.

To improve BCG tolerance without compromising efficacy, not only frequency and number of instillations, but also dose reduction was considered. Saint et al. [2] analyzed the impact of reduced BCG dose (1/3 - 1/2 dose) in 10 trials, seven of which had some form of maintenance therapy, and found that, at a mean follow-up of 40 months, the average recurrence-free survival rate was 62%, the average progression rate was 11% and disease-free specific survival rate was 90%. The authors concluded that low dose and full schedules, when maintenance therapy is used, gave similar results for recurrence and progression. The meta-analysis further confirmed that maintenance therapy was better than first induction courses as regards recurrences and better than first and second induction courses as regards progression. On the other hand, low dose schedule in first or second induction courses should be considered carefully as there were reports of 25% progression in high risk tumors, suggesting that high-risk tumors and CIS would not benefit from dose reduction [2].

Our study is the first in which this specific BCG RIVM strain was used in the form of induction with monthly maintenance protocol for one year in patients with high grade and high risk low grade NMIBC. The treatment protocol was well tolerated. However, two patients developed BCG sepsis requiring discontinuation of therapy and initiation of antituberculous treatment. The majority of complications which were encountered in our study were the less serious lower urinary tract symptoms. BCG-

RIVM was reported to have the least number of complications compared with other BCG strain (A. Frappier, Tice, Connaught and Pasteur) (10). However, Strock et al. [23] reported a 1.8% (of 858 patients), unusual solitary BCG ulceration (10 mm), exclusively in males, and seen more frequently with BCG-RIVM than Tice. We have not encountered this complication.

In our study, close surveillance, re-staging TURBT and early counseling with view to radical cystectomy for BCG failures were important tools in preventing cancer specific deaths. This is evident by the finding of pT2 in only two of seven patients and negative lymph nodes on the final histology of all cystectomy patients. Some would argue that this is an over treatment, however, evidence suggests that patients who recurred within a year of initial BCG therapy did significantly worse, with disease-free rates of 34-43% at 24 months, indicating that additional immunotherapy may not be appropriate [24]. In a more recent study, a decrease in survival was reported in patients cystectomised for pT1 disease [25] suggesting that it could be related to the more common use of intravesical therapy, thus, delaying radical surgery.

In our study five of the seven cystectomies were done within the first two year (Figure 2). Radical cystectomy was done in 12% of our patients. Our result is in concordance with that published in the literature which ranged from 9% - 26% [10,26,27].

BCG-RIVM strain was introduced into clinical practice in 1986 after its proven safety and efficacy in an animal study [28]. Over the ensuing 10 years or so, several studies were reported most notably by the Dutch South-East Cooperative Urological group and to a lesser extent by the European Organization for Research and Treatment on Cancer- Genitourinary Group (EORTC), using BCG - RIVM strain as induction courses only. However, this specific BCG strain was less frequently used in subsequently published trials compared to other BCG strains

Our interest in this specific BCG-RIVM strain stems from the fact that it is the main BCG strain used in our country (Jordan) for intravesical therapy of NMIBC. Thus, determination of its efficacy and tolerability in the clinical setting with a schedule of 'induction with maintenance' was mandatory, since such data is lacking in the literature.

Clinical evidence suggests that certain BCG strains are more effective than others [6]. Research on two bladder cancer cell lines using BCG strain S4-Jena and BCG-Tice to assess their efficacy on cancer cell lines proliferation and apoptosis showed that T24 cells were responders for S4-Jena and Tice BCG, while Cal29 cells were responders for S4-Jena only. The authors concluded that S4-Jena strain may represent an effective therapeutic agent for NMIBC [29].

A clinical study comparing BCG Tice and Connaught in Switzerland [16], showed more than two-fold more common recurrences in patients treated with BCG Tice than Connaught, prompting the authors to wonder about the worldwide clinical impact on patients, and economic burden on healthcare systems of different countries. They went on to assess the global distribution of different BCG strains used to treat bladder cancer. They obtained information from 55% (140/252) of all countries (72% of global population and 98% of industrialized countries) and showed that BCG Tice and BCG Connaught were the most commonly used BCG strains worldwide (each used in 54 countries), followed by BCG RIVM (in 28 countries), Pasteur (in 17 counties), Danish (in 6 countries), China and Tokyo (in one country each). The authors concluded that based on the observed difference in tumor recurrence for the widely use BCG Tice and Connaught in NMIBC, a large proportion of patients are at risk of an inferior treatment.

Clearly, no presumptions can be made regarding the clinical efficacy and safety of an individual BCG strain unless proven by an induction and maintenance protocol in the clinical setting.

Conclusions

Our study is the first to show the clinical efficacy and tolerability of BCG-RIVM strain in the management of high risk NMIBC when given in a schedule of induction with monthly instillations as maintenance for one year. Our maintenance protocol, achieved equivalent recurrence-free, progression-free, disease specific survival and overall survival to the more intense three-years SWOG protocol.

Only head to head comparative trials between different BCG strains in the treatment of patients with high risk NMIBC can determine their relative clinical efficacy, toxicity, appropriate dose, and ideal maintenance protocol for the individual BCG strain.

Abbreviations

BCG: Bacillus Calmette-Guerin; CI: Confidence interval; CIS: Carcinoma-in-situ; MMC: Mitomycin C; RFS: Recurrence-free survival; SE: Standard error; SWOG: South West Oncology Group; TCC: Transitional cell carcinoma; TURBT: Transurethral resection of bladder tumor; NMIBC: Non-muscle invasive bladder cancer.

Competing interests

The authors declare that they have no competing interests.

Authors' contributions

NBF: Enrollment of patients, carried out endoscopic procedures and other surgical operations, follow-up of patients and drafted the manuscript. RG: Carried out intravesical BCG instillations, participated in endoscopy procedures and other surgical operations, follow-up of patients, collection of data and participated in the manuscript drafting. MA: Participated in intravesical BCG instillations, collection of data, follow-up of patients and participated in the discussion of the manuscript draft. All authors read and approved the final manuscript.

Acknowledgements

The authors would like to extend their greatest appreciation and thanks to: Miss Dalia Al-Rimawi, Senior Statistical programmer, at King Hussein cancer Center, (e-mail: drimawi@KHCC.JO), for helping in organizing the clinical data and for the detailed statistical analysis.

Author details

[1]From the department of surgery, section of Uro-oncology, King Hussein Cancer Center, Amman, Jordan. [2]Section of Uro-oncology, King Hussein Cancer Center, Amman, Jordan. [3]Department of Surgical oncology, Amman, Jordan.

References

1. Kresowik TP, Griffith TS: **Bacillus Calmette-Guerin immunotherapy for urothelial carcinoma of the bladder.** *Immunotherapy* 2009, **1**(2):281–288.
2. Fabian S, Rodrigo Q, de Medina SGD, Laurent S, Abbou CC, Chopin DK: *Bacille Calmette-Guerin (BCG) for the treatment of superficial bladder cancer. a critical analysis of 25 years' experience with various therapeutic schedules.* www.urofrance.org/fileadmin/medias/sncuf/lettre..../25-ans-bcg.pdf.
3. Han RF, Pan JG: **Can intravesical bacillus Calmette-Guerin reduce recurrence in patients with superficial bladder cancer: a meta-analysis of randomize trials.** *Urology* 2006, **67**(6):1216–1223.
4. Per-Uno M, Per-Uno M, Sylvester RJ, Crawford DE, Martin F, Susanne K, Erkki R, Eduardo S, Di Stasi SM, Alfred Witjes J: **An individual patient data meta-analysis of the long-term out cone of randomized studies comparing intravesical mitomycin C versus bacillus calmette-guerin for non-muscle-invasive bladder cancer.** *Eur Urol* 2009, **56:**247–256.
5. Sylvester RJ, van der Meijden AP, Lamm DL: **Intravesical bacillus Calmette-Guerin reduces the risk of progression in patients with superficial bladder cancer: a meta-analysis of the published results of randomized clinical trials.** *J Urol* 2002, **168:**1964–1970.
6. Vegt PDJ, Alfred Witjes J, Witjes WPJ, Doesburg WH, Debruyne FMJ, van der Meijden APM: **A randomize study of intravesical mitomycin C, bacillus Calmette-Guerin Tice and bacillus Calmette-Guerin RIVM treatment in pTa-pT1 papillary carcinoma and carcinoma in situ of the bladder.** *J Urol* 1995, **153:**929–933.
7. Witjes WP, Witjes JA, Oosterhof GO, Debruyne MJ: **Update on the Dutch cooperative trial: mitomycin versus bacillus Calmette-Guerin- Tice versus bacillus Calmette-Guerin RIVM in the treatment of patients with pTa-pT1 papillary carcinoma and carcinoma in situ of the urinary bladder. Dutch south east cooperative urological group.** *Semin Urol Oncol* 1996, **14**(1 Suppl 1):10–16.
8. Akaza H, Hinotsu S, Aso Y, Kakizoe T, Bladder Cancer BCG, Group S: **Bacillus Calmette-Guerin treatment of existing papillary bladder cancer and carcinoma in situ of the bladder. Four year results.** *Cancer* 1995, **75:**552–559.
9. Lamm DL, Blumenstein BA, Crissman JD, Montie JE, Gottesman JE, Lowe BA, Sarosdy MF, Bohl RD, Barton Grossman H, Beck TM, Liemert JT, David Crawford E: **Maintenance bacillus Calmette-Guerin immunotherapy for recurrent TA, T1 and carcinoma in situ transitional carcinoma of the bladder: a randomized southwest oncology group study.** *J Urol* 2000, **163:**1124–1129.
10. Lamm DL: **Efficacy and safety of bacillus Calmette-Guerin immunotherapy in superficial bladder cancer.** *Clin Infect Dis* 2000, **31**(Supplement 3):S86–S90. 10.1086/314064.
11. Lamm D: **Improving patient outcomes: Optimal BCG treatment regimen to prevent progression in superficial bladder cancer.** *Eur Urol Suppl* 2006, **5:**654_659.
12. Lamm DL: **Preventing progression and improving survival with BCG maintenance.** *Eur Urol* 2000, **37**(suppl 1):9–15.
13. Christine G, Hugh M, Muhammad Shamim K, Lewis DJM: **BCG immunotherapy for bladder cancer- the effect of sub-strain difference.** *Nat Rev Urol* 2013, **10:**580_588. published on line 17 September 2013; doi:10.1038/nrurol.2013.194.
14. Gsponer JR, Bornand D, Bachmann A, Albert ML, Thalmann GN, Rentsch CA: **Intravesical treatment of non-muscle invasive bladder cancer: global distribution of BCG strains and potential health economic impact of strain differences - Switzerland as an example.** *Freitag* 2012:13:00–13:05.
15. Herr HW, Dalbagni G: **Defining bacillus Calmette-Guerin refractory superficial bladder tumors.** *J Urol* 2003, **169:**1706–1708. Pub-Med.
16. Herr HW: **Transurethral resection and intravesical therapy of superficial bladder tumors.** In *The Urology Clinics of North America*, Volume 18. Edited by Fair WR. Philadelphia: WB Saunders; 1991:525–8.
17. In-Chang C, Kim EKy, Jae Young J, Ho Kyung S, Jinsoo C, Weo Seo P, Kang Hyun L: **Adjuvant intravesical instillation for primary T1G3 bladder cancer: BCG versus MMC in Korea.** *Anticancer Res* 2012, **32:**1493–1498.
18. Koo Han Y, Tea Joon L, Sung-Goo C: **Monthly intravesical bacillus Calmette-Guerin maintenance therapy for non-muscle-invasive bladder cancer: 10-year experience in a single institute.** *Exp Ther Med* 2012, **3**(2):221–225.
19. Friedrick MG, Pichlmeier U, Schwaibold H, Conrad S, Huland H: **Long-term intravesical adjuvant chemotherapy further reduces recurrence rate compare with short-term intravesical chemotherapy and short-term therapy with bacillus Calmette-Guerin (BCG) in patients with non-muscle-invasive bladder carcinoma.** *Eur Urol* 2007, **52:**1123–1130.
20. Askeland EJ, Newton MR, O'Donnell MA, Yi L: **Bladder cancer immunotherapy: BCG and beyond.** *Adv Urol* 2012, **2012:**181987.
21. Badalament RA, Herr HW, Wong GY, Gnecco C, Pinsky CM, Whitmore WF, Fair WR, Oettgen HF: **A prospective randomized trial of maintenance versus nonmaintenance intravesical bacillus Calmette-Guerin therapy of superficial bladder cancer.** *J Clin Onco* 1987, **5:**441–449.
22. Palou J, Laguna P, Millan-Rodriguez F, Hall RR, Salvador-Bayarri J, Vincente-Rodriguez J: **Control group and maintenance treatment with bacillus Calmette-Guerin for carcinoma in situ and/or high grade bladder tumors.** *J Urol* 2001, **165**(5):1488–1491.
23. Strock V, Dotevall L, Sandberg T, Gustafsson CK, Holmang S: **Late bacille Calmette-Guerin infection with a large focal urinary bladder ulceration as a complication of bladder cancer treatment.** *BJU Int* 2011, **107**(10):1592–1597.
24. Gallagher BL, Joudi FN, Maymi JL, O'Donnell MA: **Ipact of previous bacille Calmette-Guerin failure pattern in subsequent response to bacille Calmette-Guerin plus interferon intravesical therapy.** *Urology* 2008, **71**(2):297–301.
25. Lambert EH, Pierorazio PM, Olsson CA, Benson MC, MckKiernan JM, Poon S: **The increase use of intravesical therapies for stag T1 bladder cancer coincides with decreasing survival after cystectomy.** *BJU Int* 2007, **100:**336.
26. Michael P, Florent G, Delphine A-O, Djillali S, Bernard D, Marc Z: **Intravesical bacillus Calmette-Guerin therapy for stage T1 grade 3 transitional cell carcinoma of the urinary bladder: recurence, progression and survival in a study of 57 patients.** *J Urol* 2003, **169:**2110–2212.
27. Pansadoro V, Emiliozzi P, Depaula F, Scarpone P, Pizzo M, Federico G, Martini M, Pansadoro A, Stenberg CN: **High grade superficial (G3t1) transitional cell carcinoma of the bladder treated with bacillus Calmette-Guerin (BCG).** *J Exp Clin Cancer Res* 2003, **22**(4 Suppl):223–227.
28. Mejiden APMvd, Steerenberg PA, de Jong WH, Bogman MJJ, Feitz WFJ, Hendriks BT, Debruyne FMJ, Ruitenberg EJ: **The effect of intravesical and intra-dermal application of a new BCG on dog bladder.** *Urol Res* 1986, **14**(4):207–210.
29. Katja S, Martin F, Thomas S, Inge-Marie H, Eberhard S: **BCG strain S4-Jena: an early BCG strain is capable to reduce the proliferation of bladder cancer cells by induction of apoptosis.** *Canc Cell Int* 2010, **10:**21.

Changes in the Q-tip angle in relation to the patient position and bladder filling

Jong-hyun Yun[1], Jae Heon Kim[2], Suyeon Park[3] and Changho Lee[4*]

Abstract

Background: It is hypothesized that patient position, supine or recline, and bladder filling status, empty or full, could change the Q-tip test result. This study evaluated the effect of the patient position and bladder filling status on the Q-tip angle for urethral hypermobility (UH).

Methods: There was a measurement of the Q-tip angle in the supine position and at a 45° angle in a reclining position during bladder emptying; and then the measurements were repeated while filling the bladder. We defined urethral hypermobility as the urethral angle straining or coughing minus that at rest ≥30°.

Results: All 63 female patients (mean age: 61.6 years, range: 36–81) who complained of urinary incontinence were assessed using the Q-tip angle test. The pelvic organ prolapse quantification stages of all patients were ≤ stage 1. The mean Q-tip angle with an empty bladder was 14.1 ± 9.1° in the supine position and 16.4 ± 11.1° in the reclining position ($p = 0.001$). Then mean Q-tip angle during the filling bladder state was 15.4 ± 9.7° in the supine position and 15.9 ± 11.0° in the reclining position ($p = 0.771$). The UH rate during the bladder emptying state was 11.1 % (7/63) in the supine position and 19.1 % (12/63) in the reclining position. The UH rate during the bladder filling state was 15.0 % (9/60) in the supine position and 15.3 % (9/59) in the 45° reclining position. The odds ratio (OR) was 7.03 in the reclining position for a positive Q-tip angle. The positive rate was higher in the 45° reclining position during bladder emptying than that in the other position during bladder filling.

Conclusion: The outcome of the Q-tip angle and the rate of UH changed in relation to patient position. The reclining position during bladder emptying increased the Q-tip angle, thereby resulting in a positive UH.

Keywords: Q-tip test, Stress urinary incontinence, Urethra, Urinary incontinence

Background

Urinary incontinence (UI) is the involuntary loss of urine and occurs when bladder pressure exceeds urethral closing pressure. A specific type of UI is stress urinary incontinence (SUI) is a complaint of involuntary urine leakage on effort or exertion, or on sneezing or coughing [1].

A poorly supported bladder base and urethrovesical junction (UVJ) are the main explanations for SUI; thus, urethral mobility should be assessed in all women with UI [2, 3]. The cotton swab or Q-tip test is a simple outpatient procedure used to quantify urethral mobility [4]. Although the Q-tip test was introduced more than 40 years ago, and is widely used in clinical practice, there is limited literature on its use. Furthermore, only a few studies have evaluated the Q-tip examination based on patient position and bladder filling status [5, 6].

We hypothesized that patient position (supine or recline), and bladder filling status (empty or full), would change the Q-tip test result, as patient position affects bladder pressure, and bladder filling status can change the shape of the bladder base. To verify our hypothesis, we evaluated the effects of patient position and bladder filling status of Q-tip test results for urethral hypermobility (UH).

Methods

We reviewed the medical records of women who presented to one urologist (CL) with urinary incontinence between February 2010 and March 2014. The clinical diagnosis was established based on history taking, in

* Correspondence: leech@sch.ac.kr
[4]Department of Urology, Soonchunhyang University Cheonan Hospital, Soonchunhyang University School of Medicine, 31 Soonchunhyang 6 gil, Dongnam-Gu, Cheonan, Chungcheongnam-do 330-721, South Korea
Full list of author information is available at the end of the article

particular, the chief complaints of patients. All patients underwent a pelvic examination, including a pelvic organ prolapse quantification (POP-Q) measurement and a Q-tip test performed by the same urologist (CL) in the dorsal lithotomy position. The urologist first performed the POP-Q test in the supine dorsal lithotomy position and then performed a Q-tip test. The Q-tip test was performed four times in each patient under different conditions. A sterile rubber Nelaton catheter was inserted into the bladder for emptying. Then, a sterile lubricated cotton swab (Q-tip) was introduced through the urethra into the bladder, and then withdrawn carefully until a resistance could be felt. This was considered the anatomical location of UVJ, with the length of inserted Q-tip is between 3.5 and 4.5 cm from the urethral meatus in all evaluated patients. The resting angle from the horizontal was set to 0° on a goniometer. The patient was asked to strain or cough while the maximum straining angle was measured and recorded as the Q-tip angle. This UVJ angle measurement was done in the supine position and is deemed the first measured Q-tip value. For the second Q-tip measurement value, the patient was moved to a reclining position (approximately 45°) by setting the backrest up on the examination table, and the same Q-tip measurement was repeated. Another sterile rubber Nelaton catheter was inserted, and normal saline was slowly infused using a Toomey syringe until the patient expressed a desire to void. The mean infused volume is 209.7 ± 59.4 mL (range: 50–400) and there is no significant difference of bladder filling volume between 31 MUI and 3 UUI patients versus 27 SUI patients (mean bladder filling volume 209.4 ± 68.4 vs. 210.0 ± 47.2, $p = 0.22$). The third and fourth Q-tip values for the Q-tip angle was again a measurement in the supine and reclining position. The incontinence provocation test was performed at the end of physical examination, a stress test using coughing. A positive result is indicated by efflux of the bladder solution from the meatus coinciding with the cough.

We reviewed the four Q-tip values and provocation test results on the medical records. There was an exclusion of the Q-tip angle data for patients with prolapsed pelvic organs, those over stage 1 according to the POP-Q criteria, and patients who had undergone surgery to correct incontinence. Urethral hypermobility was defined as the urethral angle straining or coughing minus that at rest ≥30°.

The statistical analysis was performed using SPSS ver. 18.0 software (SPSS Inc., Chicago, IL, USA). The paired *t*-test was used to evaluate the Q-tip angles associated with the patients' positions, and those associated with bladder filling status. The generalized linear mixed model was used to calculate the odds ratio and confidence interval. A p-value <0.05 was considered significant.

Ethics statement

This study protocol was approved by the Soonchunhyang University institutional review board of the human research and ethics committee (No. 1040875-201501-BM-002). They waived the requirement for the investigator to obtain a signed consent form.

Results

Patients

We reviewed all 75 medical records of women with urinary incontinence. Among them, we excluded the following: 4 records with pelvic organ prolapsed greater than stage 1; 2 records of previous anti-incontinence surgery; 3 records of performing evaluation two times at different visits; and 3 records of a negative Q-tip value. A total of 63 patients complaining of UI were assessed. Among them, 32 (50.8 %) had mixed urinary incontinence (MUI), 27 (42.9 %) had stress urinary incontinence (SUI), and four (6.3 %) had urgency urinary incontinence (UUI).

Among the 63 patients, 58 had provocation test results; 55.2 % (32/58) had positive provocation test results. The patients with positive provocation test results had more hypermobile urethra than the patients with negative provocation test results (Table 1). Of the 63 patients with UI, 25 (39.7 %) received a mid-urethral sling (MUS) to manage SUI. Among the 25 patients with MUS, 24 had the following Valsalva leak point pressure (VLPP) data; 33.3 % (8/24) had VLPP ≤60 cm H_2O, 41.7 % (10/24) had VLPP of 60–89 cm H_2O, and 25.0 % (6/24) had VLPP ≥90 cm H_2O. The patients with low VLPP had a tendency of more mobile urethra (Table 1).

Q-tip angle change in relation to position

We analyzed the Q-tip angle change in the 63 patients complaining of UI. The mean Q-tip angle during the bladder emptying state was 14.1 ± 9.1° in the supine position and 16.4 ± 11.1° in the reclining position ($p = 0.001$). The mean Q-tip angle during the bladder filling state was 15.4 ± 9.7° in the supine position, and 15.9 ± 11.0° in the reclining position ($p = 0.771$) (Table 2).

The proportion of patients identified with UH during the bladder emptying state (Q-tip angle ≥30°) was 11.1 % (7/63) in the supine position and 19.1 % (12/63) in the reclining position. The proportion of patients with UH during the bladder filling state was 15.0 % (9/60) in the supine position and 15.3 % (9/59) in the reclining position. The reclining position had an odds ratio of 7.03 for a positive Q-tip angle (Table 2 and Fig. 1).

Table 1 Basic characteristics of the patients ($n = 63$)

All patients ($n = 63$)			
	Age (range), years	61.6 ± 11.1 (36–81)	
	Clinical Diagnosis, n		
	Mixed urinary incontinence	32/63 (50.8 %)	
	Stress urinary incontinence	27/63 (42.9 %)	
	Urgency urinary incontinence	4/63 (6.3 %)	
			Hypermobile Urethra (Q tip ≥30)
	Provocation test positive, n	32/58 (55.2 %)	8/32 (25.0 %)
	Provocation test negative, n	26/58 (44.8 %)	3/26 (11.5 %)
MUS patients ($n = 25$)			
	Age (range), years	61.6 ± 11.0 (46–81)	
	Clinical Diagnosis, n		
	Mixed urinary incontinence	12/25 (48.0 %)	
	Stress urinary incontinence	13/25 (52.0 %)	
	BMI (kg/m^2)	25.6 ± 2.9	
	Post-hysterectomy status	3/25 (12.0 %)	
	Smoking	0/25 (0.0 %)	
			Hypermobile Urethra (Q tip ≥30)
	VLPP ≤60	8/24 (33.3 %)	50.0 % (4/8)
	VLPP 61–89	10/24 (41.7 %)	40.0 % (4/10)
	VLPP ≥90	6/24 (25.0 %)	16.7 % (1/6)

Q-tip angle change in relation to bladder filling state

The mean Q-tip angle was 14.1 ± 9.1° in the supine position during the bladder emptying state and 15.4 ± 9.7° during the bladder filling state ($p = 0.049$). The mean Q-tip angle was 16.4 ± 11.1° in the reclining position during the bladder emptying state and 15.9 ± 11.0° during the bladder filling state ($p = 0.361$) (Table 3).

The proportion of patients defined as UH during the bladder emptying state in the supine position (Q-tip angle ≥30°) was 11.1 % (7/63) and was 15.0 % (9/60) during the bladder filling state. The proportion of patients identified with UH in the reclining position was 19.1 % (12/63) during the bladder emptying state and 14.3 % (9/63) during the bladder filling state. The bladder filling status had an odds ratio of 1.45 for a positive Q-tip angle (Table 3 and Fig. 2).

Discussion

The Q-tip test was developed to measure the degree of urethral relaxation and mobility during increased intra-abdominal pressure [4, 7, 8]. When a physician performs the Q-tip test, patients are usually positioned in the supine lithotomy position, then the Q-tip is inserted into the bladder through the urethra, and the angle that the Q-tip moves from horizontal to its final position during straining is measured [5, 8]. The UH was initially defined as a Q-tip angle ≥ 20° from the horizontal position [4]. However, a Q-tip angle ≥30° appears to be widely accepted by urologists and urogynecologists [3, 9].

The Q-tip angle measures the degree of urethral mobility presented by increased intra-abdominal pressure. Abdominal pressure is approximately two times higher with the patient in the seated position than that when the patient is in the supine position [10]. Because the patient

Table 2 Comparison of mean Q-tip angles and urethral hypermobility (UH) rates in relation to patient position

	Position	Average Q-tip	*p*-value†	Q-tip ≥30°	Odds ratio	95 % CI (Confidence interval)	*p*-value††
Empty	Supine	14.1 ± 9.1	0.001	11.1 % (7/63)	7.03[a]	1.01–48.94	0.05
	Reclining	16.4 ± 11.1		19.1 % (12/63)			
Filling	Supine	15.4 ± 9.7	0.771	15.0 % (9/60)			
	Reclining	15.9 ± 11.0		15.3 % (9/59)			

[a]Reclining position had higher odds of a positive Q-tip angle, *p*-value†; by paired *t*-test, *p*-value††; by generalized linear mixed model

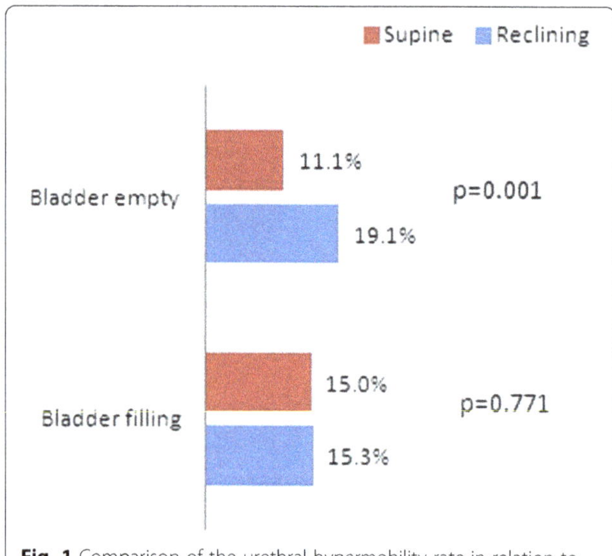

Fig. 1 Comparison of the urethral hypermobility rate in relation to patient position. Positive urethral hypermobility was defined as a Q-tip angle ≥30°

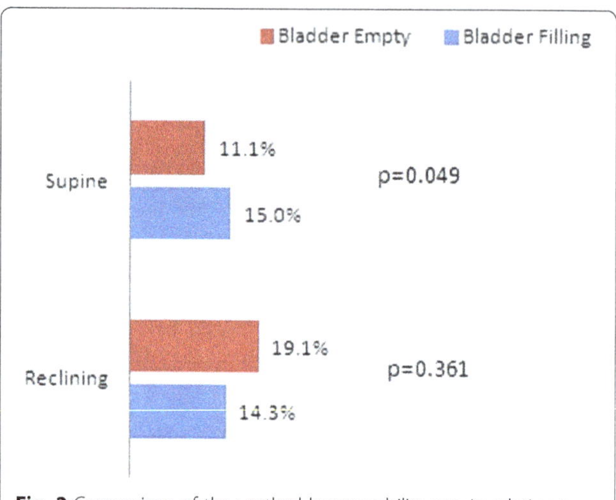

Fig. 2 Comparison of the urethral hypermobility rate in relation to bladder filling status. Positive urethral hypermobility was defined as a Q-tip angle ≥30°

position affects abdominal pressure, we hypothesized that the patient position would also affect the Q-tip angle measurement. In this study, the mean Q-tip angle was 14.1 ± 9.1° in the supine position during the empty bladder state and 16.4 ± 11.1° in the reclining position ($p = 0.001$, Table 2). We calculated the UH rate by using a 30° cut-off value to clarify whether this difference was clinically significant. The UH rate was 11.1 % in the supine position in the bladder emptying state, and 19.1 % in the reclining position. The odds ratio was 7.03 in reclining position (Table 2 and Fig. 1). Therefore, we concluded that the patient position (supine or reclining) significantly affected the change in Q-tip angle. The female urethra is more mobile in the reclining position than in the supine position because of elevated abdominal pressure in the reclining position.

The patient's bladder filling status is usually not considered when physicians measure the Q-tip angle and no reliable recommendations are available on bladder filling status while measuring the Q-tip angle [3–5, 7–9]. We hypothesized that the bladder filling status would affect the Q-tip angle measurement because it changes the shape of bladder base. Only one report has analyzed Q-tip angle measurements in patients with a symptomatically full bladder [5]. They reported no difference in either resting or straining Q-tip angle measurements when patients were tested with <150 mL of urine in their bladder as compared with patients with a symptomatically full bladder. We emptied the patient's bladder completely using a Nelaton catheter and measured the Q-tip angle in the supine and reclining positions. Then, we filled the patient's bladder until they expressed a desire to urinate, and measured the Q-tip angle again in the supine and reclining positions. The odds ratio was 1.45 for the filled bladder and there is no significant difference in the Q-tip angles between empty and full bladders (Table 3 and Fig. 2). Although these findings are supported by previous studies, the reasons are not well understood as to why bladder filling status does not affect the Q-tip angle. Moreover, although we found that the reclining position increased the Q-tip angle, this effect dissipated when we measured the Q-tip angle during the bladder filling state. We anticipated that some patients would not have an active response to straining or coughing because of worry or shyness about leaking. We believe that this may be a habitual coping method by some incontinent patients, which may explain why some patients did not show consistent Q-tip angle measurements during the bladder filling state.

Yet, an important question is: which position and bladder filling condition should be recommended for detecting

Table 3 Comparison of mean Q-tip angles and urethral hypermobility (UH) rates in relation to bladder filling status

	Position	Average Q-tip	p-value†	Q-tip ≥ 30°	Odds Ratio	95 % CI (Confidence Interval)	p-value††
Supine	Empty	14.1 ± 9.1	0.049	11.1 % (7/63)	1.45[a]	0.25–8.36	0.67
	Filling	15.4 ± 9.7		15.0 % (9/60)			
Reclining	Empty	16.4 ± 11.1	0.361	19.1 % (12/63)			
	Filling	15.9 ± 11.0		14.3 % (9/63)			

[a]Bladder filling status had higher odds of a positive Q-tip angle, *p*-value†; by paired *t*-test, *p*-value††; by generalized linear mixed model

urethral hypermobility? A good physical examination is a reflection of a patient's complaints or condition. Most incontinence events in patients with SUI occur in the standing position. Thus, the standing position might be the best position for the Q-tip test. However, previous study showed that the urethra is more mobile in the supine position than that in the standing position, and the sitting position results in a more mobile urethra than that of the supine position [6, 11]. Our current results also demonstrate that the reclining produces a more mobile urethra than that of the supine position (Table 2 and Fig. 1). A more mobile urethra has decreased Valsalva leak point pressure and is associated with the success rate of the tension-free vaginal tape procedure [12, 13]. These observations indicate that UH is an explanation for SUI but not for the female SUI mechanism.

Our study has some limitations, of which the first is its retrospective nature, which did not ensure complete data collection for all patients. Among enrolled 63 patients, we could not obtain important variables, such as body mass index (BMI), parity, and the post-hysterectomy status, except for 25 patients who had undergone an MUS. Moreover, this current study did not answer important question as to which measurement correlated with a better surgical outcome. However, the study population in this study of having an MUS is too small to answer that important question. Thus that question will have to be answered by further research.

In summary, we do not know which position more closely reflects urethral mobility in patients with SUI. The reclining position guaranteed the most mobile urethra, whereas the supine position provided a more mobile urethra than that of the standing position. We recommend an empty bladder or urine volume less than the volume when voiding is desired. According to a previous report and our result, the bladder filling status does not affect UH [5]. However, an empty bladder or a bladder with a small volume of urine was more comfortable for the examinees.

Conclusion

The outcome of Q-tip angle measurement and the rate of UH appeared to increase when patients were examined in the reclining position. However, this difference dissipated when the Q-tip angle was measured during the bladder filling state. The largest difference in Q-tip angle, indicating a positive UH, was observed in patients in the reclining position during the bladder emptying state.

Abbreviations

UH: Urethral hypermobility; UI: Urinary incontinence; SUI: Stress urinary incontinence; UVJ: Urethrovesical junction; POP-Q: Pelvic organ prolapsed quantification; MUI: Mixed urinary incontinence; UUI: Urgency urinary incontinence; MUS: Mid-urethral sling; VLPP: Valsalva leak point pressure.

Competing interests

The authors declare that they have no competing interests.

Authors' contributions

JY participated in the study design, coordination, and data analysis, performed statistical analysis of the data, prepared figures and description of figures, and helped to draft the manuscript. JHK participated in the study design, and data interpretation, and critically revised the manuscript for important intellectual content. SP participated in data analyses, performed statistical analysis of the data, and provided a statistical description of the manuscript. CL conceptualized and planned the study, provided the clinical data, participated in the study design, coordination, and data interpretation, and wrote and revised the manuscript. All authors read and approved the final manuscript.

Acknowledgements

This study was supported by Soonchunhyang University Research Fund.

Author details

[1]Department of Urology, Soonchunhyang University Gumi Hospital, Soonchunhyang University School of Medicine, Gumi, South Korea. [2]Department of Urology, Soonchunhyang University Hospital, Soonchunhyang University School of Medicine, Seoul, South Korea. [3]Department of Biostatistics, Soonchunhyang University Hospital, Seoul, South Korea. [4]Department of Urology, Soonchunhyang University Cheonan Hospital, Soonchunhyang University School of Medicine, 31 Soonchunhyang 6 gil, Dongnam-Gu, Cheonan, Chungcheongnam-do 330-721, South Korea.

References

1. Abrams P, Cardozo L, Fall M, Griffiths D, Rosier P, Ulmsten U, et al. The standardisation of terminology of lower urinary tract function: report from the Standardisation Sub-committee of the International Continence Society. Neurourol Urodyn. 2002;21(2):167–78.
2. Enhorning GE. A concept of urinary continence. Urol Int. 1976;31(1-2):3–5.
3. Kobashi KC. Evaluation of patients with urinary incontinence and pelvic prolapse. In: WA J, Kavoussi LR, Novick AC, Partin AW, PC A, editors. Campbell-Walsh urology. 10th ed. Philadelphia: Saunders; 2012. p. 1896–908.
4. Crystle CD, Charme LS, Copeland WE. Q-tip test in stress urinary incontinence. Obstet Gynecol. 1971;38(2):313–5.
5. Karram MM, Bhatia NN. The Q-tip test: standardization of the technique and its interpretation in women with urinary incontinence. Obstet Gynecol. 1988;71(6 Pt 1):807–11.
6. Handa VL, Jensen JK, Ostergard DR. The effect of patient position on proximal urethral mobility. Obstet Gynecol. 1995;86(2):273–6.
7. Bergman A, McCarthy TA, Ballard CA, Yanai J. Role of the Q-tip test in evaluating stress urinary incontinence. J Reprod Med. 1987;32(4):273–5.
8. Walters MD, Diaz K. Q-tip test: a study of continent and incontinent women. Obstet Gynecol. 1987;70(2):208–11.
9. Staskin D, Kelleher C, Avery K, Bosch R, Cotterill N, Coyne K, et al. Initial Assessment of urinary and faecal incontinence in adult male and female patients. In: Abrams P, Cardozo L, Khoury S, Wein AJ, editors. Incontinence. 4th ed. Paris: Health publication Ltd; 2009.
10. Schafer W, Abrams P, Liao L, Mattiasson A, Pesce F, Spangberg A, et al. Good urodynamic practices: uroflowmetry, filling cystometry, and pressure-flow studies. Neurourol Urodyn. 2002;21(3):261–74.
11. Caputo RM, Benson JT. The Q-tip test and urethrovesical junction mobility. Obstet Gynecol. 1993;82(6):892–6.
12. Chen Y, Wen JG, Shen H, Lv YT, Wang Y, Wang QW, et al. Valsalva leak point pressure-associated Q-tip angle and simple female stress urinary incontinence symptoms. Int Urol Nephrol. 2014;46(11):2103–8.
13. Bakas P, Liapis A, Creatsas G. Q-tip test and tension-free vaginal tape in the management of female patients with genuine stress incontinence. Gynecol Obstet Investig. 2002;53(3):170–3.

13

The diagnostic accuracy of urine-based tests for bladder cancer varies greatly by patient

Ajay Gopalakrishna[1], Thomas A. Longo[1], Joseph J. Fantony[1], Richmond Owusu[2], Wen-Chi Foo[3], Rajesh Dash[3] and Brant A. Inman[1*]

Abstract

Background: Spectrum effects refer to the phenomenon that test performance varies across subgroups of a population. When spectrum effects occur during diagnostic testing for cancer, difficult patient misdiagnoses can occur. Our objective was to evaluate the effect of test indication, age, gender, race, and smoking status on the performance characteristics of two commonly used diagnostic tests for bladder cancer, urine cytology and fluorescence in situ hybridization (FISH).

Methods: We assessed all subjects who underwent cystoscopy, cytology, and FISH at our institution from 2003 to 2012. The standard diagnostic test performance metrics were calculated using marginal models to account for clustered/repeated measures within subjects. We calculated test performance for the overall cohort by test indication as well as by key patient variables: age, gender, race, and smoking status.

Results: A total of 4023 cystoscopy-cytology pairs and 1696 FISH-cystoscopy pairs were included in the analysis. In both FISH and cytology, increasing age, male gender, and history of smoking were associated with increased sensitivity and decreased specificity. FISH performance was most impacted by age, with an increase in sensitivity from 17 % at age 40 to 49 % at age 80. The same was true of cytology, with an increase in sensitivity from 50 % at age 40 to 67 % at age 80. Sensitivity of FISH was higher for a previous diagnosis of bladder cancer (46 %) than for hematuria (26 %). Test indication had no impact on the performance of cytology and race had no significant impact on the performance of either test.

Conclusions: The diagnostic performance of urine cytology and FISH vary significantly according to the patient demographic in which they were tested. Hence, the reporting of spectrum effects in diagnostic tests should become part of standard practice. Patient-related factors must contextualize the clinicians' interpretation of test results and their decision-making.

Keywords: FISH, Cytology, Bladder cancer, Sensitivity, Specificity, Spectrum effects

Background

Bladder cancer (BC) represents 4.5 % of all new cancers in the US with over 74,000 cases and it remains the 5th most common in 2015 [1]. Typically, it presents with hematuria, and 70 % of patients with BC initially have non-muscle invasive bladder cancer (NMIBC). NMIBC has a high chance of recurrence (60–85 %) and requires long term surveillance [2]. Several guidelines exist for the management of non-muscle invasive bladder cancer, and include cystoscopy and urine-based tests for initial screening and recurrence surveillance [3–5].

Cystoscopy is the community gold standard for the detection of bladder tumors, and identifies nearly all papillary and sessile tumors [6]. However, it is invasive and a source of distress for patients. It also has a limited ability to detect occult microscopic disease or the presence of tumors in atypical locations. Microscopic disease is of particular importance in BC because of prevalent field

* Correspondence: brant.inman@duke.edu
[1]Division of Urology, Duke University Medical Center, Durham, NC 27710, USA
Full list of author information is available at the end of the article

effect [7]. While urethral cancer is a rare event, [8] upper tract tumors (UTUC) account for 5–10 % of urothelial cell carcinoma and may lead to increased morbidity and mortality if missed [9]. Therefore, guidelines recommend adjunctive tests for detection of BC [3–5]. The two most common urine-based tests are voided urine cytology and UroVysion™ (Vysis, Downers Grove, IL) fluorescence in situ hybridization (FISH) assay. Most physicians and their patients will assume that a positive urine test indicates the presence of a tumor, and will aggressively pursue a diagnosis.

The majority of physicians believe that a urine test will perform similarly in all patient populations, but this may be a false assumption. Test performance often varies across patient subgroups and is termed spectrum effects [10–12]. Although reporting spectrum effects for a given test is endorsed by the STARD initiative, it is uncommon in practice [13]. We are the first to evaluate for the existence of spectrum effects in cytology and FISH among patients being screened because of hematuria or undergoing surveillance of NMIBC. Our hypothesis is that test performance varies according to patient characteristics. We analyzed the diagnostic performance by test indication as well as four clinically significant demographic variables - age, gender, race, and smoking status. The objective of this study was to determine the presence and magnitude of spectrum effects occurring in cytology and FISH of a large contemporary cohort undergoing bladder cancer screening.

Methods

Subject selection

After approval by the Duke University Health System Institutional Review Board, all subjects who underwent cystoscopy and cytology and/or UroVysion FISH at Duke University Medical Center (DUMC) between 1/2003 to 1/2012 for either hematuria evaluation or surveillance of bladder cancer were identified. As the data for the study was obtained through retrospective chart review, a waiver of informed consent was approved by the IRB. For patients with signs or symptoms of urinary tract infection, the standard practice at our institution was to collect a urine specimen for culture, treat the patient with culture-specific antibiotics, and delay cystoscopy and urine marker testing for 2–4 weeks to avoid confounding the results.

Cystoscopy as the diagnostic gold standard for bladder tumor

White light cystoscopy, the community gold standard in diagnosis of bladder tumors, was used to determine the presence or absence of a bladder tumor [4, 14–16]. Cystoscopy was chosen over biopsy as the standard against which urine tests were compared because a biopsy is obtained only in subjects with an abnormal cystoscopy or urine test, which would subject the results to considerable verification bias [17]. Cystoscopy results were classified as positive, suspicious, or negative. A positive cystoscopy serves as a surrogate for histopathology, as nearly all visible tumors are malignant [6]. We required that cystoscopy occur within +/− 30 days of the urine-based test to serve as the gold standard.

Cytology

Urine samples received in the Cytology Preparatory Laboratory were prepared as ThinPrep slides (Cytyc Corporation, Marlborough, MA). After samples were centrifuged at 2800 rpm for 5 min, the supernatant was removed to produce a cell pellet. Cell pellets were washed with Cytolyt Solution. Two to three drops of each patient sample was transferred into PreservCyt Solution and fixed for 15 min. ThinPrep slides were then produced by loading the samples into the ThinPrep 2000 Processor. The ThinPrep slides were stained with Papanicolaou stain, cover-slipped and then screened by a cytotechnologist before being evaluated by a cytopathologist. More than one cytopathologist was involved in the analysis of the urine specimens during the study interval. After cytological evaluation, the specimens were classified into one of four categories: negative, atypical, suspicious for malignancy, or positive for malignancy.

UroVysion FISH test

Patient samples for UroVysion FISH were prepared according to manufacturer recommendations (Abbott Molecular Inc., Abbot Park, IL). The UroVysion Probe mixture contains chromosome enumeration probes (CEPs) labeled with Spectrum Red for visualization of chromosome 3, Spectrum Green for visualization of chromosome 7 and Spectrum Aqua for visualization of chromosome 17, as well as a locus specific probe for 9p21 labeled with Spectrum Gold. The slides were counterstained with DAPI and visualized with a fluorescence microscope equipped with the appropriate filters for signal enumeration of each fluorophore. A minimum of 25 morphologically abnormal cells per test were analyzed. The UroVysion FISH result was defined as meeting one or more of the following criteria: (i) ≥ 4 cells with gains of 2 or more chromosomes 3, 7, and 17 in the same cell, (ii) ≥ 10 cells with tetrasomy of chromosomes 3, 7, and 17, (iii) ≥ 10 cells showing gains of a single chromosome 3, 7, or 17, and (iv) ≥ 12 cells with homozygous loss of 9p21 locus [18].

Statistical methods

Diagnostic test performance metrics and 95 % confidence intervals (95 % CI) were calculated using logistic models: (a) a generalized estimating equation (GEE) using an exchangeable (compound symmetry) covariance structure, [19] and (b) a generalized linear mixed model (GLMM) [19]. While both models take into account clustered/correlated test results that occur due to repeated testing within subjects, they are different techniques and results are interpreted differently [20]. The GEE is a marginal model that is interpreted as "population-averaged," whereas the GLMM is a conditional model interpreted in a "subject-specific" manner [21]. Sensitivity and specificity were calculated for the overall cohort as well as by indication, age, gender, race, and smoking status subgroups. Age was analyzed as a continuous variable, but the results are presented in age decades for ease of interpretation. Indication, gender, race, and smoking status were analyzed as categorical variables. Smokers were stratified as "Never smokers," "Former smokers," or "Current smokers," as indicated in their electronic medical charts. Smoking status was available on all patients in both the cytology and FISH cohorts. A two-sided p-value of 0.05 was used to define statistical significance. Statistical analyses were conducted using R 3.1.3 with packages lme4, geepack, and BSagri installed.

Results

A total of 4023 pairs of cystoscopies and cytologies were obtained from 871 unique subjects for the cytology analysis, and 1696 pairs of UroVysion tests and cystoscopies from 827 unique subjects for the UroVysion FISH analysis. Baseline demographic characteristics of the study cohort are shown in Table 1. In patients who had positive pathology in the cytology cohort, the AJCC stage distribution was: 355 (81 %) stage 0, 33 (7.5 %) stage 1, 33 (7.5 %) stage 2, and 19 (4 %) stage 3. The grade distribution was 199 (45 %) low grade and 239 (55 %) high grade. In the FISH cohort, of patients who had positive pathology, the AJCC stage distribution was: 183 (77 %) stage 0, 24 (10 %) stage 1, 18 (8 %) stage 2, 12 (5 %) stage 3, and 1 (<1 %) stage 4. The grade breakdown was 102 (43 %) low grade and 134 (56 %) high grade.

The diagnostic performance of urine cytology is shown in Table 2 and Fig. 1. Increasing age was associated with an increase in sensitivity and decrease in specificity of urine cytology. Sensitivity increased by 17 %, from 50 % in subjects ≤40 years to 67 % in those ≥80 years. In contrast, specificity declined from 53 % in subjects ≤40 years of age to 36 % in subjects ≥80 years of age. Gender had the greatest impact on cytology performance. Subject-specific estimates of sensitivity derived from the GLMM model were dramatically higher in men than women (67 % vs 51 %), though specificity was lower (36 % vs 53 %). In subjects with a history of smoking, cytology was 10 % more sensitive and proportionally less specific compared with subjects who had never smoked. Race and indication did not significantly impact cytology test performance in either of the models.

The diagnostic performance of UroVysion FISH is shown in Table 3 and Fig. 2. Again, increasing subject age was associated with increased sensitivity and decreased specificity. Subject-specific estimates of test sensitivity obtained from the GLMM model nearly tripled from 17 % in subjects ≤40 years of age to 49 % in those ≥80 years of age. Contrarily, specificity decreased from 93 % in subjects ≤40 years of age to 74 % in those ≥80 years of age. The UroVysion FISH test was substantially less sensitive

Table 1 Clinical characteristics of the study population

	Cytology cohort	UroVysion FISH cohort
Sample size		
Unique subjects	871	827
Test-cystoscopy pairs	4023	1696
Age (years, median)	66 (IQR: 56–75)	67 (IQR: 56–76)
< 40	34 (4 %)	29 (4 %)
40–50	89 (10 %)	84 (10 %)
50–60	162 (19 %)	152 (18 %)
60–70	248 (29 %)	227 (27 %)
70–80	222 (26 %)	217 (26 %)
≥ 80	113 (13 %)	118 (14 %)
Gender		
Male	540 (62 %)	488 (59 %)
Female	328 (38 %)	339 (41 %)
Race		
White	668 (78 %)	648 (78 %)
Black	157 (18 %)	154 (19 %)
Other	26 (3 %)	25 (3 %)
Smoking status		
Current smoker	75 (9 %)	82 (10 %)
Former smoker	403 (48 %)	407 (49 %)
Never smoker	356 (43 %)	338 (41 %)
Indication for test		
Hematuria	415 (48 %)	368 (44 %)
Urothelial carcinoma	331 (38 %)	322 (39 %)
Other	125 (14 %)	137 (17 %)
Cystoscopy result		
Negative	2783 (69 %)	1324 (78 %)
Positive	752 (19 %)	185 (11 %)
Atypical/Suspicious	492 (12 %)	187 (11 %)
Urine test result		
Negative	1632 (41 %)	1210 (71 %)
Positive	375 (9 %)	486 (29 %)
Atypical/Suspicious	2016 (50 %)	-

IQR interquartile range

Table 2 Diagnostic performance of urine cytology by patient subgroup

Risk factor	Subgroup	Method	Sensitivity			Specificity			*P*-value
			Estimate (%)	LCI	UCI	Estimate (%)	LCI	UCI	
Overall	None	GLMM	62	58	66	41	38	44	0.13
		GEE	59	56	63	43	40	45	0.23
Age	40	GLMM	50	42	58	53	46	60	<0.001
	50		55	49	60	48	44	53	
	60		59	54	63	44	41	47	
	70		63	59	67	40	37	43	
	80		67	62	71	36	32	40	
	40	GEE	50	43	57	52	46	58	0.006
	50		53	48	59	49	45	53	
	60		57	53	61	45	42	48	
	70		60	57	64	42	39	44	
	80		64	60	68	38	35	42	
Smoking	Never	GLMM	56	51	62	47	42	52	0.003
	Former		66	62	71	37	33	41	
	Current		59	50	68	44	35	53	
	Never	GEE	55	50	60	47	43	51	0.005
	Former		63	59	67	39	36	43	
	Current		57	49	65	45	38	52	
Gender	Female	GLMM	51	45	57	53	48	58	<0.001
	Male		67	63	71	36	32	39	
	Female	GEE	50	45	55	52	48	56	<0.001
	Male		64	60	67	38	35	41	
Race	White	GLMM	63	59	67	40	37	44	0.34
	Black		61	53	68	43	36	50	
	Other		51	34	68	52	36	68	
	White	GEE	60	56	64	42	39	45	0.25
	Black		58	51	65	44	38	50	
	Other		49	35	63	53	39	67	
Indication	Hematuria	GLMM	63	58	69	40	35	45	0.047
	Cancer		63	59	68	40	36	44	
	Other		53	44	62	51	43	59	
	Hematuria	GEE	61	56	65	42	38	46	0.059
	Cancer		60	56	64	42	39	45	
	Other		52	45	59	51	44	57	

in women than in men (28 % vs. 44 %), though its specificity was higher (88 % vs 78 %). Test performance was similar in current and former smokers regardless of the analysis model. However, in nonsmokers, test sensitivity was approximately 15 % lower and specificity approximately 10 % higher than current and former smokers. Race was not statistically significant in the correlative models. Analysis of test performance by indication revealed significant differences. FISH was dramatically more sensitive for cancer surveillance (46 %) than for hematuria (26 %). However, it was also less specific (76 % vs 88 %).

There were 4,729 total cytologies collected, although 706 did not have a corresponding cystoscopy to perform the above analysis. During the study period, 1898 (40 %) were negative, 423 (9 %) positive, and 2408 (51 %) suspicious or atypical. When suspicious/atypical cytology results using the GLMM model were classified as positive, the sensitivity was 62 % [95 % CI: 58–66 %] and the specificity was 41 % [95 % CI: 38–44 %]. When these

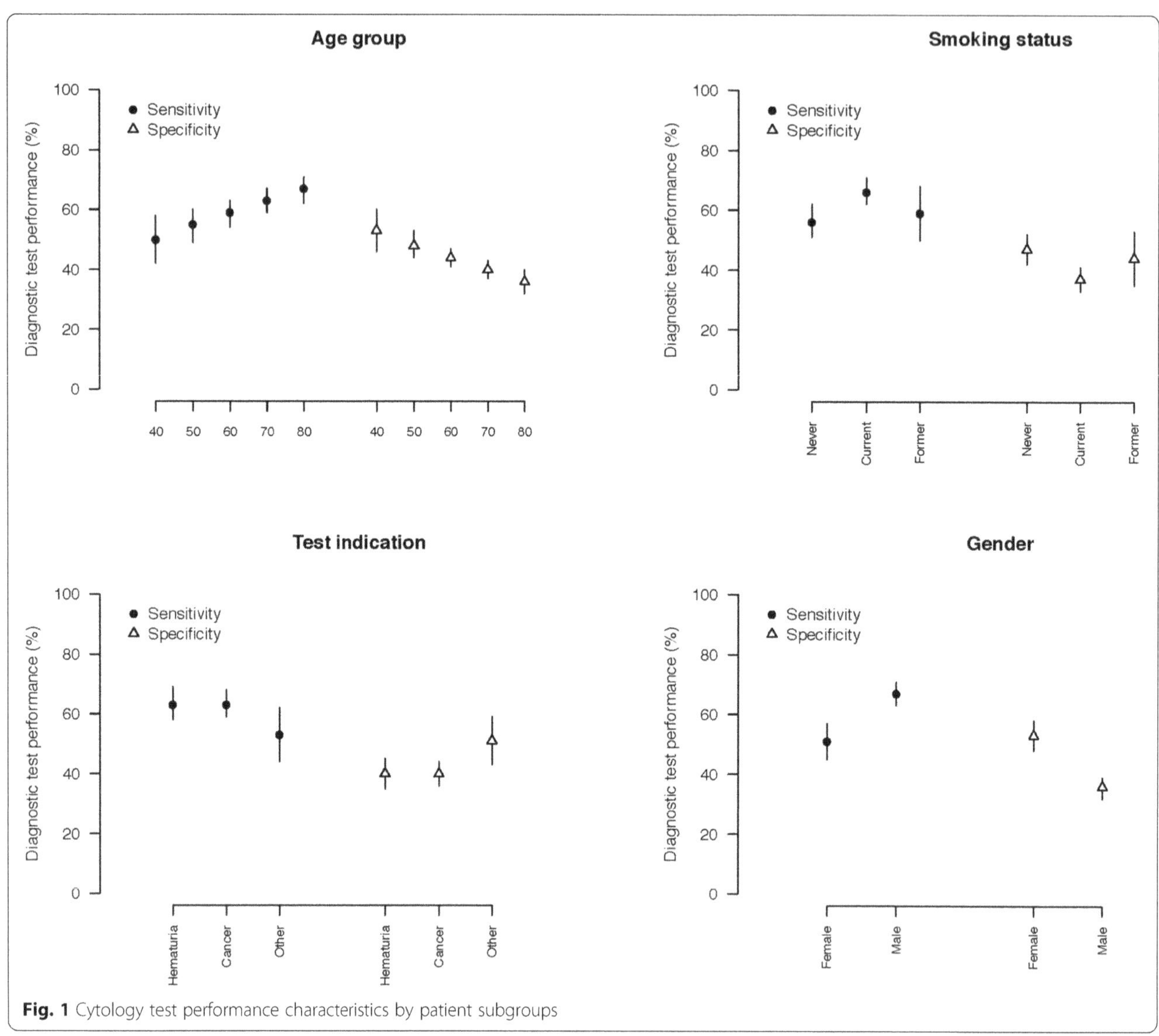

Fig. 1 Cytology test performance characteristics by patient subgroups

results were re-classified as negative, this had the effect of a large increase in specificity 100 % [95 % CI: 100-100 %] with a consequent decrease in sensitivity 0 % [95 % CI: 0-2 %].

For all the above analyses, suspicious cystoscopies were considered positive since they will generally result in intervention (e.g., bladder biopsy). To determine whether the classification of suspicious cystoscopies dramatically affected our results, we repeated the analyses with suspicious cystoscopies classified as negative and found no significant difference in our results, demonstrating that the performance of cytology and UroVysion FISH are not sensitive to how suspicious cystoscopies are classified. This stands in contrast to the large effect seen in cytology with a similar re-analysis that was mentioned above.

Discussion

Spectrum effects were first described by Mulherin et al. as inherent variations in diagnostic test performance among different subgroup populations [12]. We have shown that urine-based tests for bladder cancer (a) have poor diagnostic performance and (b) vary substantially in accuracy in different patient populations. However, the recognition of spectrum effects allows for a strategy that should result in a clinically important gain for the patient.

We stratified our cohort into four clinically relevant subgroups and found that age, male gender, and a history of smoking were all associated with increased sensitivity in both cytology and UroVysion. Smoking and aging are associated with altered cellular biology which might lead to changes detectable by cytology or UroVysion [22]. Epidemiologically, age and cigarette smoking have also been associated with more advanced disease at initial presentation [22, 23]. It is possible that the improvement in sensitivity of cytology and UroVysion is due to more advanced disease at presentation in these

Table 3 Diagnostic performance of UroVysion FISH by patient subgroup

Risk factor	Subgroup	Method	Sensitivity			Specificity			*P*-value
			Estimate (%)	LCI	UCI	Estimate (%)	LCI	UCI	
Overall	None	GLMM	39	31	46	82	79	85	<0.001
		GEE	38	32	45	77	75	80	<0.001
Age	40	GLMM	17	11	26	93	89	96	<0.001
	50		23	16	31	90	86	93	
	60		31	24	39	86	83	89	
	70		40	33	47	81	77	84	
	80		49	41	57	74	68	79	
	40	GEE	20	14	28	89	85	92	<0.001
	50		25	19	33	86	82	89	
	60		32	26	39	81	78	84	
	70		39	33	46	76	73	79	
	80		47	40	54	70	65	74	
Smoking	Never	GLMM	25	18	34	89	86	92	<0.001
	Former		46	38	54	77	72	81	
	Current		41	28	55	80	71	87	
	Never	GEE	26	34	85	85	81	88	<0.001
	Former		44	52	72	72	68	75	
	Current		40	51	76	76	68	82	
Gender	Female	GLMM	28	20	36	88	84	92	<0.001
	Male		44	36	52	78	74	82	
	Female	GEE	28	22	36	84	80	87	<0.001
	Male		43	37	37	73	69	77	
Race	White	GLMM	40	33	47	81	77	85	0.219
	Black		31	21	42	87	81	91	
	Other		37	17	61	83	65	93	
	White	GEE	39	33	46	76	73	79	0.160
	Black		31	23	41	82	76	87	
	Other		35	17	58	80	61	91	
Indication	Hematuria	GLMM	26	19	35	88	84	92	<0.001
	Cancer		46	38	54	76	71	80	
	Other		28	19	40	87	80	92	
	Hematuria	GEE	29	22	37	83	79	86	<0.001
	Cancer		44	38	52	71	67	75	
	Other		31	22	41	82	75	87	

demographics. Horstmann et al. found that age was associated with higher false positive rates in cytology and the NMP22 assay, which would translate to decreased specificity and is consistent with our results [24]. The analysis by indication also revealed increased sensitivity for UroVysion but not cytology when used for cancer surveillance compared to hematuria. This may also be a reflection of advanced disease in that population. Interestingly, Dimashkieh et al. found that both UroVysion and cytology are slightly more sensitive in the context of cancer surveillance than in hematuria [25].

Disease severity fails to explain why both tests were more sensitive in males than females. While the incidence of bladder cancer is three to four times higher in men, women tend to present with more advanced disease [26, 27]. An alternative explanation for the gender disparity we observed is that gender-specific genetic differences are affecting test performance. Recent

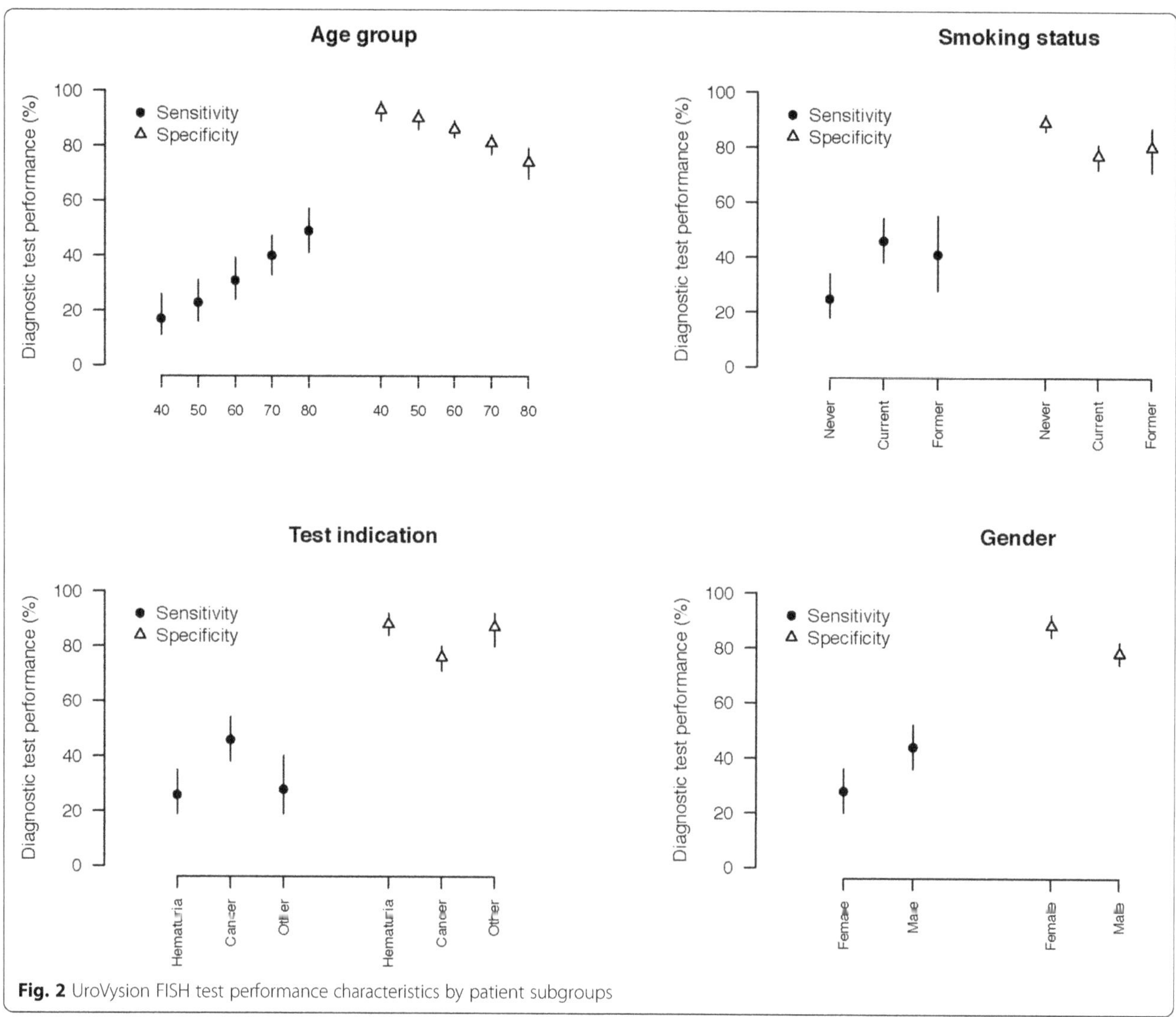

Fig. 2 UroVysion FISH test performance characteristics by patient subgroups

studies have found gender differences at a cellular level, and postulate that cells have a "sex" [28]. Shen et al. have elucidated gender differences in bladder cancer biology thought to be related to differential expression of sex steroid receptors on urothelial cells [29]. Specifically, the beta subunit of the estrogen receptor is the predominant receptor expressed in the majority of bladder cancers, and a positive correlation exists between degree of estrogen receptor expression and tumor grade and stage [29]. These gender differences in cancer biology may result in differences in cytologic morphology. Distinct patterns of chromosomal abnormalities between the genders have been described in other cancers and it is possible that the specific chromosomal aberrations detected by the UroVysion test result in improved sensitivity in men [30].

Proper stratification into relevant subgroups allows for recognition of important spectrum associations [31]. There is value in discerning between low grade and high grade lesions; high grade should be detected as early as possible, while the likelihood of missing such a tumor should be as low as possible. In high risk populations, sensitivity is more important than specificity because the consequences of a missed malignancy are great. FISH exhibits such properties in the smoking subgroup, whereas cytology does not have similar characteristics in the same population. Therefore, a clinician should give stronger consideration to FISH results than cytology results in smokers. Analogous spectrum effects can be seen for indication and cytology.

There are other patient populations were the risks of a procedure often outweigh the benefit. It is preferable for a urine test with a high specificity and low sensitivity in low grade disease to reduce the number of unnecessary invasive procedures. Age and cytology illustrate this effect because as the patient age increases, so does the specificity, with a reciprocal decrease in sensitivity. This should spare the elderly patient avoidable cystoscopies.

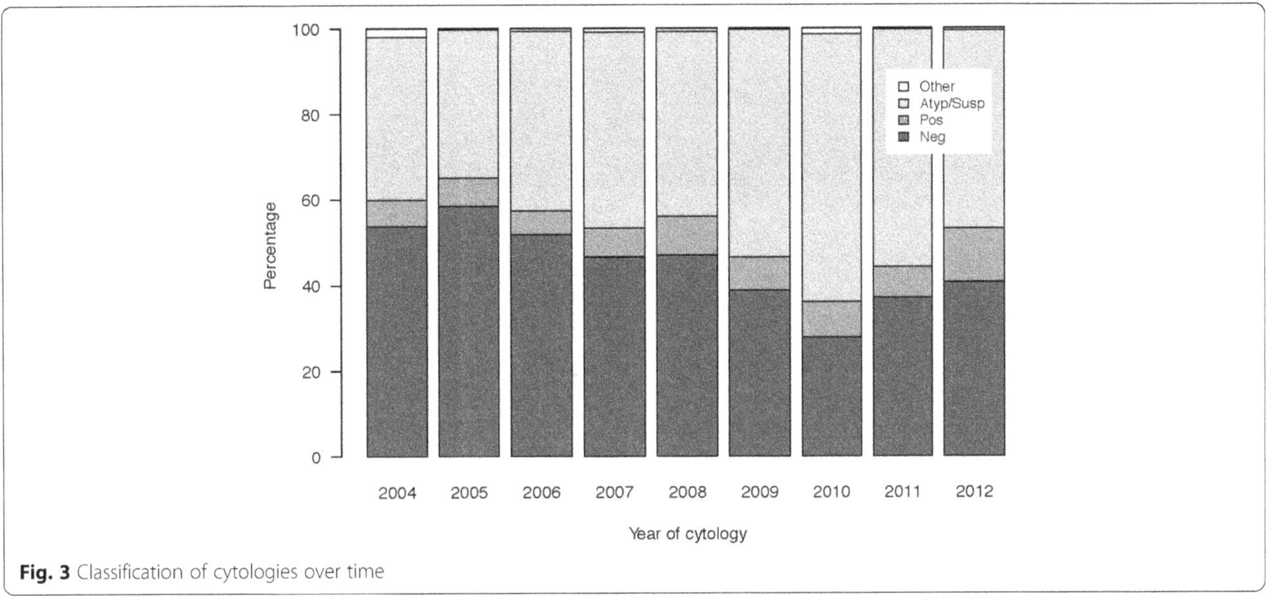

Fig. 3 Classification of cytologies over time

The tradeoff would be that some tumors may be missed for a period of time, but the literature surrounding active surveillance suggest this is safe [32].

Limitations

Our study was retrospective, and longitudinal in nature leaving us unable to control for significant variables, such as the EORTC risk scores, that predict the probability of recurrence and progression of bladder cancer. With 19 % of cystoscopies in the cytology cohort classified as positive, this cohort was at higher risk for bladder cancer than the average US population. Additionally, while the sensitivity could have been improved with narrow band imaging or fluorescent cystoscopy, these technologies were not available at our institution for the entirety of the study period. For the purposes of our analyses, suspicious lesions on cystoscopy were classified as positive. When we correlated this classification with pathology, only 59 % of pathology specimens were found to have cancer, reflecting a limitation of this classification. However, when we performed a sensitivity analysis with suspicious cystoscopies classified as negative, our results were not significantly different, indicating a minimal impact of this limitation on the interpretation of the results. The data were collected over a 10 year time frame; so indications for using the tests have changed over time as have technique of verification of test results. Furthermore, more than one cytopathologist was involved over the period examined and literature suggests high inter-observer discrepancy, but this reflects the real world. Urine cytology has a low sensitivity and is highly operator-dependent in the setting of low grade disease [33]. In experienced hands, however, specificity is about 90 % [34]. Indeed, our own data supports this conclusion, and shows an increasing percentage of reported atypical/suspicious cytologies over time (Fig. 3).

Conclusions

We are the first to show that urine-based bladder cancer tests display spectrum effects. The reporting of spectrum effects in diagnostic tests should become part of standard practice. Knowledge of these effects allows the physician to properly interpret the results and has a meaningful impact on a patient's clinical care.

Abbreviations

AJCC, American Joint Committee on Cancer; BC, Bladder cancer; CEP, Chromosome enumeration probes; DUMC, Duke University Medical Center; EORTC, European Organization for Research and Treatment of Cancer; FISH, Fluorescence in situ hybridization; GEE, Generalized estimating equations; GLMM, Generalized linear mixed models; IRB, Institutional Review Board; NMIBC, Non-muscle invasive bladder cancer; STARD, Standards for Reporting of Diagnostic Accuracy; UTUC, Upper tract urothelial carcinoma

Acknowledgements

Not applicable.

Funding

This publication was supported by the National Center for Advancing Translational Sciences, National Institutes of Health, through Duke-CTSA Grant Number 5TL1TR001116-03. Its contents are solely the responsibility of the authors and do not necessarily represent the official views of the NIH.

Authors' contributions

AG: Data collection/management, data analysis, manuscript writing/editing. JJF: Data collection/management, data analysis, manuscript writing/editing. TAL: data analysis, manuscript writing/editing. RO: Data collection/management, manuscript editing. WF: Manuscript writing/editing. RD: Data collection/management, manuscript editing. BAI: Protocol/project development, data analysis, manuscript writing/editing. All authors have read and approve of the final version of the manuscript.

Competing interests

The authors declare that they have no competing interests.

Author details

[1]Division of Urology, Duke University Medical Center, Durham, NC 27710, USA. [2]Department of Urology, University of California San Diego, San Diego, CA, USA. [3]Department of Pathology, Duke University Medical Center, Durham, NC, USA.

References

1. Siegel RL, Miller KD, Jemal A. Cancer statistics, 2015. CA Cancer J Clin. 2015;65:5–29.
2. Raghavan D, Shipley WU, Garnick MB, Russell PJ, Richie JP. Biology and management of bladder cancer. N Engl J Med. 1990;322:1129–38.
3. Network NCC. NCCN Clinical Practice Guidelines in Oncology. Bladder Cancer. V.2.2015. 2015.
4. Hall MC, Chang SS, Dalbagni G, Pruthi RS, Seigne JD, Skinner EC, et al. Guideline for the management of nonmuscle invasive bladder cancer (stages Ta, T1, and Tis): 2007 update. J Urol. 2007;178:2314–30.
5. Babjuk M, Burger M, Zigeuner R, Shariat SF, van Rhijn BW, Comperat E, et al. EAU guidelines on non-muscle-invasive urothelial carcinoma of the bladder: update 2013. Eur Urol. 2013;64:639–53.
6. van der Aa MN, Steyerberg EW, Bangma C, van Rhijn BW, Zwarthoff EC, van der Kwast TH. Cystoscopy revisited as the gold standard for detecting bladder cancer recurrence: diagnostic review bias in the randomized, prospective CEFUB trial. J Urol. 2010;183:76–80.
7. Majewski T, Lee S, Jeong J, Yoon DS, Kram A, Kim MS, et al. Understanding the development of human bladder cancer by using a whole-organ genomic mapping strategy. Lab Invest. 2008;88:694–721.
8. Swartz MA, Porter MP, Lin DW, Weiss NS. Incidence of primary urethral carcinoma in the United States. Urology. 2006;68:1164–8.
9. Roupret M, Babjuk M, Comperat E, Zigeuner R, Sylvester RJ, Burger M, et al. European Association of Urology Guidelines on upper urinary tract urothelial cell carcinoma: 2015 update. Eur Urol. 2015;68:868–79.
10. Ransohoff DF, Feinstein AR. Problems of spectrum and bias in evaluating the efficacy of diagnostic tests. N Engl J Med. 1978;299:926–30.
11. Elie C, Coste J. A methodological framework to distinguish spectrum effects from spectrum biases and to assess diagnostic and screening test accuracy for patient populations: application to the Papanicolaou cervical cancer smear test. BMC Med Res Methodol. 2008;8:7.
12. Mulherin SA, Miller WC. Spectrum bias or spectrum effect? Subgroup variation in diagnostic test evaluation. Ann Intern Med. 2002;137:598–602.
13. Bossuyt PM, Reitsma JB, Bruns DE, Gatsonis CA, Glasziou PP, Irwig LM, et al. Towards complete and accurate reporting of studies of diagnostic accuracy: the STARD initiative. Standards for Reporting of Diagnostic Accuracy. Clin Chem. 2003;49:1–6.
14. Clark PE, Agarwal N, Biagioli MC, Eisenberger MA, Greenberg RE, Herr HW, et al. Bladder cancer. J Natl Compr Canc Netw. 2013;11:446–75.
15. Kamat AM, Hegarty PK, Gee JR, Clark PE, Svatek RS, Hegarty N, et al. ICUD-EAU International Consultation on Bladder Cancer 2012: Screening, diagnosis, and molecular markers. Eur Urol. 2013;63:4–15.
16. Karl A, Adejoro O, Saigal C, Konety B. General adherence to guideline recommendations on initial diagnosis of bladder cancer in the United States and influencing factors. Clin Genitourin Cancer. 2014;12:270–7.
17. Zhou XH. Correcting for verification bias in studies of a diagnostic test's accuracy. Stat Methods Med Res. 1998;7:337–53.
18. Smith GD, Bentz JS. "FISHing" to detect urinary and other cancers: validation of an imaging system to aid in interpretation. Cancer Cytopathol. 2010;118:56–64.
19. Genders TS, Spronk S, Stijnen T, Steyerberg EW, Lesaffre E, Hunink MG. Methods for calculating sensitivity and specificity of clustered data: a tutorial. Radiology. 2012;265:910–6.
20. Fitzmaurice GM. Applied Longitudinal Analysis. Hobocken, New Jersey: Wiley; 2004.
21. Hubbard AE, Ahern J, Fleischer NL, Van der Laan M, Lippman SA, Jewell N, et al. To GEE or not to GEE: comparing population average and mixed models for estimating the associations between neighborhood risk factors and health. Epidemiology. 2010;21:467–74.
22. Taylor 3rd JA, Kuchel GA. Bladder cancer in the elderly: clinical outcomes, basic mechanisms, and future research direction. Nat Clin Pract Urol. 2009;6:135–44.
23. Chamssuddin AK, Saadat SH, Deiri K, Zarzar MY, Abdouche N, Deeb O, et al. Evaluation of grade and stage in patients with bladder cancer among smokers and non-smokers. Arab J Urol. 2013;11:165–8.
24. Horstmann M, Todenhofer T, Hennenlotter J, Aufderklamm S, Mischinger J, Kuehs U, et al. Influence of age on false positive rates of urine-based tumor markers. World J Urol. 2013;31:935–40.
25. Dimashkieh H, Wolff DJ, Smith TM, Houser PM, Nietert PJ, Yang J. Evaluation of urovysion and cytology for bladder cancer detection: a study of 1835 paired urine samples with clinical and histologic correlation. Cancer Cytopathol. 2013;121:591–7.
26. Fajkovic H, Halpern JA, Cha EK, Bahadori A, Chromecki TF, Karakiewicz PI, et al. Impact of gender on bladder cancer incidence, staging, and prognosis. World J Urol. 2011;29:457–63.
27. Garg T, Pinheiro LC, Atoria CL, Donat SM, Weissman JS, Herr HW, et al. Gender disparities in hematuria evaluation and bladder cancer diagnosis: a population based analysis. J Urol. 2014;192:1072–7.
28. Straface E, Gambardella L, Brandani M, Malorni W. Sex differences at cellular level: "cells have a sex". Handb Exp Pharmacol. 2012;(214):49–65.
29. Shen SS, Smith CL, Hsieh JT, Yu J, Kim IY, Jian W, et al. Expression of estrogen receptors-alpha and -beta in bladder cancer cell lines and human bladder tumor tissue. Cancer. 2006;106:2610–6.
30. Tabernero MD, Espinosa AB, Maillo A, Rebelo O, Vera JF, Sayagues JM, et al. Patient gender is associated with distinct patterns of chromosomal abnormalities and sex chromosome linked gene-expression profiles in meningiomas. Oncologist. 2007;12:1225–36.
31. Lachs MS, Nachamkin I, Edelstein PH, Goldman J, Feinstein AR, Schwartz JS. Spectrum bias in the evaluation of diagnostic tests: lessons from the rapid dipstick test for urinary tract infection. Ann Intern Med. 1992;117:135–40.
32. Tiu A, Jenkins LC, Soloway MS. Active surveillance for low-risk bladder cancer. Urol Oncol. 2014;32:33.e7–10.
33. Sherman AB, Koss LG, Adams SE. Interobserver and intraobserver differences in the diagnosis of urothelial cells. Comparison with classification by computer. Anal Quant Cytol. 1984;6:112–20.
34. Raitanen MP, Aine R, Rintala E, Kallio J, Rajala P, Juusela H, et al. Differences between local and review urinary cytology in diagnosis of bladder cancer. An interobserver multicenter analysis. Eur Urol. 2002;41:284–9.

A pilot prospective study to evaluate whether the bladder morphology in cystography and/or urodynamic may help predict the response to botulinum toxin a injection in neurogenic bladder refractory to anticholinergics

Ronaldo Alvarenga Álvares[1*], Ivana Duval Araújo[2] and Marcelo Dias Sanches[2]

Abstract

Background: We have observed different clinical responses to botulinum toxin A (BTX-A) in patients who had similar urodynamic parameters before the procedure. Furthermore, some bladders evaluated by cystography and cystoscopy during the procedure had different characteristics that could influence the outcome of the treatment. The aim of this study was to assess whether cystography and urodynamic parameters could help predict which patients with neurogenic detrusor overactivity (NDO) refractory to anticholinergics respond better to treatment with injection of BTX-A.

Methods: In total, 34 patients with spinal cord injury were prospectively evaluated. All patients emptied their bladder by clean intermittent catheterization (CIC) and had incontinence and NDO, despite using 40 mg or more of intravesical oxybutynin and undergoing detrusor injection of BTX-A (300 IU). Pretreatment evaluation included urodynamic, and cystography. Follow-up consisted of urodynamic and ambulatory visits four months after treatment. The cystography parameters used were bladder shape, capacity and presence of diverticula. Urodynamic parameters used for assessment were maximum cystometric capacity (MCC), maximum detrusor pressure (MDP), compliance and reflex volume (RV).

Results: After injection of BTX-A, 70% of the patients had success, with 4 months or more of continence. Before the treatment, there were significant differences in most urodynamic parameters between those who responded successfully compared to those who did not. Patients who responded successfully had greater MCC ($p = 0.019$), higher RV ($p = 0.041$), and greater compliance ($p = 0.043$). There was no significant difference in the MDP (0.691). The cystography parameters were not significantly different between these groups bladder shape ($p = 0.271$), capacity ($p > 0.720$) and presence of diverticula ($p > 0.999$). Statistical analyses were performed using SPSS (version 20.0) and included Student's t-test for two paired samples and Fisher's exact test, with a significance threshold of 0.05.

Conclusions: This study suggests that the cystography parameters evaluated cannot be used to help predict the response to injection of BTX-A in the treatment of refractory NDO. However, the urodynamic parameters were significantly different in patients who responded to the treatment, with the exception of the MDP.

Keywords: Neurogenic detrusor overactivity, Botulinum toxin A, Cystography, Urodynamic, Neurogenic bladder

* Correspondence: ronaldoalvares@sarah.br
[1]SARAH Network of Rehabilitation Hospitals, Unit Belo Horizonte, Minas Gerais, Av Amazonas 5953, Gameleira 30510-000, Brazil
Full list of author information is available at the end of the article

Background

Botulinum toxin (BTX), which was described by Van Ermengem [1] in 1897, exists as serotypes A, B, C, D, E, F and G [2]. Currently, serotypes A and B are available for clinical use. When injected into the muscle, BTX causes flaccid paralysis by inhibiting acetylcholine release at the presynaptic cholinergic junction. This effect is transient and dose-related. In smooth muscle, it was shown by Smith et al. [3] that BTX-A affects the release of acetylcholine and norepinephrine in the bladder and urethra, respectively.

The treatment of neurogenic detrusor overactivity (NDO) with an injection of BTX-A into the detrusor muscle was introduced in 2000 [4]. This therapy is a minimally invasive treatment option, and, although more invasive than oral treatment with anticholinergic, is less invasive than surgery [4]. Its safety and efficacy has been confirmed in a randomized, placebo-controlled clinical trial [5]. Some studies have evaluated the use of BTX-A injections in the detrusor muscle of patients with spinal cord injury to reduce NDO, increase bladder capacity, reduce incontinence and improve the quality of life of these patients [5,6].

In previous studies, we have observed different clinical responses to BTX-A in patients who had similar urodynamic parameters before the procedure [7]. This study was motivated by the observation that some bladders evaluated by cystography and cystoscopy during the procedure revealed different characteristics that could influence the outcome of the treatment. With respect to the morphology observed in cystography, we investigated whether differences in diverticula, shape, and capacity could influence the results of treatment. Similarly, we assessed whether the urodynamic parameters evaluated before the procedure could help predict the results of detrusor BTX-A injection for the treatment of NDO refractory to anticholinergics.

Methods

Thirty-four patients with spinal cord injury who received injections of BTX-A between January 2012 and July 2013 participated of this prospective observational study. The sample size was determined by G*Power software, version 3.1.7 [8] for two dependent groups (matched pairs). Parameters used in the calculations were as follows: effect size, 0.50; significance probability, 0.05; and power test, 0.80. Of the 34 patients, 23 were male and 11 were female. All methods and definitions were based on the standardization of terminology of lower urinary tract function, as described by Abrams et al. [9]. The study was approved by the ethics committee of Sarah Hospital in Brasilia (CAAE 24188413.3.0000.0022). Informed consent was obtained from all patients participating in the study.

The inclusion criteria for the injection of BTX-A were those patients who emptied their bladder by CIC and had urinary incontinence due to hyperactivity refractory to intravesical oxybutynin doses equal or greater than 40 mg. An evaluation was conducted before the procedure and included a clinical history, physical examination, ultrasonography of the kidneys and urinary tract, cystography and urodynamic tests (Multichannel Urodynamics - Medtronic Duet systems, version 8.20, Minneapolis). The following urodynamic parameters were measured: reflex volume (RV), maximum detrusor pressure (MDP), bladder compliance, and maximum cystometric capacity (MCC). For better assessment of compliance, only the study bladders with a capacity ≥ 150 ml were used and compliance was measured five minutes after the end of bladder filling to allow for stabilization of the detrusor pressure. During cystography, the bladder filling was stopped when the maximum capacity had been reached, urinary leakage started, or there was supra pubic discomfort. Outcome was assessed in relation to the bladder shape and capacity and the presence of diverticula. The shape of the bladder

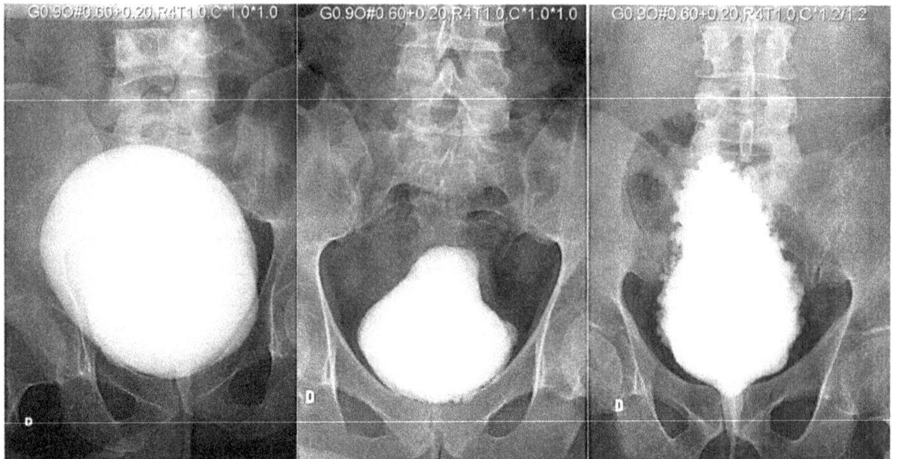

Figure 1 The shape of the bladder ("rounded" shape, "pear-shaped" or "pine").

was characterized as either "rounded" or "pear-shaped" and/or "pine" (see Figure 1). The cystometric capacity was measured in milliliters. Diverticula were characterized as absent or present, with one group consisting of patients with a diverticula number <10 and another group with a diverticula number ≥ 10 (Figure 1).

All procedures were performed in a hospital under general anesthesia. Antibiotics were administered orally, according to a urine culture, for seven days. The procedure performed on the fifth day of the antibiotic, all patients tested positive for bacteria. BTX- A (Westport Allergan Pharmaceuticals Ireland - Ireland) was diluted in sterile saline to a final concentration of 10 units/ml. Using a 19-Fr Storz cystoscope and 5 FR needle, a total of 300 IU (30 ml) was injected into 30 sites of the detrusor muscle, sparing the trigone region, as described in Schurch et al. [4]. Patients were instructed to continue using the anticholinergic medication and to gradually reduce the dose after the procedure, if it was successful and suspend its use if possible. The treatment was considered successful if the patient remained continent for four months or more, with complete absence of urinary leak, regardless of the use of the anticholinergic medication. Clinical and urodynamic control assessments were performed 4 months after treatment. Statistical analyses were performed using SPSS (version 20.0) and included Student's t-test for two paired samples and Fisher's exact test with a significance threshold of 0.05. Before each t-test, the hypothesis of equality of variances was checked using Levene's test. Differences between the groups were compared with the Mann–Whitney U test for two independent samples.

Results

Of the 34 patients, 23 were male and 11 were female. The mean age was 31.2 ± 10.3 years (mean ± standard deviation), with a range 19–55 years. There were 28 paraplegic and 6 tetraplegic patients and 25 traumatic and 9 non-traumatic cases. The mean time since SCI was 5.9 ± 4.4 years, with a maximum of 19 years and a minimum of 1 year. The patients tolerated all of the procedures and showed no acute complications related to the injections. Thirty patients (88.2%) were completely continent after the procedure. Six of these patients, however, showed little clinical response at four months and were considered unsuccessful. Four patients (11.8%) remained incontinent four months after treatment, although there were improvements in most urodynamic parameters and urinary losses. Twenty-four (70%) patients remained continent for more than 4 months and were considered successful. Twelve patients (35.2%) had an acontractile detrusor bladder after surgery. After four months, the following changes in the urodynamic parameters were observed: increased MCC (P <0.001), increased RV (p <0.001) and decreased MDP (p <0.001).

Table 1 Urodynamic assessment before and after botulinum toxin injection

	Before (n = 34)	After (n = 34)	*p-value**
Cystometric capacity (ml)	309 ± 155	492 ± 193	<0.001
Detrusor overactivity (cmH_2O)	70 ± 27	41 ± 20	< 0.001
Reflex volume (ml)	228 ± 99	381 ± 229	<0.001
Compliance (ml/cmH_2O)	32 ± 21	29 ± 18	=0.366

*Paired, two-sided Student's t-test.

The compliance did not change significantly (p = 0.366) (Table 1). There were significant differences in most of the pretreatment urodynamic parameters in patients with a successful response compared with those with an unsuccessful response. The MCC (p = 0.019), RV (0.041) and compliance (p = 0.043) were higher in patients with a successful response. The MDP was not significantly different between groups (p = 0.691) (Table 2).

Regarding cystography, before the procedure, 24 patients (70%) had no diverticula, eight patients had between 1 and 10 diverticula and 2 patients had more than 10 diverticula. By Fisher's exact test, there was no association between the response and the presence of diverticula (p > 0.999), bladder shape (p <0.271) or bladder capacity (p = 0.720) (Table 3).

After 4 months of follow-up, twenty patients (58.8%) had reduced the dose of anticholinergics, five (14.7%) had discontinued their use and nine (26.5%) had not changed the dose (Table 4). Among the 24 patients with successful results, only 5 had discontinued the use of anticholinergics. However, 16 of these patients were able to decrease the dose of the anticholinergic drugs after the procedure (Table 5).

Discussion

BTX-A injections into the detrusor muscle provide a clinically significant improvement in patients with NDO refractory to anticholinergics and are very well tolerated (5;6). In this study, continence was observed over a period of more than 4 months in 70% of the patients undergoing treatment with BTX-A. In studies with similar populations of patients, the percentage of patients with continence after injection of the toxin ranged from 42 to 87% [10]. Karsenty et al. reported that anticholinergic agents may be discontinued in 28% to 58% of patients after treatment

Table 2 Urodynamic parameters before botulinum toxin injection

Urodynamic parameters	Success (n = 24)	Unsuccess (n = 10)	*p-value**
Cystometric capacity (ml)	335 ± 157	246 ± 138	0.019
Detrusor overactivity (cmH_2O)	68 ± 27	72 ± 26	0.691
Reflex volume (ml)	243 ± 95	193 ± 103	0.041
Compliance (ml/cmH_2O)	37 ± 23	20 ± 10	0.043

*Mann–Whitney U Test for two independent samples.

Table 3 Results and cystography parameters

		Success	Unsuccess	p-value*
Capacity (ml)		351,0 ± 259,3 ml	315,8 ± 212 ml	P = 0,720
Forma	"Rounded" (n = 22)	17 (77%)	5 (23%)	P = 0,271
	"pear-shaped"/ "pine" (n = 12)	7 (58%)	5 (42%)	
Diverticula	Absent (n = 24)	17 (71%)	7 (29%)	p > 0,999
	Present (n = 10)	7 (70%)	3 (30%)	

*Mann–Whitney U Test for two independent samples.

with BTX-A and the dose can be substantially reduced in the remaining patients [10]. In this study, after 4 months of follow-up, twenty patients (58.8%) had reduced the dose of anticholinergics, five (14.7%) discontinued the use and nine (26.5%) did not change the dose of medication (Table 4). Among the 24 patients with successful results, only 5 had discontinued the use of anticholinergics. However, 16 patients were able to decrease the dose of anticholinergic drugs after the procedure (Table 5). We note that some of these patients did not reduce the dose because they were afraid that the urinary losses would return after being continent. According to previous studies, some factors that may be related to the efficacy of BTX-A injections into the detrusor muscle include, for example, whether the doses of anticholinergics used before the procedure were considered high (refractory bladder) [7], what the optimal dose of BTX-A is [11,12], the formulations used [13,14] and the injection technique [11]. These factors may explain some of the differences observed in the results across different studies. The results obtained in this study were similar to earlier studies. Among patients presenting with NDO that is refractory to anticholinergic agents, there was a percentage with unsuccessful results.

Although it has been reported that alterations can occur in the detrusor muscle of the NDO [15,16], it was postulated that the morphology of the bladder (shape and presence of diverticula) could be a result of these alterations, and could, in turn, influence the response to BTX-A injections. These changes in bladder shape are most likely the result of smooth muscle hypertrophy and changes in the connective tissue matrix that do not respond to conservative treatment. However, the present study did not demonstrate that the cystography parameters could predict which cases would be more likely to have a better response to BTX-A injections.

Table 4 Anticholinergic use after botulinum toxin injection (Total)

Use of anticholinergics	N° patients
Not decreased	9 (26,5%)
Decreased	20 (58,8%)
Suspended	5 (14,7%)
Total	34 (100%)

Table 5 Anticholinergic use after botulinum toxin injection (success)

Use of anticholinergics	N° patients
Not decreased	3 (12,5%)
Decreased	16 (66,6%)
Suspended	5 (20,8%)
Total	24 (100%)

Regarding urodynamic parameters, we observed in this study that the bladders that had better compliance, greater capacity and increased reflex volume before treatment showed a better response to treatment. Furthermore, there was no significant change in compliance after surgery ($p = 0.366$), suggesting that compliance is related to alterations in the bladder wall, is unresponsive to drug therapy, and is, therefore, directly related to the treatment response. This is in contrast to a study conducted by Klaphajone J [17], in which a small number of patients did not show this relationship.

Conclusion

This study suggests that the cystography parameters evaluated cannot be used to predict the response to BTX-A injection for the treatment of refractory NDO. It was observed in the urodynamic parameters, that patients whose bladders had higher cystometric capacity, greater reflex volume and greater compliance showed better results after treatment. The bladder compliance showed no significant improvement after the procedure, which is an important factor to be noted. A larger study with a multivariate analysis would be appropriate to clarify the results of this work.

Abbreviations

NDO: Neurogenic detrusor overactivity; BTX-A: Botulinum toxin A; BTX: Botulinum toxin; CIC: Clean intermittent catheterization; RV: Reflex volume; MDP: Maximum detrusor pressure; MCC: Maximum cystometric capacity.

Competing interests

The authors declare that they have no competing interests.

Author's contributions

RAA conceived of the study and carried out the acquisition, analysis and interpretation of data and was involved in drafting the manuscript. IDA provided substantial contributions to the conception and design and revised the manuscript critically for important intellectual content. MDS participated in the study design and coordination. All authors read and approved the final manuscript.

Acknowledgements
We thank Luiz Sergio Vaz for fundamental help during the statistical analysis and all fellow nurses who participated in data collection, especially Veronique, Solange, Luiza and Maria Cristina.
We thank Dr Márcio Josbete for his help and critical revision of the intellectual content.

Author details
[1]SARAH Network of Rehabilitation Hospitals, Unit Belo Horizonte, Minas Gerais, Av Amazonas 5953, Gameleira 30510-000, Brazil. [2]Federal University of Minas Gerais - UFMG, Rua Alfredo Balena, 190, 30130-100, Brazil.

References

1. van Ermengem E: **Classics in infectious diseases. A new anaerobic bacillus and its relation to botulism. E. van Ermengem. Originally published as "Ueber einen neuen anaeroben Bacillus und seine Beziehungen zum Botulismus" in Zeitschrift fur Hygiene und Infektionskrankheiten 26: 1–56, 1897.** *Rev Infect Dis* 1979, **1**(4):701–719.
2. Comella CL, Pullman SL: **Botulinum toxins in neurological disease.** *Muscle Nerve* 2004, **29**(5):628–644.
3. Smith CP, Franks ME, McNeil BK, Ghosh R, de Groat WC, Chancellor MB, Somogyi GT: **Effect of botulinum toxin A on the autonomic nervous system of the rat lower urinary tract.** *J Urol* 2003, **169**(5):1896–1900.
4. Schurch B, Stohrer M, Kramer G, Schmid DM, Gaul G, Hauri D: **Botulinum-A toxin for treating detrusor hyperreflexia in spinal cord injured patients: a new alternative to anticholinergic drugs? Preliminary results.** *J Urol* 2000, **164**(3 Pt 1):692–697.
5. Schurch B, De SM, Denys P, Chartier-Kastler E, Haab F, Everaert K, Plante P, Perrouin-Verbe B, Kumar C, Fraczek S, Brin MF: **Botulinum toxin type a is a safe and effective treatment for neurogenic urinary incontinence: results of a single treatment, randomized, placebo controlled 6-month study.** *J Urol* 2005, **174**(1):196–200.
6. Schurch B, Denys P, Kozma CM, Reese PR, Slaton T, Barron RL: **Botulinum toxin A improves the quality of life of patients with neurogenic urinary incontinence.** *Eur Urol* 2007, **52**(3):850–858.
7. Alvares RA, Silva JA, Barboza AL, Monteiro RT: **Botulinum toxin A in the treatment of spinal cord injury patients with refractory neurogenic detrusor overactivity.** *Int Braz J Urol* 2010, **36**(6):732–737.
8. Faul F, Erdfelder E, Lang AG, Buchner A: **G*Power 3: a flexible statistical power analysis program for the social, behavioral, and biomedical sciences.** *Behav Res Methods* 2007, **39**(2):175–191.
9. Abrams P, Cardozo L, Fall M, Griffiths D, Rosier P, Ulmsten U, Van Kerrebroeck P, Victor A, Wein A: **The standardisation of terminology in lower urinary tract function: report from the standardisation sub-committee of the International Continence Society.** *Urology* 2003, **61**(1):37–49.
10. Karsenty G, Denys P, Amarenco G, De SM, Game X, Haab F, Kerdraon J, Perrouin-Verbe B, Ruffion A, Saussine C, Soler JM, Schurch B, Chartier-Kastler E: **Botulinum toxin A (Botox) intradetrusor injections in adults with neurogenic detrusor overactivity/neurogenic overactive bladder: a systematic literature review.** *Eur Urol* 2008, **53**(2):275–287.
11. Smaldone MC, Ristau BT, Leng WW: **Botulinum toxin therapy for neurogenic detrusor overactivity.** *Urol Clin North Am* 2010, **37**(4):567–580.
12. Ginsberg D, Gousse A, Keppenne V, Sievert KD, Thompson C, Lam W, Brin MF, Jenkins B, Haag-Molkenteller C: **Phase 3 efficacy and tolerability study of onabotulinumtoxinA for urinary incontinence from neurogenic detrusor overactivity.** *J Urol* 2012, **187**(6):2131–2139.
13. Del PG, Filocamo MT, Li M, V, Macchiarella A, Cecconi F, Lombardi G, Nicita G: **Neurogenic detrusor overactivity treated with english botulinum toxin a: 8-year experience of one single centre.** *Eur Urol* 2008, **53**(5):1013–1019.
14. Gomes CM, de Castro Filho JE, Rejowski RF, Trigo-Rocha FE, Bruschini H, de Barros Filho TE, Srougi M: **Experience with different botulinum toxins for the treatment of refractory neurogenic detrusor overactivity.** *Int Braz J Urol* 2010, **36**(1):66–74.
15. Haferkamp A, Dorsam J, Resnick NM, Yalla SV, Elbadawi A: **Structural basis of neurogenic bladder dysfunction. III. Intrinsic detrusor innervation.** *J Urol* 2003, **169**(2):555–562.
16. Haferkamp A, Dorsam J, Resnick NM, Yalla SV, Elbadawi A: **Structural basis of neurogenic bladder dysfunction. II. Myogenic basis of detrusor hyperreflexia.** *J Urol* 2003, **169**(2):547–554.
17. Klaphajone J, Kitisomprayoonkul W, Sriplakit S: **Botulinum toxin type A injections for treating neurogenic detrusor overactivity combined with low-compliance bladder in patients with spinal cord lesions.** *Arch Phys Med Rehabil* 2005, **86**(11):2114–2118.

15

miR-221 facilitates the TGFbeta1-induced epithelial-mesenchymal transition in human bladder cancer cells by targeting STMN1

Jun Liu, Jian Cao and Xiaokun Zhao*

Abstract

Background: Distant metastasis is the major cause of cancer-related death, and epithelial-to-mesenchymal transition (EMT) has a critical role in this process. Accumulating evidence indicates that EMT can be regulated by microRNAs (miRNAs). miR-221, as oncogenes in several human cancers, was significantly up-regulated in bladder cancers. However, the role of miR-221 in the progression of bladder cancer metastasis remains largely unknown.

Methods: We used qRT-PCR and western blot to accurately measure the levels of miR-221, STMN1 and EMT markers in TGFβ1 induced EMT of bladder cancer cells. miR-221 inhibitors were re-introduced into bladder cancer cells to investigate its role on tumor metastasis which was measured by MTT, wound healing, transwell invasion and adherent assays. Luciferase reporter assay was used to reveal the target gene of miR-221.

Results: miR-221 expression was greatly increased by TGFβ1 in bladder cancer cell. miR-221 inhibition reversed TGFβ1 induced EMT by sharply increasing the expression of the epithelial marker E-cadherin and decreasing the expression of the mesenchymal markers vimentin, Fibroactin and N-cadherin. Furthermore, miR-221 expression is positively correlated with malignant potential of bladder cancer cell through promoting loss of cell adhesion and prometastatic behavior. Luciferase reporter assay revealed that miR-221 negatively regulates STMN1 expression by direct targeting to the 3'UTR region of STMN1.

Conclusions: Our study demonstrated that miR-221 facilitated TGFβ1-induced EMT in human bladder cancer cells by targeting STMN1 and represented a promising therapeutic target in the process of metastasis.

Keywords: miR-221, Bladder cancer, EMT, STMN1, TGFβ1

Background

Bladder cancer is one of the most common worldwide malignancies. In developed countries, bladder cancer (BC) is the fifth most commonly diagnosed tumor and the second most common cause of death among genitourinary tumours [1]. So it is urgent to understand the molecular and cellular mechanisms of metastasis for investigating the development of bladder cancer. Currently, there is a theory considering Epithelial–Mesenchymal Transition (EMT) as the first step of metastasis [2]. Previous studies showed that EMT was a complex and reversible process initiated by specific substances so that epithelial cells gain mesenchymal characteristics in cervical and breast cancers [3-6]. Recent advances have fostered a more detailed understanding of molecular mechanisms and networks governing EMT in tumor progression [7]. Although several growth factors participate in EMT, TGFβ is the most studied. Upon TGFβ1 treatment, epithelial cell changed from a cuboidal to an elongated spindle shape with enhanced expressions of Snail1 & Twist1 and subsequently decreased expression of E-cadherin [8]. Accumulating studies showed that TGFβ could consequently promote cancer progression through the induction of EMT, during which tumor cells become more invasive and metastatic [9]. However, whether miRNA are involved in regulating TGFβ -induced EMT in BC remains obscure.

MicroRNA (miRNA), a class of naturally occurring, 17–25 nucleotide small noncoding small RNA, regulates the expression of genes through binding to the 3′ untranslated

* Correspondence: xiaokunzhao2014@163.com
Department of Urology, 2nd xiangya Hospital, Central South University, NO.139 Middle Renmin Road, 410011 Changsha, Hunan, China

regions (3′ UTR) of target mRNAs. Recently, growing evidence suggests that aberrant expression of microRNAs (miRNAs) is a common phenomenon in bladder cancer and miRNAs can be key players in diverse physiological and pathological processes, such as embryonic development, tumorigenesis, metastasis, metabolism and apoptosis [10]. Recently, miRNAs have also been demonstrated to be involved in the process of epithelial–mesenchymal transition (EMT) by modulation of EMT-related genes [11]. MiR-7 reverses the EMT of breast cancer stem cells by downregulating the STAT3 pathway [12]. MicroRNA-451 induces EMT in docetaxel-resistant lung adenocarcinoma cells by targeting proto-oncogene c-Myc [13]. More interestingly, a recent study has shown that miRNA192 were upregulated by TGF- β 1 in mouse mesangial cells, and miRNA192 plays a pivotal role in diabetic nephropathy, mediated via controlling TGF-β1-induced collagen I expression by downregulating E-box repressors [14]. miRNA-200 and miRNA-205 were downregulated during TGF β mediated EMT and regulated EMT by targeting the E-cadherin transcriptional repressors ZEB1 and SIP1[15].

miR-221 has been shown to participate in both the onset and progression of various malignant tumors, including ovarian cancer [16,17]. For example, Qin J demonstrated that miR-221 is an oncogenic miRNA and regulates CRC migration and invasion through targeting reversion-inducing cysteine-rich protein with Kazal motifs (RECK) [18]. miR-221 is a critical modulator in the Hepatocellular carcinoma signaling pathway, and miR-221 silencing inhibits liver cancer malignant properties in vitro and in vivo [19]. Recent studies showed that Human microRNAs miR-221 was significantly up-regulated in bladder cancers [20]. Lu et al. revealed that miR-221 was significantly up-regulated in bladder cancer and miR-221 silencing predisposed T24 cells to undergo apoptosis induced by TRAIL [21]. However, to the best of our knowledge, the specific role of miR-221 in the TGFβ1-induced EMT in bladder cancer and the mechanisms underlying its effects remain unknown. Because EMT is of particular significance as a marker of tumor invasion and metastasis and TGFβ1 treatment represents a classical induction approach for in vitro EMT research, we believe that elaborating both the specific roles of miR-221 in TGFβ1-induced EMT models of bladder cancer and the latent molecular mechanisms will enlarge our theoretical understanding of human bladder cancer and provide future clinical approaches to treating this disease.

Methods

Cell culture and TGFβ1 treatment

Human bladder cancer cell lines (RT4 and T24) (Shanghai Cell Bank, China) were propagated in DMEM (Invitrogen) supplemented with 10% FCS at 37°C in 5% CO_2 cell culture incubator. In the TGFβ1 (Sigma Aldrich, St. Louis, MO) treatment, the cells were serum starved overnight and treated with 2.5 ng/ml TGFβ1 for 24 hours. The medium containing TGFβ1 was replaced every 24 hours (The Clinical Research Ethics Committee of Central South University approved the research protocols, and written informed consent was obtained from the participants).

microRNA and transient transfection

miR-221 mimics, control mimics, miR-221 inhibitors, and control inhibitors were purchased from RiboBio (Guangzhou, China). RT4 and T24 cells were seeded into 6-well plates until 50%–60% confluent and then transiently transfected with 60 nM control or miR-221 mimics or with 120 nM control or miR-221 inhibitors using the X-treme GENE siRNA Transfection Reagent (Roche, Indianapolis, IN, USA) according to the manufacturer's instructions. After 48 hours of miRNA transfection, the cells were harvested for further study.

Quantitative real-time PCR

Total RNA was isolated using TRIzol reagent (Invitrogen, Carlsbad, CA, USA) according to the manufacturer's recommendations. For mRNA detection, first-strand cDNA was synthesized using a PrimeScript RT reagent kit (Perfect Real Time; Takara, Dalian, China). Quantitative real-time PCR was performed using a SYBR Premix Ex Taq™ II kit (Takara, Dalian, China) on a CFX96 real-time PCR system (Bio- Rad, Hercules, CA, USA). The PCR conditions were as follows: 95°C for 30 s, followed by 40 cycles of 95°C for 5 s and 60°C for 34 s. β-Actin was used as an internal control to normalize the results. For miRNA detection, miR-221 levels were determined using a TaqMan microRNA kit (Applied Biosystems) and normalized to small nuclear RNA (Rnu6), which served as a control; the data were expressed as the log 2 fold change in respective miR/U6 snRNA levels. Primers for miR-221 and U6 reverse transcription and amplification were designed by and purchased from RiboBio Co., Ltd. (Guangzhou, China).

Western blot analysis

Whole cell extracts were prepared with a cell lysis reagent (Sigma-Aldrich, St. Louis, MO, USA) according to the manual, and then, the protein was quantified by a BCA assay (Pierce, Rockford, IL, USA). Then, the protein samples were separated by SDS-PAGE (10%) and detected by Western blot using polyclonal (rabbit) anti-STMN1, anti-Fibroactin, anti-N-Cadherin, anti-E-Cadherin and anti-Vimentin antibody (Santa Cruz Bio-technology, Santa Cruz, CA, USA, 1:1000). Goat anti-rabbit IgG (Pierce, Rockford, IL, USA) secondary antibody conjugated to horseradish peroxidase and ECL detection systems (SuperSignal West Femto, Pierce) were used for detection.

Cell survival assay

The 3-(4,5-dimethylthiazal-2-yl)-2,5-diphenyl-tetrazolium bromide (MTT) assay was used to estimate cell viability [22]. Briefly, cells were plated at a density of 1×10^4 cells per well in 96-well plates. After exposure to specific treatment, the cells were incubated with MTT at a final concentration of 0.5 mg/ml for 4 h at 37°C. After the removal of the medium, 150 mM DMSO solutions were added to dissolve the formazan crystals. The absorbance was read at 570 nm using a multi-well scanning spectrophotometer reader. Cells in the control group were considered 100% viable.

Invasion assay

Cells were cultivated to 80% confluence on the 12-well plates. Then, we observed the procedures of cellular growth at 24 h. All the experiments were repeated in triplicate. The transwell invasion chambers were used to evaluate cell invasion. Then cells invasing cells across the membrane were counted under a light microscope.

Adhesion assay

Cells were pretreated with or without different concentrations of excisanin A for 24 h. The cells were suspended in serum-free DMEM medium to form a single-cell suspension and were seeded into 96-well plates precoated with Matrigel™ (BD Biosciences, Franklin Lakes, NJ, USA). The wells were incubated at 37°C for 50 min and washed three times with PBS to remove the non-adherent cells. Cell viability was determined via the MTT assay described above.

Wound healing assay

For the wound healing assay, cells were seeded in 12-well plates and grown to 90% confluence. Monolayers in the center of the wells werescraped with pipette tips and washed with PBS. Subsequently, the cellswere cultured in serum-free DMEM medium in the absence or presenceof different concentrations of excisanin A for 24 h. Cell movement intothe wound area was monitored and photographed at 0 and 24 h usinga light microscope. The migration distance between the leading edge ofthe migrating cells and the edge of the wound was compared as previous work [23].

Luciferase reporter assay

HEK293 cells (1×10^4 cells/well) were plated in a 48-well plate and cotransfected with 50 n M of either miR-221 or microRNA control (miRcontrol), 20 ng of either pGL3-STMN1-3′-UTR-WT or pGL3-STMN1-3′-UTR-Mutation, and 2 ng of pRL-TK (Promega, Madison, WI, USA) using Lipofectamine TM 2000 (Invitrogen). The pRL-TK vector was cotransfected as an internal control to correct the differences in both transfection and harvest efficiencies. HEK293 cells were collected 48 h after transfection and assays were performed by using the dual luciferase reporter assay system (Promega).

Statistical analysis

All experiments were performed at least in triplicate, and each experiment was independently performed at least 3 times. Data are presented as the means ± standard deviation (SD) and were analyzed using SPSS 19.0. Statistical significance was assessed using the two-tailed unpaired Student's t-test. Differences were considered statistically significant when the P value was <0.05.

Results

MiR-221 and expression in TGFβ1-induced EMT

In preliminary experiments, we tested various TGFβ1 concentrations and incubation durations for their ability to induce EMT in RT4 and T24 cells. Based on these experiments, we determined the dose of 2.5 ng/ml and the duration of 24 hours as appropriate conditions for EMT stimulation by TGFβ1. To explore whether miR-221 is involved in TGFβ1-induced EMT in human bladder cancer cells, we first attempted to determine the expression level of miR-221 before/after TGFβ1 treatment. Surprisingly, compared with control group, miR-221 expression was significantly increased in both RT4 and T24 cells incubated with TGFβ1(Figure 1A). As shown in Figure 1B and C, STMN1 was significantly decreased by TGFβ1 treatment at both the mRNA and protein levels. These results suggested that miR-221 and STMN1 involved in TGFβ1-induced EMT of bladder cancer cells.

STMN1 is negatively regulated by MiR-221 in TGFβ1-induced EMT

We performed a bioinformatic analysis using mircoRNA.org and predicted that STMN1 was the possible target gene of miR-221. To confirm this speculation, 3′ UTR luciferase reporter assay was used in this study. As shown in Figure 2A, co-transfection of miR-221 suppressed the luciferase activity of the reporter containing wild-type STMN1 3′ UTR sequence, but failed to inhibit that of mutated STMN1 by dual-luciferase reporter assay. These result suggested that miR-221 directly binds to the STMN1 3′UTR. Furthermore, we employed miR-221 mimics and inhibitors to specifically overexpress and knock down the endogenous expression of miR-221 in RT4 and T24 cells. As shown in Figure 2B and C, STMN1 expression was significantly decreased by transfection with miR-221 mimics and was greatly increased by transfection with miR-221 inhibitors at both the mRNA and protein level. Therefore, miR-221 negatively regulates STMN1 expression in bladder cancer cells. Together, these results demonstrated that miR-221 directly binds to its complementary sequence motif in the STMN1 3′UTR, thus negatively regulating STMN1 expression.

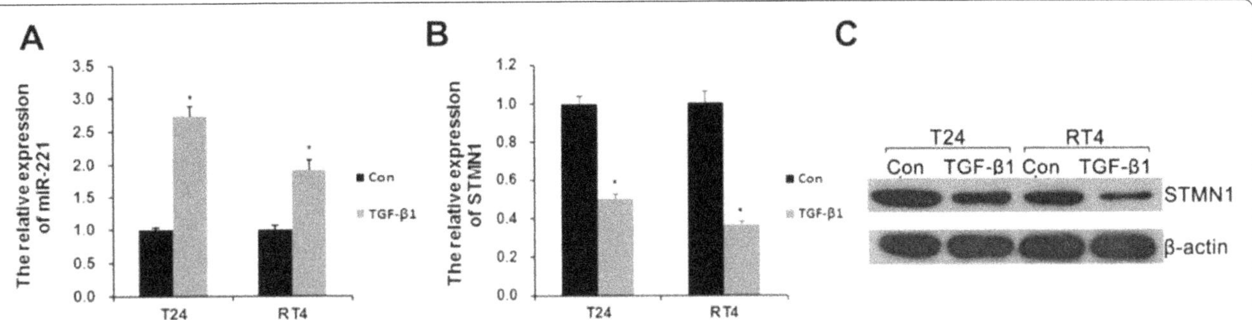

Figure 1 The expression level of miR-221 and STMN1 before/after TGFβ1 treatment. **A**, qRT-PCR analysis indicated miR-221 expression in TGFβ1-induced EMT in both RT4 and T24 cells. qRT-PCR analysis **(B)** and western blot analysis **(C)** indicated STMN1 expression in TGFβ1-induced EMT in both RT4 and T24 cells. Error bars represent ± S.E. and $^*p < 0.05$ versus control.

MiR-221 expression is positively correlated with malignant potential of bladder cancer cell

Enhanced cellular malignant capacity, including cell survival, migration and invasion abilities, is the functional hallmarks of an EMT process. Because incubation with TGFβ1 resulted in increasing miR-221 levels in both RT4 and T24 cells, we silenced miR-221 to test whether miR-221 is involved in motility changes in bladder cancer cells, aiming to examine the specific role of miR-221 in TGFβ1-induced EMT. The cell line RT4 and T24, which constitutively expresses high levels of miR-221, was transfected with miR-221 siRNA to knock down its endogenous miR-221 expression or with a scrambled siRNA as a control. As shown in Figure 3, MTT results showed that significantly increase of cell survival was observed in TGFβ1 group compared with control group and significantly attenuation of cell invasion was observed in TGFβ1 + anti-miR-221 group compared with TGFβ1 group and TGFβ1 + anti-Con group. These result indicated that TGFβ1 greatly promoted the cell survival in bladder cancer, and TGFβ1-induced cell survival was reversed by miR-221 inhibition.

Transwell invasion assay showed that significant increase of bladder cancer cell invasion was observed in TGFβ1 group compared with control group and significant attenuation of bladder cancer cell invasion was observed in TGFβ1 + anti-miR-221 group compared with TGFβ1 group and TGFβ1 + anti-Con group. These results indicated that TGFβ1-induced cell invasion was reversed by miR-221 inhibition (Figure 4). As shown by the representative images presented in Figure 5, wound healing generated results that were similar to those obtained using the transwell assay. The cell migration rates of cells in miR-221 inhibition groups were shown to be

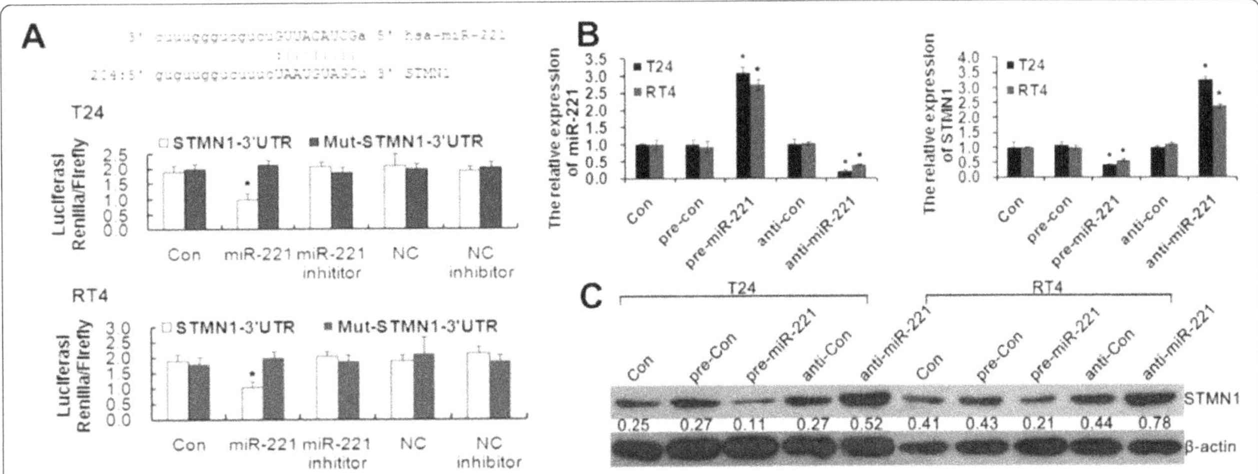

Figure 2 miR-221 negatively regulates STMN1 expression. **(A)** Luciferase reporter assay with co-transfection of wild-type or mutant STMN1 and miR-221 mimics or miR-221 inhibitor or negative–control or inhibitor negative-control or blank control in H9c2 cells. **(B)** qRT-PCR analyses were performed to examine the effects of miR-221 on expression of STMN1. **(C)** Western blotting was performed to determine effects of miR-221 on expression of STMN1 protein in T24 and RT4 cells. Error bars represent ± S.E. and $^*p < 0.01$ versus control.

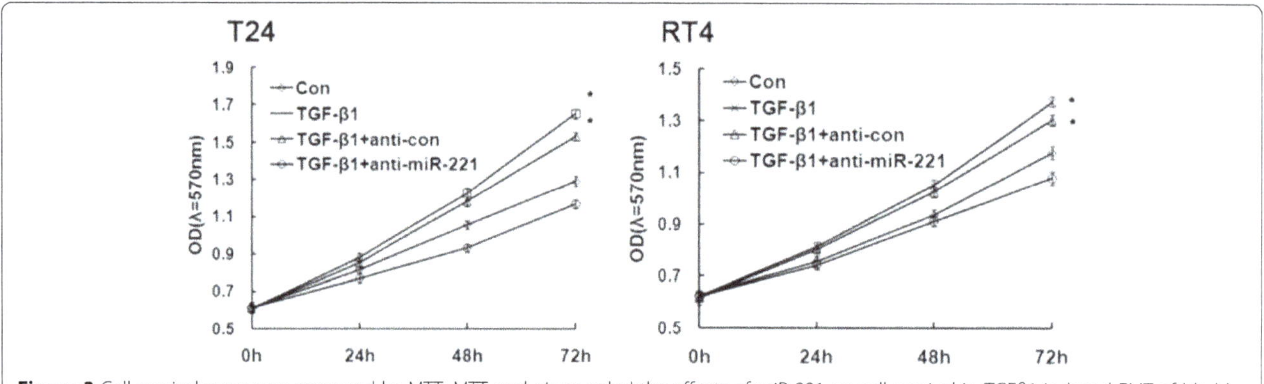

Figure 3 Cell survival curve was measured by MTT. MTT analysis revealed the effects of miR-221 on cell survival in TGFβ1-induced EMT of bladder cancer. Error bars represent ± S.E. and *p < 0.05 versus control.

significantly lower than control group, as evaluated using a wound-healing assay. In contrast, miR-221 inhibition decreased the migration and invasion of bladder cancer cells, perhaps through the reversal of EMT. In conclusion, miR-221 plays an important role in mediating the malignant potential of metastatic bladder cancer cells. In conclusion, these results demonstrated that miR-221 promoted the migration and invasion of bladder cancer cells, possibly through the induction of EMT. Cell adherent assay (Figure 6) generated results that were similar to those obtained using the transwell migration assay, suggesting that inhibition of miR-221 resulted in an attenuation of TGFβ1-induced invasion and adherent capacity.

MiR-221 inhibition attenuated TGFβ1-induced EMT in bladder cancer cells

To further assess the effects of miR-221 on TGFβ1-induced EMT, we transfected control and miR-221 inhibitor into T24 and RT4 cells, and then cells were treated with TGFβ1, and detected the effects of miR-221 on TGFβ1-induced EMT in bladder cancer cells. Western blotting analyses (Figure 7) showed that TGFβ1 treatment sharply decreased the expression of the epithelial marker E-cadherin and increased the expression of the mesenchymal markers vimentin, Fibroactin and N-cadherin. However, combination of miR-221 inhibition and TGFβ1 reversed the suppression of epithelial genes and the upregulated expression

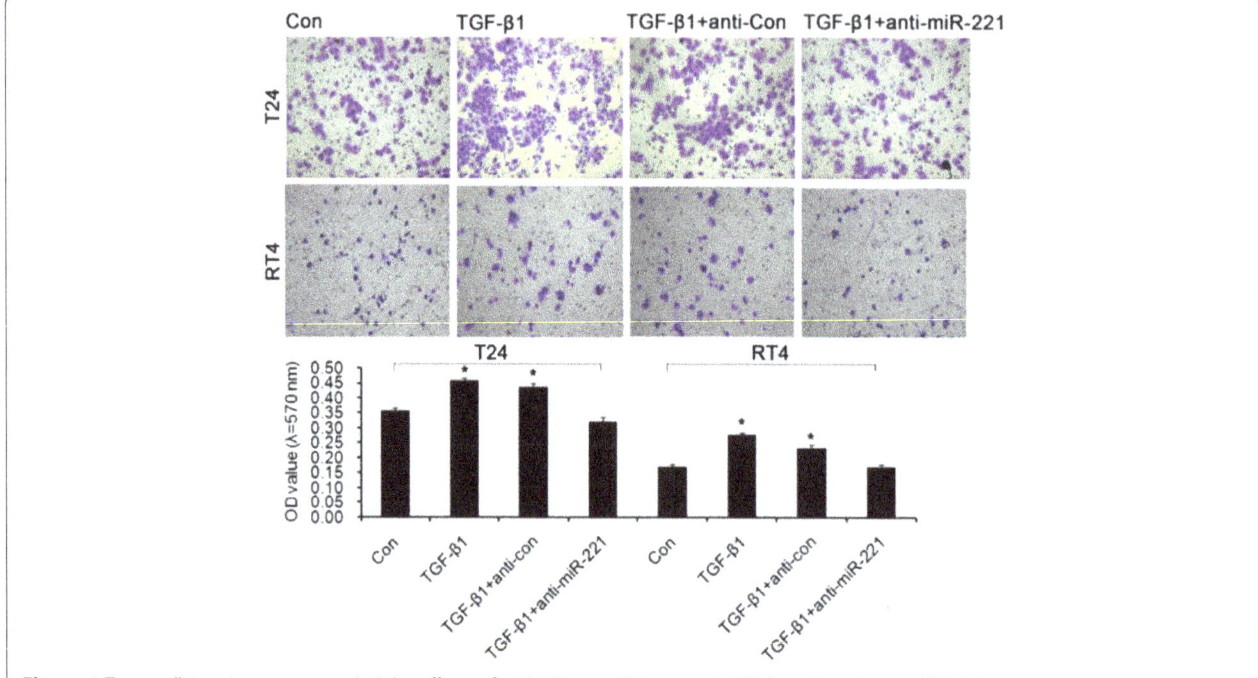

Figure 4 Transwell invasion assay revealed the effects of miR-221 on cell invasion in TGFβ1-induced EMT of bladder cancer. Error bars represent ± S.E. and *p < 0.05 versus control.

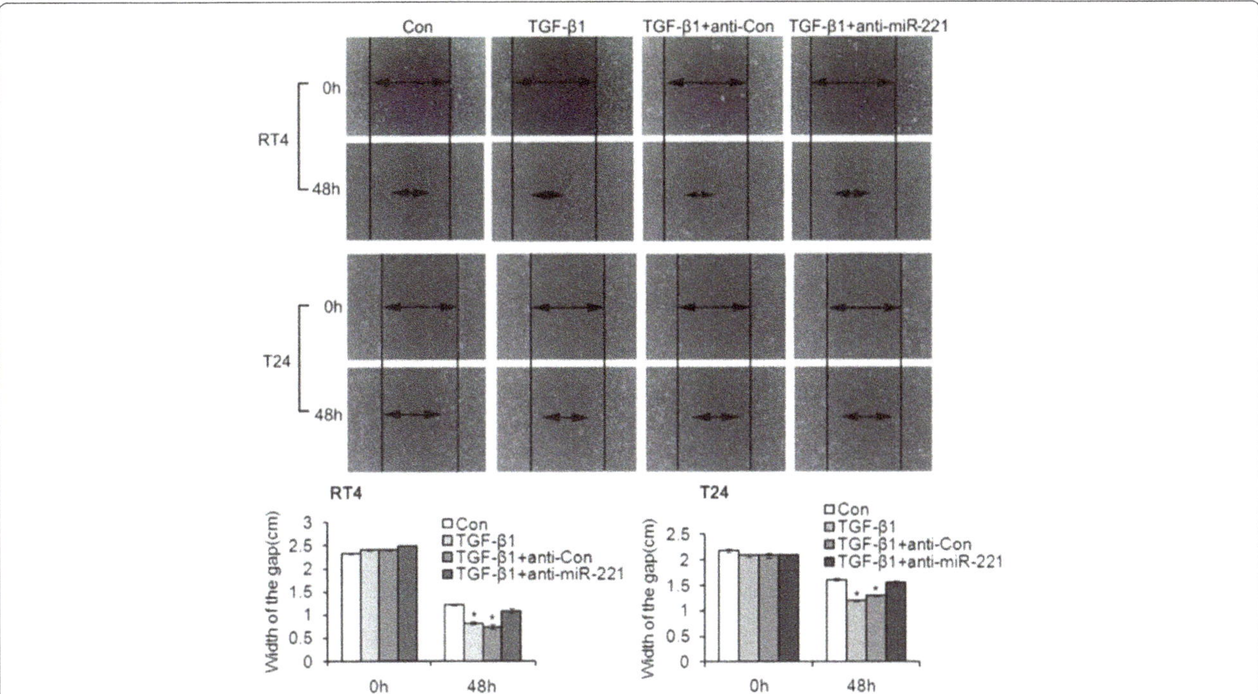

Figure 5 Wound healing assay revealed the effects of miR-221 on cell migration in TGFβ1-induced EMT of bladder cancer. Error bars represent ± S.E. and *p < 0.05 versus control.

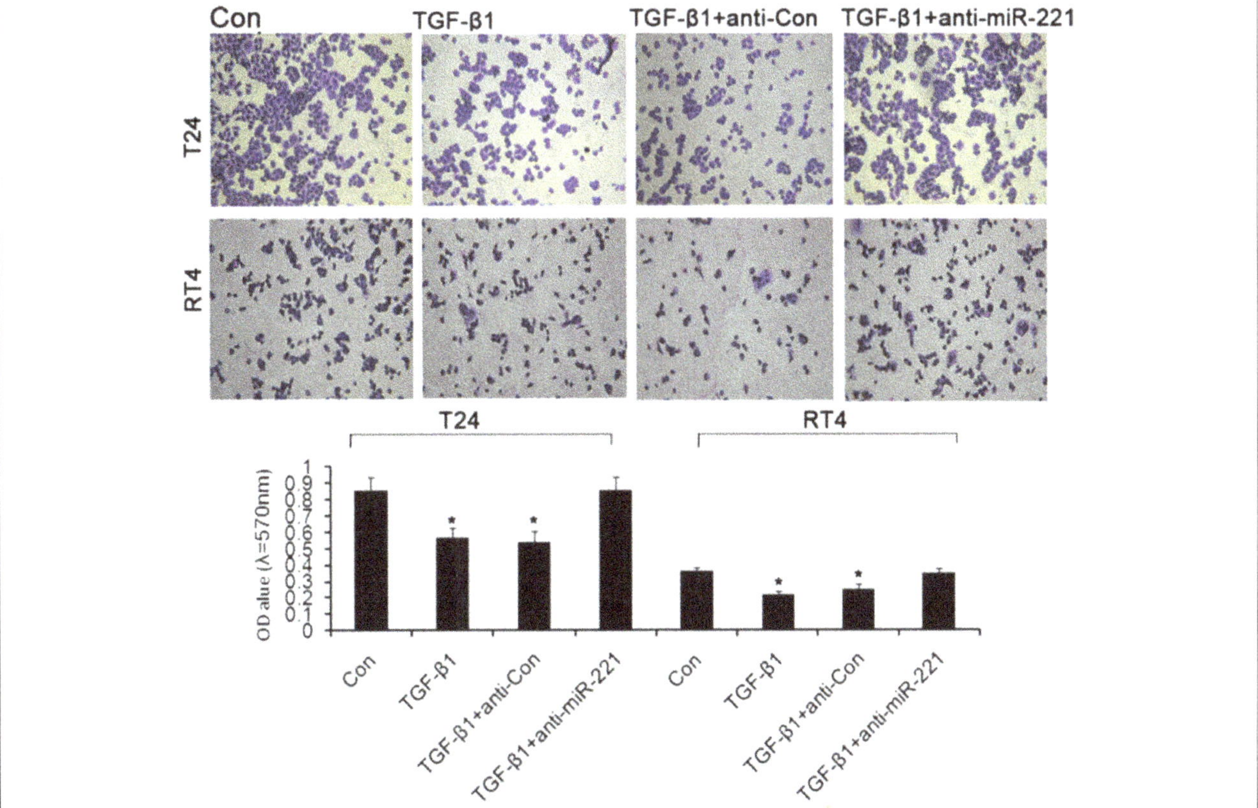

Figure 6 Adhesion assay revealed the effects of miR-221 on cell adhesion in TGFβ1-induced EMT of bladder cancer. Error bars represent ± S.E. and *p < 0.05 versus control.

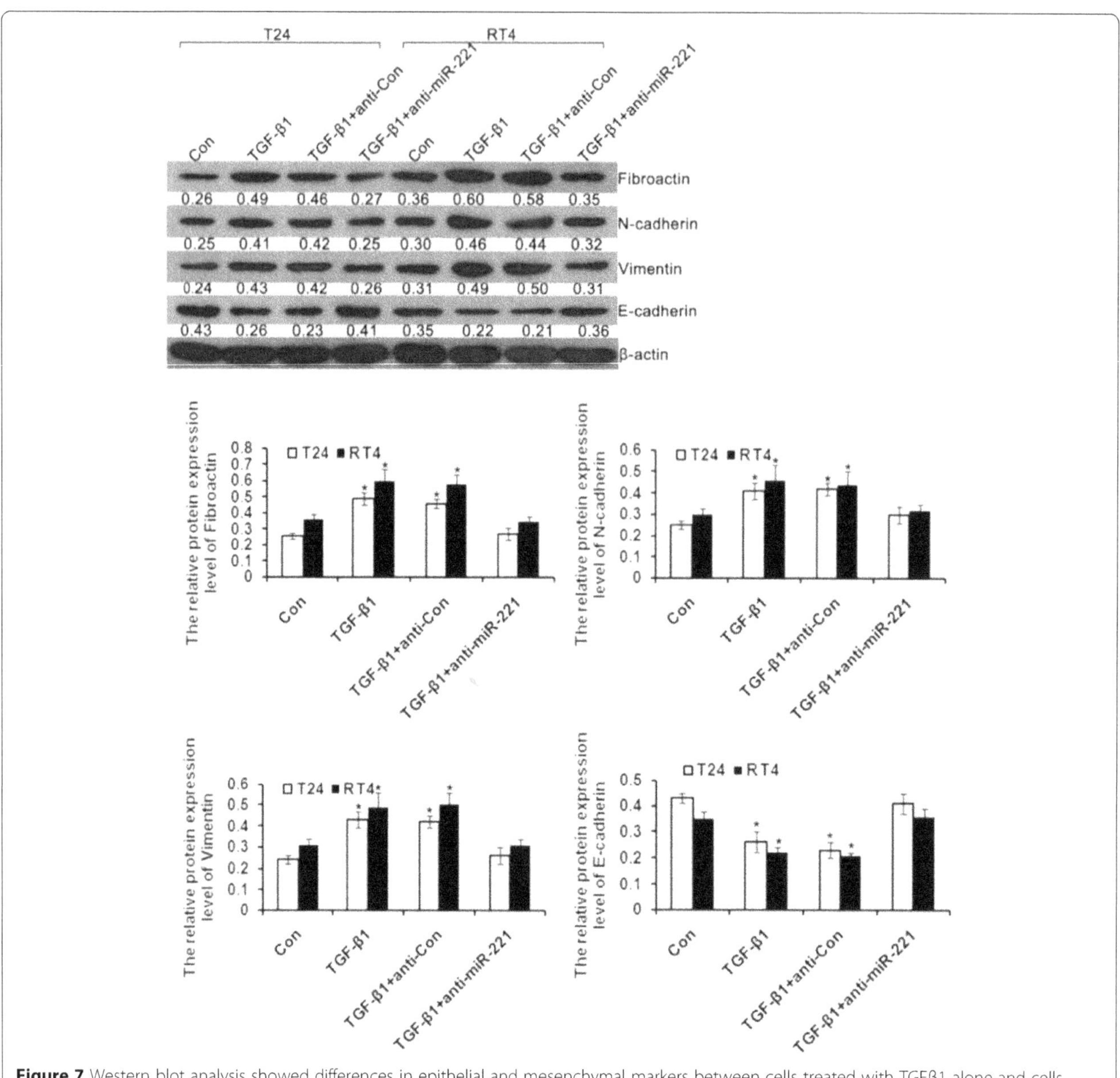

Figure 7 Western blot analysis showed differences in epithelial and mesenchymal markers between cells treated with TGFβ1 alone and cells treated with both TGFβ1 and miR-221 inhibitor. Error bars represent ± S.E. and *, $p < 0.05$ versus control.

of mesenchymal genes compared to treatment with TGFβ1 alone. In conclusion, miR-221 inhibition attenuated TGFβ1-induced EMT in bladder cancer cells.

Discussion

In the present study, we found that miR-221 expression is specifically upregulated in TGFβ1-responsive bladder cancer cells and contributes significantly to the development of the EMT phenotype. The EMT is characterized by changes in morphology, the loss of intercellular junctions, increased motility, decreased proliferation, and alterations in gene expression. Our study demonstrated that miR-221 knockdown inhibits these TGFβ1-induced changes. Similarly to our observations, miR-221 is also found to promote EMT in other types of human cancer cells, such as breast cancer cells [24,25]. Taken together, these findings confirm the involvement of miR-221 in TGFβ1-mediated EMT. Moreover, dysregulation of miR-221 is frequently found in various human cancers, including ovarian cancer, prostate cancer, endometrial cancer, and breast cancer, and is associated with features of cancerous progression and metastasis [23]. In our study, miR-221 inhibition decreased cell survival, migration and invasion capacities and enhanced adhesion capacities in bladder cancer cells. In conclusion, these results demonstrated that the expression of miR-221 is positively correlated with bladder cancer cell metastasis and further corroborate the connection between miR-221 expression and EMT features in human bladder cancer cells. Therefore, targeting miR-221 might represent a feasible and attractive option for the future clinical treatment and prevention of human bladder cancer.

Recently, accumulating evidence indicated that miRNAs play key roles in carcinogenesis by modulating gene expression on posttranscriptional level. Our data further support this conclusion that upregulated miR-221 suppressed expression of STMN1 in bladder cancer cells, further promoted the progressive and metastatic potential of human bladder cancer. The microtubule-destabilising protein, stathmin 1/oncoprotein 18 (STMN1), has an important role during mitosis, influencing cell cycle progression [26,27]. In addition, STMN1, as an oncoprotein, is involved in tumour metastasis, cell invasion and migration [28-30] and is a considered therapeutic cancer target [31]. Recently, Williams K, et al showed that inactivation of STMN1 is key to promoting oncogenesis and EMT [32]. loss-of-STMN1 compromises cell-cell adhesion, which is followed by EMT, increased cell migration, and metastasis via cooperative activation of p38 and through TGF-β1-independent and -dependent mechanisms [32]. In this study, STMN1 was downregulated by TGFβ1 in bladder cancer. By employing the Dual Luciferase Reporter Assay System, we report for the first time that miR-221 suppressed STMN1 expression by targeting STMN1 3′UTR in bladder cancer. Collectively, these findings confirm that miR-221 plays a significant role in cancer development and progression by directly targeting STMN1.

Conclusion

Taken together, our findings demonstrate for the first time that miR-221 can facilitate the TGFβ1-induced EMT process in human bladder cancer cells by suppressing STMN1. Moreover, miR-221 levels are also correlated with pathological mesenchymal behaviors, such as decreased cell adherent capacity and increased cell survival, migration and invasion in human bladder cancer cells. Further studies targeting STMN1 and the mechanism of miR-221 regulation by TGFβ1 induction will provide promising and feasible options for the treatment and prevention of human bladder cancer.

Abbreviations

TGFβ1: Transforming growth factor beta 1; STMN1: Stathmin 1; EMT: Epithelial-to-mesenchymal transition; BC: Bladder cancer.

Competing interests

The authors declare that they have no competing interests.

Authors' contributions

XZ conceived the project; JL designed the experiments and carried out the majority of the experiments; JC helped to culture cells; all authors discussed the results; JL and XZ wrote the manuscript. All authors read and approved the final manuscript.

References

1. Parkin DM. The global burden of urinary bladder cancer. Scand J Urol Nephrol Suppl. 2008;218:12–20.
2. Chaffer CL, Weinberg RA. A perspective on cancer cell metastasis. Science. 2011;331(6024):1559–64.
3. Ha GH, Kim JL, Breuer EK. TACC3 is essential for EGF-mediated EMT in cervical cancer. PLoS One. 2013;8(8):e70353.
4. Creighton CJ, Chang JC, Rosen JM. Epithelial-mesenchymal transition (EMT) in tumor-initiating cells and its clinical implications in breast cancer. J Mammary Gland Biol Neoplasia. 2010;15(2):253–60.
5. Cheng R, Sun B, Liu Z, Zhao X, Qi L, Li Y, et al. Wnt5a suppresses colon cancer by inhibiting cell proliferation and epithelial-mesenchymal transition. J Cell Physiol. 2014;229(12):1908–17.
6. Nauseef JT, Henry MD. Epithelial-to-mesenchymal transition in prostate cancer: paradigm or puzzle? Nat Rev Urol. 2011;8(8):428–39.
7. Huber MA, Kraut N, Beug H. Molecular requirements for epithelial-mesenchymal transition during tumor progression. Curr Opin Cell Biol. 2005;17(5):548–58.
8. Zavadil J, Bottinger EP. TGF-beta and epithelial-to-mesenchymal transitions. Oncogene. 2005;24(37):5764–74.
9. Levy L, Hill CS. Alterations in components of the TGF-beta superfamily signaling pathways in human cancer. Cytokine Growth Factor Rev. 2006;17(1-2):41–58.
10. Itesako T, Seki N, Yoshino H, Chiyomaru T, Yamasaki T, Hidaka H, et al. The microRNA expression signature of bladder cancer by deep sequencing: the functional significance of the miR-195/497 cluster. Plos One. 2014;9(2):e84311.
11. Hu Y, Tang H. MicroRNAs regulate the epithelial to mesenchymal transition (EMT) in cancer progression. MicroRNA. 2014;3(2):108–17.
12. Zhang H, Cai K, Wang J, Wang X, Cheng K, Shi F, et al. MiR-7, inhibited indirectly by LincRNA HOTAIR, directly inhibits SETDB1 and reverses the EMT of breast cancer stem cells by downregulating the STAT3 pathway. Stem Cells. 2014;32(11):2858–68.
13. Chen D, Huang J, Zhang K, Pan B, Chen J, De W, et al. MicroRNA-451 induces epithelial-mesenchymal transition in docetaxel-resistant lung adenocarcinoma cells by targeting proto-oncogene c-Myc. Eur J Cancer. 2014;50(17):3050–67.
14. Kato M, Zhang J, Wang M, Lanting L, Yuan H, Rossi JJ, et al. MicroRNA-192 in diabetic kidney glomeruli and its function in TGF-beta-induced collagen expression via inhibition of E-box repressors. Proc Natl Acad Sci U S A. 2007;104(9):3432–7.
15. Gregory PA, Bert AG, Paterson EL, Barry SC, Tsykin A, Farshid G, et al. The miR-200 family and miR-205 regulate epithelial to mesenchymal transition by targeting ZEB1 and SIP1. Nat Cell Biol. 2008;10(5):593–601.
16. Sun T, Wang X, He HH, Sweeney CJ, Liu SX, Brown M, et al. MiR-221 promotes the development of androgen independence in prostate cancer cells via downregulation of HECTD2 and RAB1A. Oncogene. 2014;33(21):2790–800.
17. Dentelli P, Traversa M, Rosso A, Togliatto G, Olgasi C, Marchio C, et al. miR-221/222 control luminal breast cancer tumor progression by regulating different targets. Cell Cycle. 2014;13(11):1811–26.
18. Qin J, Luo M. MicroRNA-221 promotes colorectal cancer cell invasion and metastasis by targeting RECK. FEBS Lett. 2014;588(1):99–104.
19. He XX, Guo AY, Xu CR, Chang Y, Xiang GY, Gong J, et al. Bioinformatics analysis identifies miR-221 as a core regulator in hepatocellular carcinoma and its silencing suppresses tumor properties. Oncol Rep. 2014;32(3):1200–10.
20. Gottardo F, Liu CG, Ferracin M, Calin GA, Fassan M, Bassi P, et al. Micro-RNA profiling in kidney and bladder cancers. Urol Oncol. 2007;25(5):387–92.
21. Lu Q, Lu C, Zhou GP, Zhang W, Xiao H, Wang XR. MicroRNA-221 silencing predisposed human bladder cancer cells to undergo apoptosis induced by TRAIL. Urol Oncol. 2010;28(6):635–41.
22. Liu B, Che W, Xue J, Zheng C, Tang K, Zhang J, et al. SIRT4 prevents hypoxia-induced apoptosis in H9c2 cardiomyoblast cells. Cell Physiol Biochem. 2013;32(3):655–62.
23. Liang CC, Park AY, Guan JL. In vitro scratch assay: a convenient and inexpensive method for analysis of cell migration in vitro. Nat Protoc. 2007;2(2):329–33.
24. Hwang MS, Yu N, Stinson SY, Yue P, Newman RJ, Allan BB, et al. miR-221/222 targets adiponectin receptor 1 to promote the epithelial-to-mesenchymal transition in breast cancer. PLoS One. 2013;8(6):e66502.
25. Stinson S, Lackner MR, Adai AT, Yu N, Kim HJ, O'Brien C, et al. miR-221/222 targeting of trichorhinophalangeal 1 (TRPS1) promotes epithelial-to-mesenchymal transition in breast cancer. Sci Signal. 2011;4(186):t5.

26. Baldassarre G, Belletti B, Nicoloso MS, Schiappacassi M, Vecchione A, Spessotto P, et al. p27(Kip1)-stathmin interaction influences sarcoma cell migration and invasion. Cancer Cell. 2005;7(1):51–63.
27. Rana S, Maples PB, Senzer N, Nemunaitis J. Stathmin 1: a novel therapeutic target for anticancer activity. Expert Rev Anticancer Ther. 2008;8(9):1461–70.
28. Akhtar J, Wang Z, Yu C, Li CS, Shi YL, Liu HJ. STMN-1 is a potential marker of lymph node metastasis in distal esophageal adenocarcinomas and silencing its expression can reverse malignant phenotype of tumor cells. BMC Cancer. 2014;14:28.
29. Byrne FL, Yang L, Phillips PA, Hansford LM, Fletcher JI, Ormandy CJ, et al. RNAi-mediated stathmin suppression reduces lung metastasis in an orthotopic neuroblastoma mouse model. Oncogene. 2014;33(7):882–90.
30. Hsu HP, Li CF, Lee SW, Wu WR, Chen TJ, Chang KY, et al. Overexpression of stathmin 1 confers an independent prognostic indicator in nasopharyngeal carcinoma. Tumour Biol. 2014;35(3):2619–29.
31. Nemunaitis J. Stathmin 1: a protein with many tasks. New biomarker and potential target in cancer. Expert Opin Ther Targets. 2012;16(7):631–4.
32. Williams K, Ghosh R, Giridhar PV, Gu G, Case T, Belcher SM, et al. Inhibition of stathmin1 accelerates the metastatic process. Cancer Res. 2012;72(20):5407–17.

16

Histologic and functional outcomes of small intestine submucosa-regenerated bladder tissue

Yiming Wang[1,2] and Limin Liao[1,2*]

Abstract

Background: Intestinal bladder augmentation has more disadvantages. One of the most promising alternative methods is tissue engineering in combination with surgical construction. Small intestine submucosa (SIS) is commonly used materials in tissue engineer. The aim of this study is determine the histologic and functional characteristics of SIS as bladder wall replacement in a rabbit augmentation model.

Methods: 18 New Zealand adult male rabbits, weight 2.5 ± 0.5Kg, were used in this study. The rabbits were divided into 3 groups of 6 based on the number of days post-operative (A, 4 weeks; B, 12 weeks; C, 24 weeks). All of the animals underwent urodynamic testing under anesthesia before cystoplasty with SIS patch. The cystometrograms were repeated 4, 12, and 24 weeks after surgery with the same method. SIS-regenerated bladder strips (10 × 3 × 3 mm) and normal bladder strips (10 × 3 × 3 mm) from the same bladder were obtained at 4, 12, and 24 weeks for in vitro detrusor strip study. The frequency and amplitude of the strip over 15 min was recorded. The regenerated tissue and normal tissue underwent histologic and immunocytochemical analysis. The results were quantified as optical density (OD) values.

Results: Histologically, the SIS-regenerated bladders of group C (24 weeks post-operation) resembled normal bladder in that all 3 layers (mucosa with submucosa, smooth muscle, and serosa) were present. In the in vitro detrusor strip study, there were no significant differences in autorhythmicity and contractility between regenerated and normal tissues in group C ($p > 0.05$). Immunohistochemical analysis indicated that the quantity of A-actin grew to a normal level. Urodynamic testing showed that compliance remained stable in all groups post-operatively, and the volume increased 24 weeks post-operatively.

Conclusion: Regenerated tissue has similar histologic and functional characteristics. SIS seems to be a viable material in the reconstruction of the rabbit urinary bladder.

Keywords: Small intestine submucosa, Regenerated bladder, Bladder augmentation, Urodynamics

Background

Bladder augmentation is used to reduce the high bladder pressure that develops in patients with neurogenic bladder to protect the upper urinary system [1]. Gastrointestinal segment augmentation cystoplasty is associated with a number of complications, such as mucus production, stone formation, leakage and rupture, fibrosis, electrolyte imbalance, and development of bowel obstruction. [2,3]. All of these complications, which adversely affect the quality of life, give patients pause when offered a renal rescue operation. In view of these disadvantages, alternative patches have been investigated [4]. One of the most promising alternative methods is tissue engineering in combination with surgical construction [5-7].

Small intestine submucosa (SIS) is an acellular, non-immunogenic, biodegradable, xenogeneic, collagen-based material that is derived from the submucosal layer of porcine small intestine [8]. SIS has demonstrated regenerative capacities in multiple organ systems, including the aorta, vena cava, ligaments, tendons, abdominal wall, and skin [9,10]. The aim of our study was to determine the functional and histologic characteristics of SIS (Cook-SIS

* Correspondence: lmliao@263.net
[1]Department of Urology, China Rehabilitation Research Center, 10 Jiaomen Beilu, Beijing 100068, Fentai District, China
[2]Department of Urology of Capital Medical University, Center of Neural Injury and Repair, Beijing Institute for Brain Disorders, 10 Youanmenwai Xitoutiao, Beijing 100069, Fentai District, China

Technology, [Indiana, USA]) as bladder wall replacement in a rabbit augmentation model.

Methods

After approval of the ethics committee of the China Rehabilitation Research Center, 18 New Zealand adult male rabbits, weight 2.5 ± 0.5 Kg, were used in this study. All the animals were in good health. The rabbits were divided into 3 groups of 6 based on the number of days post-operative (A, 4 weeks; B, 12 weeks; C, 24 weeks). The abdominal regions of the rabbits were shaved after anesthesia with 2% phenobarbital (30 mg/kg). The abdomen was opened through a midline incision and the bladder was exposed. The anterior wall of the bladder was opened longitudinally through a 3-cm incision in the midline of the bladder body. The SIS patch (1.0 × 2.0 cm) was grafted onto the host bladder with a 5/0 vicryl interrupted suture (Figure 1a). Four 5/0 silk marking stitches were placed outside the bladder wall near the corners of the patch. Perivesical fat was fixed over the bladder wall to cover the graft and the abdominal wall was closed anatomically. A single dose of ceftriaxone was administered (500 mg intramuscular). Neither urinary diversion nor urethral catheterization was used. The rabbits were housed and fed in separate cages.

Urodynamic test

All of the animals underwent urodynamic testing under anesthesia with 2% Phenobarbital (30 mg/kg) before cystoplasty. Cystometrograms (CMGs) were carried out with a 5 F double-lumen urodynamic catheter placed through the urethra and a continuous infusion (10 ml/min) of sterile saline via the catheter. The saline infusion was stopped at the first sign of overflow incontinence. Then the CMGs were repeated twice, the averaged maximal capacity was recorded. Bladder compliance was calculated as the change in volume divided by the change in pressure. The CMGs were repeated 4, 12, and 24 weeks after surgery with the same method. Data are expressed as the mean ± standard error of the mean.

In vitro detrusor strip study

The entire bladder was removed post-operatively after CMGs at 4, 12, and 24 weeks and placed in Krebs solution continually bubbled with 95% O_2 and 5% CO_2. This solution contained the following compounds in g/L: NaCl, 6.92; KCl, 0.35; KH_2PO_4, 0.16; $MgSO_4.7H_2O$, 0.29; $NaHCO_3$, 2.1; $CaCl_2$, 0.35; and glucose, 2.0. SIS-regenerated bladder strips (10 × 3 × 3 mm) and normal bladder strips (10 × 3 × 3 mm) from the same bladder were obtained. Silk ligatures were used to mount the

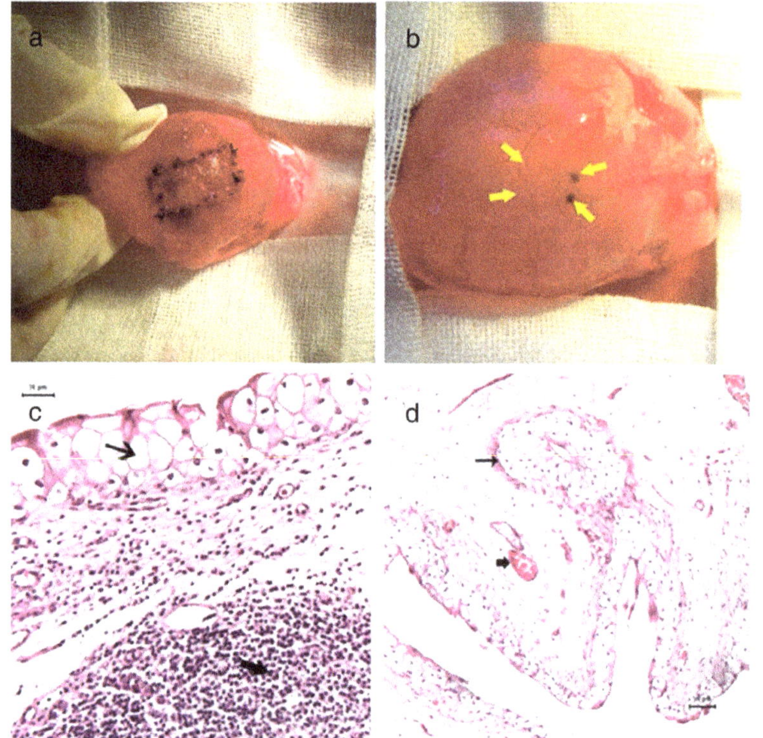

Figure 1 Macroscopic and HE evaluation. a. The SIS patch (1.0 × 2.0 cm) was already grafted onto the host bladder. **b**. Regenerated tissue in the arrows 24 weeks post-operation. **c**. Thin arrow marked the regenerated transitional epithelium in the region of the SIS graft. Coarse arrow marked the infiltrated inflammatory cells (×20). **d**. Thin arrow marked the regenerated transitional epithelium. Coarse arrow marked the new vessels (×10).

strips vertically between two suspension clasps in organ bath chambers. The tissue was continually immersed in Krebs solution at 37°C. Tension on the strips was measured using a force-displacement transducer. Tension (1 g) was applied to the strips. The frequency and amplitude of the strip over 15 min was recorded. Data are expressed as the mean ± standard error of the mean.

Histologic and immunocytochemical analyses

As controls for each rabbit, a full thickness bladder fragment was excised distal from the grafted area. Formalin-fixed specimens from the grafted and normal areas of the bladder were embedded in paraffin. Five μm sections were cut and stained with hematoxylin and eosin (HE). A-actin (BIOSS Inc., Massachusetts, USA) was also used for immunohistochemical evaluation of smooth muscle regeneration. The main steps of immunohistochemistry methods: (1) Put the slide with paraffin section in drying oven 2 hours, 60°C. (2) Put it in xylene 15 min, 3 times. (3) Then in ethanol, from 100% to 95%, then 90%, 80%, 70%, each 5 min. (4) Wash with water one time, 5 min, then transform into PBS (0.01 M, pH 7.4), wash 5 min, 3 times. (5) Antigen retrieval: put the slide into citrate buffer (0.01 M, pH 6.0), keep the solution in boiling water for 10-15 min, cool down to room temperature (6) Wash with PBS (0.01 M, pH 7.4) 5 min, 3 times (7) Block endogenous peroxidase by 3% H2O2 for 30 min (8) Wash with PBS (0.01 M, pH 7.4) 5 min, 3 times (9) Incubation with blocking buffer (normal goat serum or 3% BSA) at 37°C for 20 min (10) Discarding the goat serum and droping the primary antibody A-actin (BIOSS Inc, USA) with diluted in PBS (0.01 M PBS, pH 7.4,1:100–500), incubating the sections overnight at 4°C (11) Wash with PBS (3X5 min) (12) Add secondary antibody, Goat Anti-rabbit IgG, (BIOSS Inc, USA) incubating the sections for 20 min at 37°C (13) Wash with PBS (3X5 min) (14) Add Avidin/HRP, incubating the sections for 20 min at 37°C (15) Wash with PBS (3X5 min) (16) Colouration with 3,3-diaminobenzidin (DAB), Observe by microscope, stop colouration with the distilled water at the right time (17) Dehydration in ethanol, from 70% to 80%, then 90%, 95%, 100%, each 5 min, then transform into xylene 10 min, 3 times (18) Cover with coverslip by neutral gums. The preparations were observed under a light microscope. For the convenience of analysis, the results were quantified as optical density (OD) values. Using analysis software (Leica Qwin, v2.3; Leica Inc. Solms, Germany) with the same parameters (exposure time, 22 ms; light intensity, 60%), the mean OD of A-actin was measured.

Statistical analysis

In this study, self-control was approached. Quantitative data were compared using t-tests. All statistical analyses used SPSS 13.0 (SPSS, Inc., Chicago, IL, USA).

Results

Macroscopic evaluation

All rabbits were euthanized. The outer and inner surfaces of the bladder, perivesical fat, kidneys, and ureters were evaluated macroscopically. The kidneys and ureters were grossly normal without evidence of hydronephrosis. There were no diverticula in any group. There was no extravasation or contractions in the graft regions. The material was degraded in groups B and C, but not degraded on the inner surface in group A. Regenerated tissue covered the outer surface of the region of the graft, which was indistinguishable from the normal host bladder at the outer and inner surfaces in group C (Figure 2b).

Microscopic evaluation

Continuation of host transitional epithelium in the region of the SIS graft was observed under light microscopy in all groups. Inflammatory cells infiltrated regenerated epithelium 4 weeks after surgery (group A; Figure 1c), and nearly disappeared 12 weeks post-operatively (group B). Detrusor was formed 12 weeks post-operatively (group B). These layers were indistinguishable from normal bladder 24 weeks post-operatively (group C).

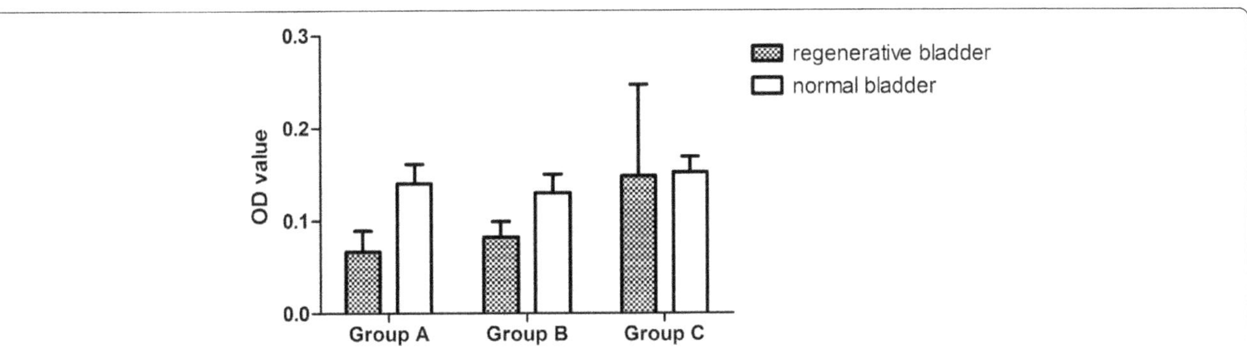

Figure 2 Compare of OD value. The OD value of regenerated tissue was 0.067 ± 0.022 in group A, 0.082 ± 0.017 in group B, and 0.148 ± 0.099 in group C. Compared with normal bladder (0.140 ± 0.021 in group A, 0.130 ± 0.020 in group B, 0.152 ± 0.017 in group C), groups A and B were significantly different with normal bladder ($p < 0.05$), while there was no significant difference in group C and normal bladder ($p > 0.05$).

Table 1 Comparisons between regenerated and normal bladder and results of urodynamic testing

	Group A		Group B		Group C	
	Pre-op	Post-op	Pre-op	Post-op	Pre-op	Post-op
Bladder volume (ml)	40.30 ± 7.6*	26.11 ± 4.8*	55.7 ± 27.2	60.4 ± 24.7	48.98 ± 27.8*	57.80 ± 27.7*
	P = 0.021		P = 0.111		P = 0.001	
Compliance (ml/cmH_2O)	2.74 ± 1.57	2.36 ± 0.71	4.9 ± 2.04	5.1 ± 1.54	6.88 ± 4.07	6.2±3.86
	P = 0.653		P = 0.272		P = 0.732	

*P < 0.05 was considered statistically significant.

Immunohistochemical evaluation

Detrusor was present and well-visualized with A-actin staining. The detrusor component was scarce in group A, while the detrusor fiber was more evident in group B than in group A, but smaller in number and size compared with normal tissue (P = 0.001). There was no significant difference in the OD value of A-actin staining in group C and normal bladder (P = 0.759) (Figure 2).

Urodynamic test

Pre-operatively, the bladder capacities in groups A, B, and C were 40.30 ± 7.6, 55.7 ± 27.2, and 48.98 ± 27.8 ml, respectively. Post-operatively, the capacities were 26.11 ± 4.8, 60.4 ± 24.7, and 57.80 ± 27.7 ml, respectively. There was a significant decrease in the bladder volume of group A, and no significant difference in group B; however, the bladder volume was significantly increased in group C (24 weeks post-operation; P = 0.001). The bladder compliance of groups A, B, and C pre-operatively was not significantly different post-operation (Table 1).

In vitro detrusor strip study

Regenerated detrusor strips in group A had visible slight vibration waves, the frequency and amplitude of which could not be measured; the group A strips were significantly different from normal detrusor strips. In group B, the frequency (min-1) of regenerated detrusor strips was 2.88 ± 0.49 (min-1) and the amplitude was 0.13 ± 0.014 (g), which was significantly different from normal detrusor strips. The frequency (3.64 ± 0.98) and amplitude (4.35 ± 1.25) of regenerated detrusor strips in group C were not significantly different compared with normal detrusor strips (Table 2).

Discussion

To create a target volume and functional regenerated bladder are challenges in tissue engineering. We chose SIS as materials used for bladder regeneration; using SIS with the help of host tissues gives successful results [6]. In recent years, bladder regeneration using SIS has been reported in rat and dog models [11,12]; however, research involving functional bladder regeneration of rabbits has seldom been reported. We showed that regenerated bladder tissue has similar function in vitro strip studies with normal tissue and as part of new bladder post-operation compared with pre-operative bladder.

We chose male rabbits as our study animals because the external urethral orifice of male rabbits is easier to identify than the urethra in female rabbits. Urodynamic testing was carried out after opening the abdomen under anesthesia to remove the influence of abdominal pressure. We did not choose cystometry via cystostomy as has been previously reported [13]. We attempted to maintain the complete bladder, as excessive damage to the bladder tissue might adversely impact the results. The bladder volume of group A (26.11 ± 4.8 ml) was decreased significantly compared with the pre-operative volume (P = 0.021). Encrustration of the bladder was observed all cases in group A (4 weeks post-operation). It has been suggested that encrustration is a result of high urate levels in rabbits [14]. And the encrustration all disappeared at last [15]. We suggest that encrustation might be the patch which was not degraded because encrustation was not noted in group B or C. Furthermore, we found that in group A the region of the patch surrounded by a large area of inflammatory polyp hyperplasia. All of these observations could be the result of decreased bladder capacity in group A.

Table 2 Comparisons between regenerated and normal bladder tissues and the results of the detrusor strip study

	Group A		Group B		Group C	
	Normal	Regenerated	Normal	Regenerated	Normal	Regenerated
Frequency (min^{-1})		—	4.80 ± 1.20*	2.88 ± 0.49*	3.64 ± 0.98	4.35 ± 1.25
			(p = 0.005)		(P = 0.442)	
Amplitude (g)		—	0.47 ± 0.083*	0.13 ± 0.014*	0.67 ± 0.09	0.50 ± 0.25
			(p = 0.000)		(p = 0.051.)	

*P < 0.05 was considered statistically significant.

The bladder volume was significantly increased 24 weeks post-operation (group C; P = 0.001). In the current study, the reduction in bladder capacity was transient and the bladder capacity was eventually expanded.

Furthermore, the results showed that compliance post-operation was similar with compliance pre-operation in group C (p = 0.051). The regenerated bladder tissue did not reduce the original normal bladder compliance. Moreover, in the in vitro detrusor strip study, regenerated tissue had a slight contraction wave in group A. Based on HE staining, group A showed scattered *de novo* tissue formation of muscle fibers, thus muscle regeneration began to emerge in the patch area 4 weeks post-operation, albeit a small number and discontinuous. Therefore, a smaller contraction wave was recorded in group A. The regenerated strips were similar to normal muscle strips with a spontaneous contraction frequency and amplitude in group C, which were not statistically different (frequency, p = 0.442; amplitude, p = 0.051). Regenerated smooth muscle bundles were also observed in regenerated tissue by HE staining in which the arrangement was also similar to normal tissue with a vertical outer ring-type arrangement.

Sandusky et al. [16] has offered two explanations regarding the smooth muscle regeneration process: (1) normal smooth muscle tissue growth from the patch edge inward; and (2) *de novo* smooth muscle is derived from peripheral cells, which includes the epithelium of capillaries. The author believes that both explanations might exist, but further trials are needed. SIS may also promote muscle regeneration. Many studies have identified the structure, and demonstrated the useful biological properties in tissue regeneration since discovery in 1987 [6,13]. Based on the results of urodynamic testing and the in vitro detrusor strip study, we conclude that along with SIS functional bladder was regenerated.

Some studies [17] have reported that the patch area is infiltrated by a large number of fibroblasts and inflammatory cell, 1–4 weeks after transport. These cells secrete all types of materials, such as TGF-β, that can determine tissue regeneration.

Actin is one of the primary contractile proteins in bladder smooth muscle cells. Currently, A-actin is considered to be the main phenotype indicator in contractile smooth muscle cells [18]. Immunohistochemical studies have shown that A-actin stains brown. The OD was used for statistical analysis; higher OD values indicated increased expression of A-actin. The OD value increased with time post-operation. The OD value reached a level similar to normal tissue in group C (24 weeks post-operation).

Conclusion

We conclude that histologic and functional regeneration of bladder in rabbit can be achieved with SIS. Therefore, SIS seems to be a viable material in the reconstruction of the rabbit urinary bladder. Advanced and more detailed researches on whether or not regeneration of normal tissue can be accomplished from a pathologic organ should be carried out.

Competing interests

The authors declare that they have no competing interests.

Authors' contributions

YW performed the animal experiments and drafted the manuscript. LL contributed to the conception and design of the study, analysis interpretation of data, and helped to draft the manuscript. Both authors read and approved the final manuscript.

Authors' information

YW is MD and urologist in the department of urology of China Rehabilitation Research Center (CRRC). LL, MD & PhD, is chairman of the department of urology of CRRC, and a professor of urology and vice-chairman of urologic department of Capital Medical University in Beijing. His main interests are neurourology, urodynamics and incontinence. He is a committee member of the neurourology promotion committee of the international continence society (ICS), and was chairman of 42nd ICS annual meeting in Beijing. Yiming Wang and Limin Liao are co-first authors.

Acknowledgment

This work was supported by China National Technology R&G Program (2012BAI34B02).

References

1. Chen JL, Kuo HC: **Long-term outcomes of augmentation enterocystoplasty with an ileal segment in patients with spinal cord injury.** *J Formos Med Assoc* 2009, **108**:475–480.
2. Gilbert SM, Hensle TW: **Metabolic consequences and long-term complications of enterocystoplasty in children: a review.** *J Urol* 2005, **173**:1080–1086.
3. Badylak SF, Lantz GC, Coffey A, Geddes LA: **Small intestinal submucosa as a large diameter vascular graft in the dog.** *J Surg Res* 1989, **47**:74–80.
4. Atala A, Vacanti JP, Peters CA, Mandell J, Retik AB, Freeman MR: **Formation of urothelial structures in vivo from dissociated cells attached to biodegradable polymer scaffolds in vitro.** *J Urol* 1992, **148**:658–662.
5. Oberpenning F, Meng J, Yoo JJ, Atala A: **De novo reconstitution of a functional mammalian urinary bladder by tissue engineering.** *Nat Biotechnol* 1999, **17**:149–155.
6. Dedecker F, Grynberg M, Staerman F: **Small intestinal submucosa (SIS): prospects in urogenital surgery.** *Prog Urol* 2005, **15**:405–410.
7. Becker C, Jakse G: **Stem cells for regeneration of urological structures.** *Eur Urol* 2007, **51**:1217–1228.
8. Aiken SW, Badylak SF, Toombs JP, Shelbourne KD, Hiles MC, Lantz GC, Van Sickle D: **Small intestinal submucosa as an intra-articular ligamentous repair material: a pilot study in dogs.** *Vet Comp Orthopedics Traumatol* 1994, **7**:124–128.
9. Badylak SF, Voytik SL, Kokini K, Shelbourne KD, Klootwyk T, Kraine MR, Tullius R, Simmons C: **The use of xenogeneic small intestinal submucosa as a biomaterial for Achilles' tendon repair in a dog model.** *J Biomed Mater Res* 1995, **29**:977–985.
10. Lantz GC, Badylak SF, Hiles MC, Co€ey AC, Geddes LA, Kokini K, Sandusky GE, Mor€ RJ: **Small intestinal submucosa as a vascular graft: a review.** *J Invest Surg* 1993, **6**:297–310.
11. Kropp BP, Eppley BL, Prevel CD, Rippy MK, Harruff RC, Badylak SF, Adams MC, Rink RC, Keating MA: **Experimental assessment of small intestinal submucosa as a bladder wall substitute.** *Urology* 1995, **46**:396–400.
12. Lai JY, Chang PY, Lin JN: **Bladder autoaugmentation using various biodegradable scaffolds seeded with autologous smooth muscle cells in a rabbit model.** *J Pediatr Surg* 2005, **40**(12):1869–1873.
13. Kropp BP, Cheng EY, Lin HK, Zhang Y: **Reliable and reproducible bladder regeneration using seeded distal small intestinal submucosa.** *J Urol* 2004, **172**:1710–1713.

14. Ayyildiz A, Akgül KT, Huri E, Nuhoğlu B, Kiliçoğlu B, Ustün H, Gürdal M, Germiyanoğlu C: **Use of porcine small intestinal submucosa in bladder augmentation in rabbit: long-term histological outcome. Biomaterials.** *ANZ J Surg* 2008, **78:**1–2.
15. Nuininga JE, van Moerkerk H, Hanssen A, Hulsbergen CA, Oosterwijk-Wakka J, Oosterwijk E, de Gier RP, Schalken JA, van Kuppevelt TH, Feitz WF: **A rabbit model to tissue engineer the bladder.** *Biomaterials* 2004, **25:**1657–1661.
16. Sandusky GJ, Badylak SF, Morff RJ, Johnson WD, Lantz G: **Histologic findings after in vivo placement of small intestine submucosal vascular grafts and saphenous vein grafts in the carotid artery in dogs.** *Am J Path01* 1992, **140:**317–324.
17. Stelnicki EJ, Chin GS, Gittes GK, Longaker MT: **Fetal wound healing: where do we go from here?** *Semin Pediatr Surg* 1999, **8:**124–130.
18. Owens GK: **Regulation of differentiation of vascular smooth muscle cells.** *Physiol ReV* 1995, **75:**487–517.

Regulation of urinary bladder function by protein kinase C in physiology and pathophysiology

Joseph A. Hypolite and Anna P. Malykhina*

Abstract

Background: Protein kinase C (PKC) is expressed in many tissues and organs including the urinary bladder, however, its role in bladder physiology and pathophysiology is still evolving. The aim of this review was to evaluate available evidence on the involvement of PKC in regulation of detrusor contractility, muscle tone of the bladder wall, spontaneous contractile activity and bladder function under physiological and pathophysiological conditions.

Methods: This is a non-systematic review of the published literature which summarizes the available animal and human data on the role of PKC signaling in the urinary bladder under different physiological and pathophysiological conditions. A wide PubMed search was performed including the combination of the following keywords: "urinary bladder", "PKC", "detrusor contractility", "bladder smooth muscle", "detrusor relaxation", "peak force", "detrusor underactivity", "partial bladder outlet obstruction", "voltage-gated channels", "bladder nerves", "PKC inhibitors", "PKC activators". Retrieved articles were individually screened for the relevance to the topic of this review with 91 citations being selected and included in the data analysis.

Discussion: Urinary bladder function includes the ability to store urine at low intravesical pressure followed by a subsequent release of bladder contents due to a rapid phasic contraction that is maintained long enough to ensure complete emptying. This review summarizes the current concepts regarding the potential contribution of PKC to contractility, physiological voiding, and related signaling mechanisms involved in the control of both the storage and emptying phases of the micturition cycle, and in dysfunctional voiding. Previous studies linked PKC activation exclusively with an increase in generation of the peak force of smooth muscle contraction, and maximum force generation in the lower urinary tract. More recent data suggests that PKC presents a broader range of effects on urinary bladder function including regulation of storage, emptying, excitability of the detrusor, and bladder innervation.

Summary: In this review, we evaluated the mechanisms of peripheral and local regulation of PKC signaling in the urinary bladder, and their impact on different phases of the micturition cycle under physiological and pathophysiological conditions.

Keywords: Detrusor smooth muscle, Micturition, Nerves, Contractility, Signaling pathways, Bladder pathophysiology

* Correspondence: Anna.Malykhina@ucdenver.edu
Division of Urology, Department of Surgery, University of Colorado Denver, Anschutz Medical Campus, 12700 E 19th Ave. Mail Stop C317, Aurora, CO 80045, USA

Background

Physiological contractions of the detrusor smooth muscle (DSM) involve the ability to generate and maintain contractile force during the emptying phase of the micturition cycle [1–13]. Initial animal studies suggested that PKC plays a minimal role in DSM contractility [14–19]. This conclusion was based on the failure of PKC to make a significant contribution to maximal force generation in response to muscarinic receptor agonists [14, 16, 18]. Subsequent investigations provided evidence that PKC likely has dual effects on bladder function regulating both contractility and relaxation of the detrusor [3, 7, 8, 20, 21]. For instance, it was determined that low levels of PKC stimulation could inhibit spontaneous contractions and lower basal resting tone of DSM *in vitro*, thereby, likely contributing to bladder storage [8], while high levels of PKC activity contributed to an increase and maintenance of total DSM force (integral force) required for bladder emptying [22].

Stimulation of muscarinic receptors triggers activation of phospholipase C (PLC)/PKC downstream signaling associated with smooth muscle contractility via G-protein-coupled receptors [15, 16, 23, 24]. Animal studies confirmed that the same pathway is present in the urinary bladder [15], and that PKC is involved in a variety of cellular events that regulate DSM contractility. Among these are the effects on the smooth muscle itself [3, 7, 8, 17, 25–30], expression and function of ion channels [8, 26, 31–33], and intrinsic bladder nerves assessed by *in vitro* contractility studies on isolated DSM strips during electric field stimulation (EFS) [22, 34, 35]. In this review, we summarized current data on the involvement of PKC signaling in modulation of bladder function with focus on the contractile force of DSM, relaxation of the muscle during filling phase, as well as the ability of the detrusor to develop and maintain muscle tone throughout the micturition cycle under physiological and pathophysiological conditions.

Methods

This is a non-systematic review of the published literature which summarizes the available animal and human data on the role of PKC signaling in the urinary bladder under different physiological and pathophysiological conditions. A wide PubMed search was performed including the combination of the following keywords: "urinary bladder", "PKC", "detrusor contractility", "bladder smooth muscle", "detrusor relaxation", "peak force", "detrusor underactivity", "partial bladder outlet obstruction", "voltage-gated channels", "bladder nerves", "PKC inhibitors", "PKC activators". Retrieved articles were individually screened for the relevance to the topic of this review with 91 citations being selected and included in the analysis.

Table 1 summarizes the effects of a variety of PKC inhibitors, activators, and cholinergic agonists on PKC signaling and contractility of DSM.

Discussion

The aim of this review was to evaluate the available evidence on the involvement of PKC in regulation of detrusor contractility, muscle tone of the bladder wall, spontaneous contractile activity and bladder function under physiological and pathophysiological conditions.

Modulation of DSM excitability and ion channel activity by PKC

Bladder smooth muscle cells express a variety of ion channels controlling cell excitability. Voltage-gated calcium channels (VGCC), large- (BK), and small- (SK) conductance Ca^{2+}-activated potassium channels, and ATP-sensitive potassium channels (K_{ATP}) are the main channels involved in the control of detrusor excitability and excitation-contraction coupling [4, 15, 26, 32, 36].

Voltage gated calcium channels

Several types of VGCC are expressed in the detrusor [15] with L-type VGCC being the main ion channel responsible for the onset of action potentials in DSM cell, as well as for the contractile response of the detrusor to muscarinic receptor stimulation [37–42]. VGCC have also been shown to mediate spontaneous contractions in DSM cells [4]. Recent studies determined that one of the PKC activators, phorbol-12,13-dibutyrate (PDBu), inhibited voltage-dependent spontaneous contractions in isolated DSM strips from rabbit and rat bladders at low concentrations [8, 22]. Additionally, PKC activation by PDBu inhibited receptor-induced phasic activity in the bladders of newborn mice but not in adult bladders [29]. Inhibition of DSM spontaneous contractility by PKC activator, PDBu, was also observed in isolated muscle strips of the human DSM (unpublished observations from our laboratory) and rat DSM [22]. Utilizing whole-cell patch clamp technique, Kajioka et al. (2002) demonstrated an increase in the amplitude and current density of L-type Ca^{2+} channels upon depolarization in pig and human bladders [43]. Interestingly, in the same study, carbachol significantly diminished the amplitude of VGCC current which was sensitive to nifedipine. The mechanisms of the opposing actions of carbachol on VGCC are not entirely clear. It is well established that initial phasic contraction of DSM in response to carbachol stimulation is associated with membrane depolarization and opening of VGCC [15]. However, this initial massive increase in intracellular calcium is followed by subsequent closing of VGCC and a decrease in intracellular Ca^{2+} due to its storage in the intracellular stores [44]. These subsequent changes are associated with a quiescent state of the muscle after initial

Table 1 Effects of PKC signaling on bladder function

PKC Drugs	Tissue	Methods	Physiological condition	Species	Effect on bladder function	Reference
PBBu (PKC activator, 1nM–50nM)	Muscle strips	*In vitro*	Normal	Rabbit, Rat	Inhibition of spontaneous contraction	[8] [22]
PDBu (100nM-1 μM)	Muscle strips	*In vitro*	Normal	Rabbit	Increased contractility	[8, 25, 28]
PDBu (100nM-1 μM)	Muscle strips	*In vitro*	Normal	Rat	Increased nerve sensitivity, force maintenance	[8, 22, 31]
PDBu (1 μM)	Bladder	*In vivo* (cystometry)	Normal	Rat	Bladder emptying, and frequency of urination	[22]
PDBu	Muscle strip	*In vitro*	Normal	Rabbit	Activation of ROCK, Increased DSM tone	[28]
PDBu	Muscle strips	*In vitro*, EFS	Normal	Rat	Increased peak force and area; increased release of acetylcholine.	[30]
PDBu	Bladder myocytes	*In vitro*	Normal	Mice	Increased Cav1.2 current	[33]
PDBu	α-toxin muscle strips	*In vitro*	Normal	Guinea pig	Increased Ca^{2+} sensitivity	[80]
PDBu (0.001–3 μM)	Muscle strips	*In vitro*	Obese PBOO	Mice	Increased contractility	[26] [60]
PDBu	Muscle strips	*In vitro*	PBOO	Rabbit	Decreased contraction and PKC activity	[25, 27]
PMA (PKC activator)	DSM cells & Muscle strips	*In vitro*, Patch-clamp recordings	Normal	Guinea pig	Inhibition of K_{ATP} and BK currents; increased DSM contraction	[22, 31, 47]
Bim-1 (PKC inhibitor)	Muscle strips Bladder	*In vitro* *In vivo*	Normal Normal	Rabbit Rat	Increased spontaneous contractions; decreased force maintenance; decreased peak force; decreased void; increased non-voiding contractions	[8, 22, 24]
Ro318220 (PKC inhibitor)	Muscle strips Bladder	*In vitro* *In vivo*	Normal Normal	Rat Rat	Inhibition of force maintenance; Increased non-voiding contractions; decreased void volume	[22]
GF109203X (PKC inhibitor)	Muscle strips	*In vitro*	Normal	Guinea pig; rat	Inhibition of Ca^{2+} sensitization	[17]
Carbachol	DSM cells	*In vitro*, Patch-clamp recordings	Unknown	Human	Inhibition of BK channels	[76]
Carbachol	DSM	*In vitro*	Unknown	Human	Increased Ca++ sensitivity of contractile filaments	[68]

phasic contraction, and, likely, underlie the absence of spontaneous contractile activity during relaxation phase after muscarinic stimulation (Fig. 1). This action may be mediated by carbachol-induced activation of PKC [24] at low or resting calcium concentration, since PKC stimulation by PDBu was reported to activate BK channels resulting in inhibition of spontaneous contractions [8, 22]. Interestingly, pre-incubation of the DSM strips *in vitro* with the PKC inhibitor, Bim-1, before carbachol stimulation preserved spontaneous contractility during relaxation phase (Fig. 1).

Effects of PKC activation on BK channels

The storage phase of the micturition cycle requires a quiescent smooth muscle that can accommodate increasing volumes at low intravesical pressure. Potassium channels contribute to this process by helping maintain the resting membrane potential via regulation of both the intracellular calcium concentration, and calcium entry into the cell from extracellular sources [32, 36, 45]. Several types of potassium channels are expressed in DSM, and are known to be involved in this regulation. Among them, BK and K_{ATP} channels were shown to be regulated by PKC. PKC was

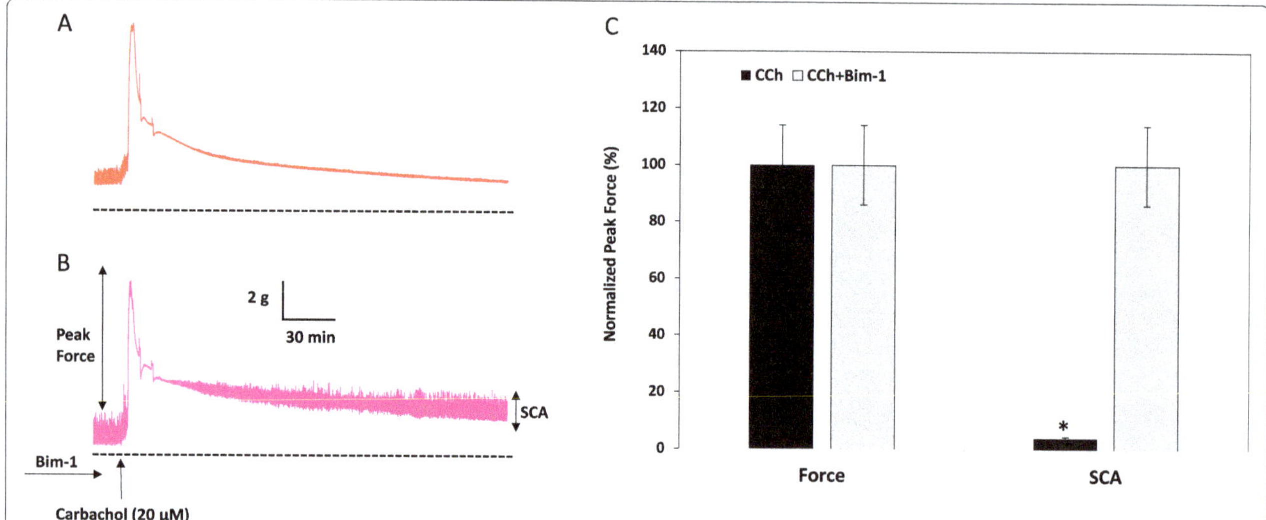

Fig. 1 Effects of carbachol (CCh) on the contractile force and spontaneous contractions in DSM *in vitro*. Isolated muscle strips from rabbit bladders were mounted in organ baths with Tyrode's buffer (equilibrated with $95\%O_2/5\%CO_2$) and allowed to develop spontaneous contractions. The muscle strip shown in **a** was treated with 20 μM of carbachol while the muscle strip in **b** was first pre-incubated with Bim-1 (28 nM), a PKC inhibitor, for 45 min prior to adding carbachol. Treatment with carbachol increased peak muscle force and reduced the amplitude of spontaneous contraction (SCA) by 96 ± 14 %, ($n = 4$, $p < 0.05$ in **a**), however, carbachol had no effect on spontaneous contraction amplitude (SCA) after PKC inhibition with Bim-1 (**b**). **c** Normalized amplitude of the peak force of the contractile response to CCh. Maximal amplitude was taken as 100 %. Light bars show the effects of carbachol on peak force and SCA without Bim-1. Dark bars show the effect of carbachol on peak force and SCA with Bim-1 application

shown to be involved in the regulation of BK channels expressed in DSM tissue of rabbit [8] and guinea pig [31] bladders. Hypolite et al. (2013) reported that low levels of PKC stimulation by the PKC activator, PDBu, inhibited spontaneous myogenic contractions, and reduced basal DSM tone in rabbit DSM, which was dependent on activation of BK channels [8]. Additionally, PDBu was unable to inhibit spontaneous contractions in the presence of the BK channel blocker, iberiotoxin, suggesting that the mechanism of PDBu-induced inhibition of spontaneous contractions was via activation of BK channels. Utilizing whole-cell patch clamp recordings in guinea pig DSM cells, Hristov et al. (2014) confirmed that PKC does regulate BK channel activity, however, these authors reported that PKC stimulation with PMA increased muscle force along with amplitude of spontaneous contractions [31]. The variability in the responses to PKC stimulation reported by the abovementioned studies could be attributed to different species (guinea pigs *vs* rabbits), or the use of distinct PKC activators (PDBu versus PMA), as well as slightly different methodological approaches.

Modulation of K_{ATP} channels by PKC

Similar to BK channels, K_{ATP} channels also participate in the control of detrusor excitability across a broad spectrum of mammalian species including guinea pigs [46, 47], humans [48], and rats [49]. Activation of these channels induces DSM relaxation in response to K_{ATP} channel openers pinacidil [50], and cromakalim [51]. Activation of M_3 receptors can induce inhibition of these channels in smooth muscle cells via PKC signaling pathways [52]. Stimulation of muscarinic receptors by carbachol was shown to inhibit K_{ATP} currents by 60.7 %, while activators of PKC inhibited K_{ATP} channels by 74 % [52]. Additionally, PKC blockers used before stimulation with muscarinic receptor agonists, significantly reduced carbachol-induced inhibition of K_{ATP} currents confirming that muscarinic-dependent inhibition of K_{ATP} currents is mediated via PKC pathways [52]. This speculation is consistent with *in vitro* studies showing that the PKC inhibitor, Bim-1, reduced both intrinsic basal tone, and maintained force [8], while awake cystometry performed in rats revealed that inhibition of PKC resulted in increased frequency of urination, and decreased void volume [22]. Schematic presentation of the ion channels involved in regulation of BSM excitability and contractility as well as downstream signaling including PKC pathways is depicted in Fig. 2.

The link between muscarinic receptors and PKC signaling in the control of detrusor contractility

Muscarinic receptor type 3 (M_3) signaling via $G_{q/11}$ G-protein-coupled receptors includes activation of PLC/PKC as determined for several types of smooth muscle [23] including the DSM of the bladder [16, 53–55]. Initial experiments in the urinary bladder established that inhibition of PLC/PKC pathway by a number of specific inhibitors had no significant effect on maximal contractility of rat bladder

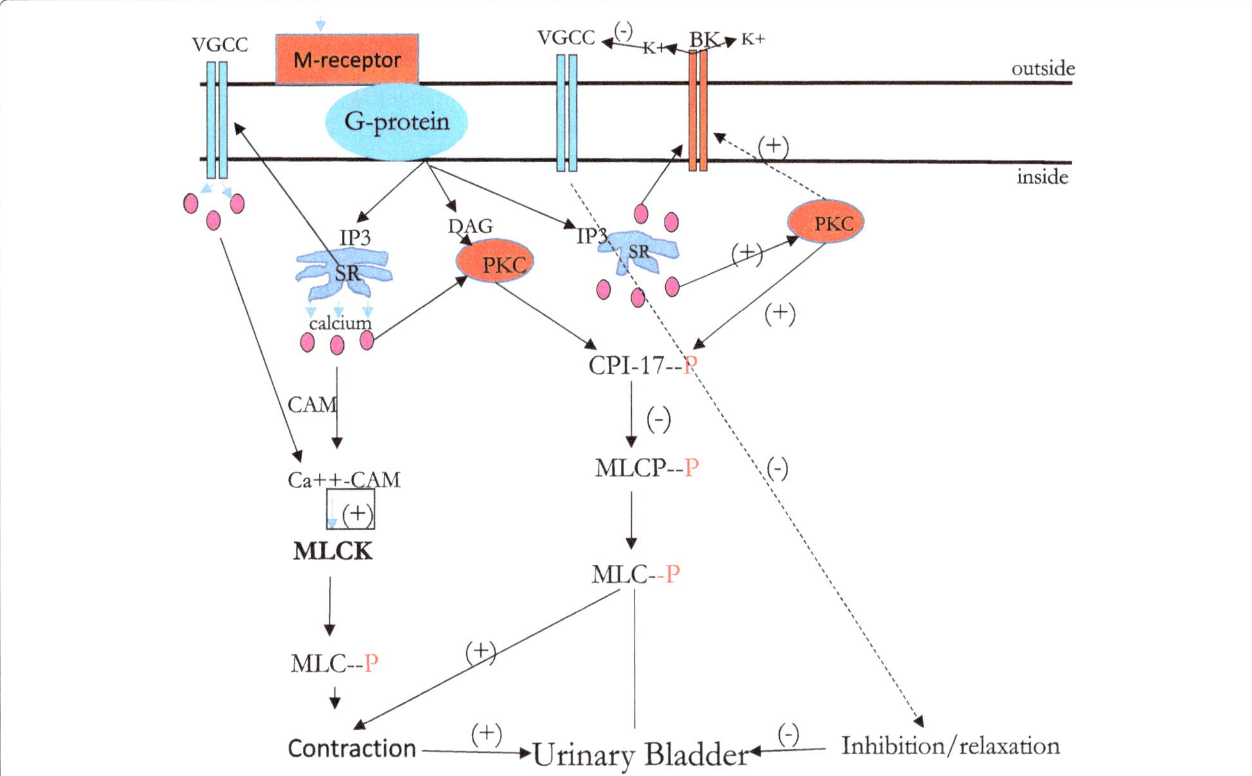

Fig. 2 Schematic presentation of the PKC signaling pathways involved in the regulation of urinary bladder function. Abbreviations are spelled out in the text of the manuscript. (+) Activation of the pathways, (–) means Inhibition, (P) is Phosphorylation. Broken arrows indicate potential pathways for PKC-induced inhibition of DSM tone via activation of BK channels

muscle strips in response to carbachol stimulation leading to the conclusion that PLC/PKC-dependent signaling via M_3 receptors does not significantly contribute to DSM contractility [16]. This data was further buttressed by the studies showing that direct inhibition of PKC had no significant effect on the peak contractile force in response to both carbachol and EFS stimulation [8, 14].

An exception to the above findings was the observation that one of the PKC inhibitors, Bim-1, did reduce maximal force in response to carbachol upon application of a higher concentration of the inhibitor [24]. Another PKC inhibitor, GF 109203X (1 μM), was also reported to reduce peak force in control bladders by 29 % [56]. Subsequent studies clarified that inhibition of PKC with Bim-1, at lower concentrations, did not significantly affect electric field stimulation (EFS)-induced maximal amplitude of DSM contractions, however, significantly reduced the integral, or total force [8, 22]. The integral (total) force is calculated as the area under the curve of a single recorded contraction, and represents the ability of DSM to maintain muscle force required for physiological bladder emptying [8]. The effects of Bim-1 observed *in vitro* were further confirmed *in vivo* by cystometric recordings in unanesthetized rats [22]. During urodynamic recordings (cystometry), the urinary bladder was slowly infused with a solution containing Bim-1, causing the voided urine volumes to decline progressively in comparison with infusion of saline in the control group. These *in vivo* results supported the importance of PKC for muscle force maintenance associated with bladder emptying.

Additional studies confirmed the involvement of PKC in the maintenance of muscle force at the molecular and biochemical level [24]. Stimulation of muscarinic receptors in the smooth muscle results in inhibition of myosin light chain (MLC) phosphatase activity, an increase in MLC phosphorylation and, therefore, contractile force. One of the underlying pathways for inhibition of MLC phosphatase activity is protein kinase C (PKC)-catalyzed phosphorylation of CPI-17 protein [57, 58]. Wang and co-authors evaluated phosphorylation of protein complex Thr(38)-CPI-17, the downstream target of PKC signaling, and established that PKC activation increased Thr(38)-CPI-17 phosphorylation throughout the phasic and tonic portions of carbachol stimulation confirming that PKC is involved in maintaining the contractile force in the detrusor [24].

Limited contribution of the PLC/PKC pathway to the peak amplitude of the contractile response in DSM seems to be physiologically justified as the maximal contractile force of smooth muscle is predominantly controlled by calcium/calmodulin-dependent activation of myosin light chain kinase (MLCK) followed by subsequent phosphorylation of the myosin light chain (MLC) [59]. Since stimulation of DSM by muscarinic receptor agonists leads to a rapid rise in intracellular calcium followed by an equally rapid decline of the calcium to almost basal levels [44], it is highly likely that PKC-induced calcium sensitization via Gq_{11} receptors [3] plays a major role in the maintenance phase of the contraction that is critical for bladder emptying. This mechanism may partly explain why inhibition of PKC significantly reduces DSM force maintenance, and bladder emptying, without significantly affecting peak force generation [14, 22].

Role of PKC in regulation of spontaneous contractions in the urinary bladder

Protein kinase C is also involved in other aspects of DSM contractility, including the inhibition of basal DSM tone, and spontaneous myogenic contractions [8, 22]. For instance, PDBu, a PKC activator, inhibits spontaneous contractions, and basal myogenic tone at low levels of application (1–50 nM) whereas high concentrations of the drug increase the sensitivity to EFS stimulation *in vitro*, and also trigger micturition contractions *in vivo* confirming a dual, concentration-dependent activation profile of PKC effects in DSM [22]. The ability of PKC to modulate basal DSM tone, and inhibit spontaneous contractions at low levels of stimulation may have physiological implications for bladder storage function, while its contribution to the maintenance of DSM force and nerve-mediated contractions may be important for bladder emptying.

Spontaneous myogenic contractions of DSM have been recorded *in vivo* and *in vitro* in several species including rabbit [8, 11], rat [60], guinea pig [31], pig [40], and humans [61]. The mechanism of these contractions involves calcium entry into the smooth muscle cells via VGCC [40, 43, 62, 63] to trigger action potential generation, while the repolarization phase is thought to be mediated mainly by opening of calcium-activated potassium channels and exit of potassium ions from the smooth muscle cells leading to muscle relaxation [64]. Early reports suggested that spontaneous large-amplitude contractions recorded *in vitro* in isolated DSM strips were likely an artifact with no significant functional role [11]. Subsequent studies suggested that these contractions participate in the maintenance of an intrinsic DSM tone by helping the smooth muscle adjust its length and shape in response to bladder filling [4]. They have also been reported to be associated with peripheral sensory processing that informs the need to void as the bladder approaches capacity [6].

The inhibitory effect of the PKC activator, PDBu, on spontaneous contractions was linked to activation of BK channels, subsequent hyperpolarization of the membrane, and restriction of calcium entry via VGCC [8, 65]. Freshly isolated DSM strips from the rabbit bladder exhibit high amplitude spontaneous contractions which decline over several hours, however, the amplitude of contractions remains at a high level in the presence of PKC inhibitor Bim-1 [8]. This observation suggests that endogenous PKC signaling likely maintains the amplitude of spontaneous contractions at a low, physiological level under normal physiological conditions. This assumption is supported by the fact that commercially available PKC activator, PDBu, at low levels of stimulation (1–50 nM), accelerated the decline in amplitude of spontaneous contractions over time *in vitro* [8]. PDBu was also reported to inhibit carbachol-induced phasic contractions in neonatal bladders associated with the effects on T-type channels [29], and was also observed to inhibit spontaneous contractions in rat DSM [22].

Effects of calcium on PKC activity

Protein kinase C conveys both calcium-dependent [66–68], and calcium-independent [3, 68, 69] effects on DSM contractility *in vitro* mediated via inhibition of MLCP. It is still unknown if these separate effects are mediated by different PKC isoforms. However, the ability of PKC to mediate both of these actions in DSM may be well suited to urinary bladder storage and emptying function. The storage phase requires the maintenance of basal intrinsic DSM tone at low calcium concentrations which can be mediated, in part, by calcium-independent contractile effects of PKC involved in an increase in tone during the storage phase. This process may be aided by the stretch of the bladder wall associated with an up-regulation of the proteins involved in calcium sensitization [70] and contributing to the basal tone during the early phase of the micturition cycle. However, as the bladder continues to expand, it is likely that enhanced stretch-induced calcium release [71], and calcium-dependent PKC activity increase wall tension further as the bladder approaches capacity. This dual, calcium-independent and dependent, flexibility of PKC may be vital in helping ensure that wall tension rises in a controlled fashion so as to prevent steep increases in bladder pressure during the storage phase of the micturition cycle. PKC-dependent effects have been observed in DSM in response to EFS, which activates the intramural nerves, suggesting that PKC-dependent regulation of neuronal function in DSM is also a distinct possibility [65, 72–74].

PKC signaling in the human bladder

In comparison to extensive animal data, very little information is available regarding the effects of PKC on human bladder contractility and relaxation. Early studies using human tissues suggested that PKC did not significantly contribute to human bladder contractions

[14]. However, only the peak amplitude of contraction (maximum force) was evaluated in the presence of various PKC inhibitors, and no difference was found in peak force generation in comparison to the absence of inhibitors. Since bladder emptying requires both, the generation of peak force and the ability to maintain force, it is possible that PKC could play a more significant role in force maintenance in the human DSM in addition to force generation.

A recent study [75] provided evidence that carbachol, a muscarinic receptor agonist, could indirectly inhibit large conductance Ca^{2+}-activated potassium (BK) channels in human DSM cells leading to increased excitability [76]. This is an interesting finding as the ongoing studies in our laboratory using human DSM indicate that carbachol can induce a significant increase in phasic contractions in some human DSM isolated strips, but not in all of them (unpublished data). It is possible that PKC could be an important secondary messenger between muscarinic receptors and BK channels in the human detrusor. Therefore, further studies are warranted to comprehensively characterize the role of PKC in the regulation of cholinergic activity in the human DSM under normal and pathologic conditions.

Regulation of bladder function by PKC under pathophysiological conditions

The role of PKC in bladder pathophysiology is largely related to DSM contractile dysfunction and dysfunctional voiding associated with partial bladder outlet obstruction (PBOO), and detrusor overactivity (DO). Initial studies, using a PBOO model in rabbits, reported that PKC signaling under pathophysiological conditions was uncoupled from its downstream targets and produced little or no force in response to PKC activator, PDBu [27]. Chang et al. [25] also determined that decreased force generation in decompensated PBOO bladders in response to PKC activator, PDBu, was associated with reduced expression of PKC and increased frequency of urination in the obstructed bladders. It should be noted, however, that a broad range of contractile and metabolic dysfunctions were linked to decompensated bladder function in PBOO models [77, 78]. Further studies confirmed a deficit in the PKC pathway in guinea pig DSM after PBOO [79]. Partial bladder outlet obstruction causes two phenotypes of bladder dysfunction referred to as compensated and decompensated bladders [25, 77]. Compensated bladders are characterized mainly by increased smooth muscle hypertrophy, however, residual urine and frequency of micturition have been reported in compensated bladders associated with PKC dysfunction [25, 80, 81]. Decompensated bladders develop an increase in extracellular matrix including collagen and connective tissue resulting in a loss of bladder compliance, decreased contractility, and a substantial loss of bladder emptying function [25, 77, 78, 80–83]. Changes in PKC expression and activity in a PBOO model seem to be dependent on the species and degree of obstruction. Thus, in the rabbit model of PBOO, decompensated bladders revealed a reduction in PKC expression, activity and force generation associated with reduced bladder emptying and frequency of urination, while compensated bladders exhibited increased PKC expression [25]. However, in the rat bladders with PBOO, PKC expression was reduced in both compensated, and decompensated bladders [81]. Additionally, recent *in vivo* studies established that inhibition of PKC during cystometric recordings in awake rats induced bladder decompensation characterized by an increase in non-voiding contractions (DO), and a significant decrease in void volume [22].

Increased PKC-mediated frequency of urination along with DO have also been reported in the absence of PBOO. In a model of obesity associated with insulin resistance, PKC expression was significantly higher in the bladders of obese mice [26] which showed increased contractility to PDBu, increased frequency, and non-voiding contractions. The changes in the voiding cycle were reversed by metformin treatment which restored high PKC expression in the urinary bladders. High levels of PKC stimulation in rat bladders [22], and high level of expression in compensated rabbit bladders [25] were associated with enhanced nerve-mediated contractions, and frequency of urination, respectively. Thus, a high level of PKC activity and expression may lower the threshold for activation of intramural nerves leading to neurogenic frequency of urination in both diabetic, and compensated bladders. It was established that the protein adiponectin, expressed in adipose tissue, contributed to the increased expression of calcium-dependent PKC-α and enhanced contractile force of DSM in adiponectin-sense transgenic mice [67]. Additionally, carbachol-induced phosphorylation of PKC-α was also elevated in these animals in comparison with WT mice suggesting that adiponectin increases calcium dependency of DSM contractions mediated by PKC-α expression.

It was previously shown that reduced expression of PKC in decompensated rabbit bladders was associated with increased frequency, decreased void, and consequently large residual volumes [25]. Additional cystometric studies in awake rats also revealed that pharmacological inhibition of PKC by Bim-1, and Ro318220 induced an increase in non-voiding contractions, frequency, and decreased void volume [22]. Interestingly, both inhibitors of PKC significantly reduced the ability to maintain muscle force of DSM but did not affect the sensitivity of force generation in response to EFS-mediated nerve stimulation. These data indicate that resting and low levels of PKC activity do not have a significant effect on nerve-mediated contractions in DSM. The ability to maintain DSM force is largely a function of the smooth muscle, and involves calcium sensitization mechanisms mediated by PKC, and Rho-kinase in a calcium-independent manner [3, 8, 24, 68]. Therefore, the frequency of micturition induced by reduced expression of PKC in decompensated rabbit bladders, and pharmacologic inhibition during cystometry in rat bladders are largely myogenic. The inability to maintain muscle force due to significantly low levels of PKC activity results in reduced bladder emptying, increased residual volumes, and an overall shortening of the micturition cycle leading to voiding frequency [22].

Partial bladder outlet obstruction, well known for its prevalence in aging males and often secondary to benign prostatic hyperplasia, has also been shown to alter structural proteins within the bladder wall leading to reduced compliance, DO, and frequency of urination. Among the structural proteins altered in PBOO are smooth muscle myosin (SMM) [84] collagen [85], caldesmon [80] and connective tissue [86]. A change in the ratio and organization of smooth muscle to non-smooth muscle elements is generally believed to lead to stiffening of the bladder wall, and a reduction in compliance resulting in a reduced storage capacity, and frequency of urination [77, 80, 85, 87]. However, significant changes in structural elements such as connective tissue, and collagen may represent some of more severe consequences of acute bladder outlet obstruction, associated with bladder decompensation, and may not represent some of the more subtle changes in bladder function that occur due to changes in regulatory proteins and associated with bladder compensation [3, 25, 88, 89].

Figure 3 highlights the changes which characterize a milder form of dysfunction in compensated bladders such as decreased relaxation and increased DSM tone in response to the PKC activator, PDBu. Low levels of PKC stimulation which induce inhibition in normal DSM (panel A1) resulted in increased force in compensated DSM (panel A2). Additionally, moderate to high levels of PKC stimulation caused a modulated rise in tension in normal bladder DSM (panel B1), but a linear increase in the compensated DSM (panel B2). A failure to relax sufficiently and a linear, instead of a modular, increase in DSM tone are the contributing factors to a higher bladder pressure and bladder dysfunction observed in compensated bladders in comparison with normal and sham-operated controls.

Study limitations

We acknowledge that our study has several limitations. First, we were not able to find any direct data on the role of PKC signaling in detrusor underactivity nor whether PKC pathways could be pharmacologically targeted to improve this condition. Second, we could

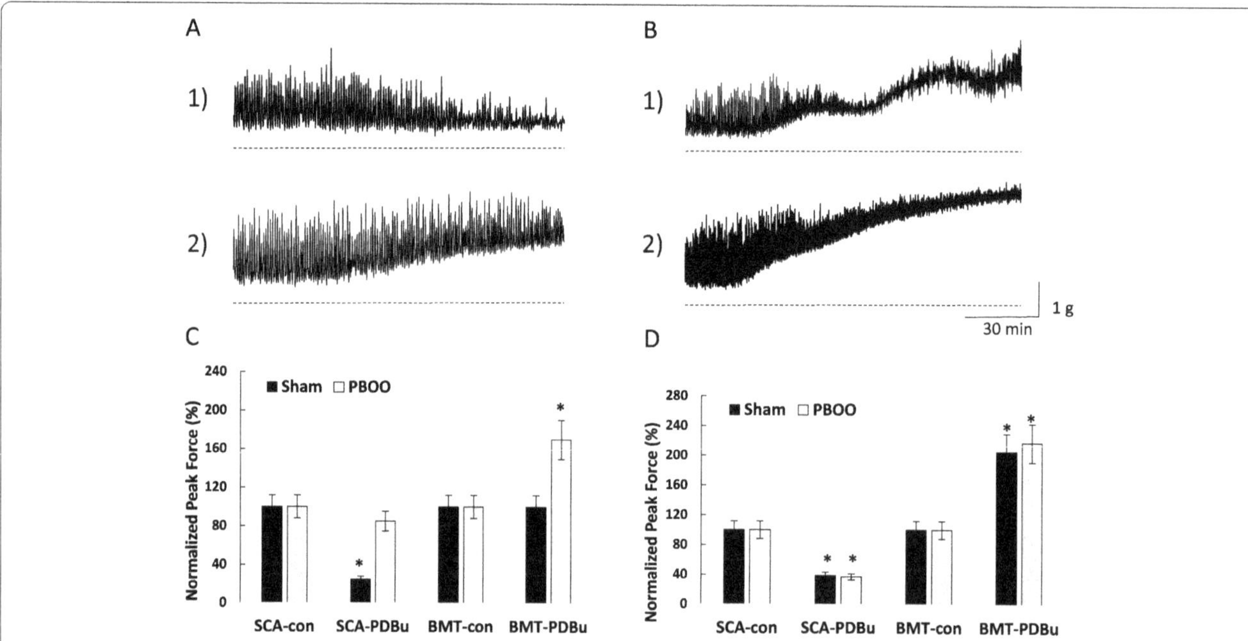

Fig. 3 Low and high levels of PKC stimulation by PDBu differentially affect DSM tone and spontaneous contractions. **a** Representative isolated muscle strips showing the effect of low (20nM) PDBu stimulation on sham (*upper trace*) and PBOO (*lower trace*) DSM strips from rabbits. Summary data is presented in **c. b** Representative isolated muscle strips showing the effect of high (100 nM) PDBu stimulation on sham (*upper trace*) and PBOO (*lower trace*). Summary data is presented in **d**. Low PDBu stimulation caused a significant inhibition of spontaneous contraction amplitude (SCA) of the sham muscle strips but only a minor effect in PBOO strips, however low PDBu caused a significant increase in basal DSM tone in the PBOO strips. High PDBu stimulation caused a significant increase in basal DSM tone for both sham and PBOO, however, there was a qualitative difference in the profile of the contractions. The force increase in the sham bladders displayed a biphasic effect whereas an increase in PBOO muscle strips tended to be more linear. High PDBu also significantly reduced the amplitude of spontaneous contractions for both sham and PBOO muscle strips

not find sufficient information on the role of PKC pathways in sensory and efferent innervation of the lower urinary tract. This could be especially important for understanding the role of PKC in other pathological urologic conditions such as chronic pelvic pain (CPP) and bladder pain syndrome (BPS) [90, 91]. For example, a high level of PKC expression and/or activity has been suggested to play a role in feline interstitial cystitis [73], a naturally occurring bladder pain and dysfunctional voiding in cats. It would be of interest to determine whether or not PKC is overexpressed in these bladders, since high PKC stimulation was shown to increase bladder wall tension, and enhance neuronal sensitivity and contractility [8, 22, 25, 28]. Third, future studies focused on the role of PKC in the bladder urothelium are required to clarify the role of epithelial PKC in micturition.

Conclusions

PKC function in the urinary bladder extends far beyond its contribution, or the lack thereof, to maximum force generation in response to agonists, either directly, or in response to EFS. Data indicate that PKC is involved in the regulation of normal bladder function, and that PKC dysfunction is associated with DO, reduced contractility, and decreased void volume. Relaxation and modulation of spontaneous myogenic, and NVC via PKC-dependent activation of BK and K_{ATP} channels may also be one of its primary functions in support of bladder storage. Both *in vitro*, and *in vivo* studies reveal that PKC may be involved in regulating neuronal activity at the peripheral level in a concentration-dependent manner that may function in a complementary way to facilitate voiding. Finally, the demonstration that PKC dysfunction coexists with pathological changes such as PBOO, DO and is associated with reduced contractility and bladder emptying is further evidence of a significant and important role for PKC in the regulation of urinary bladder function.

Abbreviations

Bim-1: Bisindilylmaleimide1; BK: Large conductance calcium-activated potassium channel; BSM: Bladder smooth muscle; BPS: Bladder pain syndrome; Ca^{++}: Calcium; CPP: Chronic pelvic pain; CNS: Central nervous system; DSM: Detrusor smooth muscle; DO: Detrusor overactivity; EFS: Electrical field stimulation; IF: Integral force; M_3: Muscarinic; MLCP: Myosin light chain phosphorylation; NVC: Non-voiding contractions; OAB: Overactive bladder; PBOO: Partial bladder outlet obstruction; PDBu: Phorbol-12,13-dibutyrate; PF: Peak force; PLC: Phospholipase C; PMA: Phorbol-12,13-myristate; PKC: Protein kinase C; ROK: Rho-associated kinase; VGCC: Voltage gated calcium channels; SK: Small conductance ca^{++}-activated potassium channels; SMM: Smooth muscle myosin; THR: Threonine.

Competing interests

The authors declare that they have no competing interests.

Authors' contributions

JAH - conception and design, analysis and interpretation of the data, drafting of the manuscript. APM - general supervision, critical revision for intellectual content. All authors have made a significant contribution to the paper, and have read and approved the final draft.

Acknowledgments

The study has been supported by the NIH/NIDDK grant DK095817.

References

1. Andersson KE. Changes in bladder tone during filling: pharmacological aspects. Scand J Urol Nephrol Suppl. 1999;201:67–72. discussion 76–99.
2. Andersson KE. Detrusor myocyte activity and afferent signaling. Neurourol Urodyn. 2010;29(1):97–106.
3. Boopathi E, Hypolite JA, Zderic SA, Gomes CM, Malkowicz B, Liou HC, et al. GATA-6 and NF-kappaB activate CPI-17 gene transcription and regulate Ca2+ sensitization of smooth muscle contraction. Mol Cell Biol. 2013;33(5):1085–102.
4. Brading AF. Spontaneous activity of lower urinary tract smooth muscles: correlation between ion channels and tissue function. J Physiol. 2006;570(Pt 1):13–22.
5. Drake MJ, Harvey IJ, Gillespie JI. Autonomous activity in the isolated guinea pig bladder. Exp Physiol. 2003;88(1):19–30.
6. Gillespie JI. Modulation of autonomous contractile activity in the isolated whole bladder of the guinea pig. BJU Int. 2004;93(3):393–400.
7. Hypolite JA, Chang S, LaBelle E, Babu GJ, Periasamy M, Wein AJ, et al. Deletion of SM-B, the high ATPase isoform of myosin, upregulates the PKC-mediated signal transduction pathway in murine urinary bladder smooth muscle. Am J Physiol Renal Physiol. 2009;296(3):F658–665.
8. Hypolite JA, Lei Q, Chang S, Zderic SA, Butler S, Wein AJ, et al. Spontaneous and evoked contractions are regulated by PKC-mediated signaling in detrusor smooth muscle: involvement of BK channels. Am J Physiol Renal Physiol. 2013;304(5):F451–462.
9. Hypolite JA, Wein AJ, Haugaard N, Levin RM. Role of substrates in the maintenance of contractility of the rabbit urinary bladder. Pharmacology. 1991;42(4):202–10.
10. Levin RM, Hypolite J, Longhurst PA, Wein AJ. Comparison of the contractile and metabolic effects of muscarinic stimulation with those of KCl. Pharmacology. 1991;42(3):142–50.
11. Levin RM, Ruggieri MR, Velagapudi S, Gordon D, Altman B, Wein AJ. Relevance of spontaneous activity to urinary bladder function: an in vitro and in vivo study. J Urol. 1986;136(2):517–21.
12. Wein AJ. Physiology of micturition. Clin Geriatr Med. 1986;2(4):689–99.
13. Zhao Y, Wein AJ, Levin RM. Role of calcium in mediating the biphasic contraction of the rabbit urinary bladder. Gen Pharmacol. 1993;24(3):727–31.
14. Schneider T, Fetscher C, Krege S, Michel MC. Signal transduction underlying carbachol-induced contraction of human urinary bladder. J Pharmacol Exp Ther. 2004;309(3):1148–53.
15. Frazier EP, Peters SL, Braverman AS, Ruggieri Sr MR, Michel MC. Signal transduction underlying the control of urinary bladder smooth muscle tone by muscarinic receptors and beta-adrenoceptors. Naunyn Schmiedebergs Arch Pharmacol. 2008;377(4–6):449–62.
16. Frazier EP, Braverman AS, Peters SL, Michel MC, Ruggieri Sr MR. Does phospholipase C mediate muscarinic receptor-induced rat urinary bladder contraction? J Pharmacol Exp Ther. 2007;322(3):998–1002.
17. Durlu-Kandilci NT, Brading AF. Involvement of Rho kinase and protein kinase C in carbachol-induced calcium sensitization in beta-escin skinned rat and guinea-pig bladders. Br J Pharmacol. 2006;148(3):376–84.
18. Fleichman M, Schneider T, Fetscher C, Michel MC. Signal transduction underlying carbachol-induced contraction of rat urinary bladder. II. Protein kinases. J Pharmacol Exp Ther. 2004;308(1):54–8.
19. An JY, Yun HS, Lee YP, Yang SJ, Shim JO, Jeong JH, et al. The intracellular pathway of the acetylcholine-induced contraction in cat detrusor muscle cells. Br J Pharmacol. 2002;137(7):1001–10.
20. Aburto T, Jinsi A, Zhu Q, Deth RC. Involvement of protein kinase C activation in alpha 2-adrenoceptor-mediated contractions of rabbit saphenous vein. Eur J Pharmacol. 1995;277(1):35–44.
21. Dessy C, Kim I, Sougnez CL, Laporte R, Morgan KG. A role for MAP kinase in differentiated smooth muscle contraction evoked by alpha-adrenoceptor stimulation. Am J Physiol. 1998;275(4 Pt 1):C1081–1086.

22. Hypolite JA, Chang S, Wein AJ, Chacko S, Malykhina AP. Protein kinase C modulates frequency of micturition and non-voiding contractions in the urinary bladder via neuronal and myogenic mechanisms. BMC Urol. 2015;15(1):34.
23. Caulfield MP, Birdsall NJ. International Union of Pharmacology. XVII. Classification of muscarinic acetylcholine receptors. Pharmacol Rev. 1998;50(2):279–90.
24. Wang T, Kendig DM, Smolock EM, Moreland RS. Carbachol-induced rabbit bladder smooth muscle contraction: roles of protein kinase C and Rho kinase. Am J Physiol Renal Physiol. 2009;297(6):F1534–1542.
25. Chang S, Hypolite JA, Mohanan S, Zderic SA, Wein AJ, Chacko S. Alteration of the PKC-mediated signaling pathway for smooth muscle contraction in obstruction-induced hypertrophy of the urinary bladder. Lab Invest. 2009;89(7):823–32.
26. Leiria LO, Sollon C, Calixto MC, Lintomen L, Monica FZ, Anhe GF, et al. Role of PKC and CaV1.2 in detrusor overactivity in a model of obesity associated with insulin resistance in mice. PLoS One. 2012;7(11):e48507.
27. Stanton MC, Austin JC, Delaney DP, Gosfield A, Marx JO, Zderic SA, et al. Partial bladder outlet obstruction selectively abolishes protein kinase C induced contraction of rabbit detrusor smooth muscle. J Urol. 2006;176(6 Pt 1):2716–21.
28. Wang T, Kendig DM, Trappanese DM, Smolock EM, Moreland RS. Phorbol 12,13-dibutyrate-induced, protein kinase C-mediated contraction of rabbit bladder smooth muscle. Front Pharmacol. 2012;2:83.
29. Ekman M, Andersson KE, Arner A. Receptor-induced phasic activity of newborn mouse bladders is inhibited by protein kinase C and involves T-type Ca2+ channels. BJU Int. 2009;104(5):690–7.
30. Somogyi GT, Tanowitz M, Zernova G, de Groat WC. M1 muscarinic receptor-induced facilitation of ACh and noradrenaline release in the rat bladder is mediated by protein kinase C. J Physiol. 1996;496(Pt 1):245–54.
31. Hristov KL, Smith AC, Parajuli SP, Malysz J, Petkov GV. Large-conductance voltage- and Ca2 + –activated K+ channel regulation by protein kinase C in guinea pig urinary bladder smooth muscle. Am J Physiol Cell Physiol. 2014;306(5):C460–470.
32. Petkov GV. Central role of the BK channel in urinary bladder smooth muscle physiology and pathophysiology. Am J Physiol Regul Integr Comp Physiol. 2014;307(6):R571–584.
33. Huster M, Frei E, Hofmann F, Wegener JW. A complex of Ca(V)1.2/PKC is involved in muscarinic signaling in smooth muscle. FASEB J. 2010;24(8):2651–9.
34. Liu SH, Lin-Shiau SY. Protein kinase c regulates purinergic component of neurogenic contractions in mouse bladder. J Urol. 2000;164(5):1764–7.
35. Weng TI, Chen WJ, Liu SH. Bladder instillation of Escherichia coli lipopolysaccharide alters the muscle contractions in rat urinary bladder via a protein kinase C-related pathway. Toxicol Appl Pharmacol. 2005;208(2):163–9.
36. Petkov GV. Role of potassium ion channels in detrusor smooth muscle function and dysfunction. Nat Rev Urol. 2012;9(1):30–40.
37. Schneider T, Hein P, Michel MC. Signal transduction underlying carbachol-induced contraction of rat urinary bladder. I. Phospholipases and Ca2+ sources. J Pharmacol Exp Ther. 2004;308(1):47–53.
38. Wuest M, Hiller N, Braeter M, Hakenberg OW, Wirth MP, Ravens U. Contribution of Ca2+ influx to carbachol-induced detrusor contraction is different in human urinary bladder compared to pig and mouse. Eur J Pharmacol. 2007;565(1–3):180–9.
39. Zderic SA, Sillen U, Liu GH, Snyder 3rd MC, Duckett JW, Gong C, et al. Developmental aspects of excitation contraction coupling of rabbit bladder smooth muscle. J Urol. 1994;152(2 Pt 2):679–81.
40. Buckner SA, Milicic I, Daza AV, Coghlan MJ, Gopalakrishnan M. Spontaneous phasic activity of the pig urinary bladder smooth muscle: characteristics and sensitivity to potassium channel modulators. Br J Pharmacol. 2002;135(3):639–48.
41. Uchida W, Masuda N, Shirai Y, Shibasaki K, Satoh N, Takenada T. The role of extracellular Ca2+ in carbachol-induced tonic contraction of the pig detrusor smooth muscle. Naunyn Schmiedebergs Arch Pharmacol. 1994;350(4):398–402.
42. Masters JG, Neal DE, Gillespie JI. The contribution of intracellular Ca2+ release to contraction in human bladder smooth muscle. Br J Pharmacol. 1999;127(4):996–1002.
43. Kajioka S, Nakayama S, McMurray G, Abe K, Brading AF. Ca(2+) channel properties in smooth muscle cells of the urinary bladder from pig and human. Eur J Pharmacol. 2002;443(1–3):19–29.
44. Levin RM, Hypolite J, Ruggieri MR, Longhurst PA, Wein AJ. Effects of muscarinic stimulation on intracellular calcium in the rabbit bladder: comparison with metabolic response. Pharmacology. 1989;39(2):69–77.
45. Herrera GM, Heppner TJ, Nelson MT. Regulation of urinary bladder smooth muscle contractions by ryanodine receptors and BK and SK channels. Am J Physiol Regul Integr Comp Physiol. 2000;279(1):R60–68.
46. Bonev AD, Nelson MT. ATP-sensitive potassium channels in smooth muscle cells from guinea pig urinary bladder. Am J Physiol. 1993;264(5 Pt 1):C1190–1200.
47. Gopalakrishnan M, Whiteaker KL, Molinari EJ, Davis-Taber R, Scott VE, Shieh CC, et al. Characterization of the ATP-sensitive potassium channels (KATP) expressed in guinea pig bladder smooth muscle cells. J Pharmacol Exp Ther. 1999;289(1):551–8.
48. Buckner SA, Milicic I, Daza A, Davis-Taber R, Scott VE, Sullivan JP, et al. Pharmacological and molecular analysis of ATP-sensitive K(+) channels in the pig and human detrusor. Eur J Pharmacol. 2000;400(2–3):287–95.
49. Ha JH, Lee KY, Kim WJ. Actions of potassium channel openers in rat detrusor urinae. J Korean Med Sci. 1993;8(1):53–9.
50. Edwards G, Henshaw M, Miller M, Weston AH. Comparison of the effects of several potassium-channel openers on rat bladder and rat portal vein in vitro. Br J Pharmacol. 1991;102(3):679–86.
51. Malmgren A, Andersson KE, Sjogren C, Andersson PO. Effects of pinacidil and cromakalim (BRL 34915) on bladder function in rats with detrusor instability. J Urol. 1989;142(4):1134–8.
52. Bonev AD, Nelson MT. Muscarinic inhibition of ATP-sensitive K+ channels by protein kinase C in urinary bladder smooth muscle. Am J Physiol. 1993;265(6 Pt 1):C1723–1728.
53. Frayer SM, Barber LA, Vasko MR. Activation of protein kinase C enhances peptide release from rat spinal cord slices. Neurosci Lett. 1999;265(1):17–20.
54. Braverman AS, Doumanian LR, Ruggieri Sr MR. M2 and M3 muscarinic receptor activation of urinary bladder contractile signal transduction. II. Denervated rat bladder. J Pharmacol Exp Ther. 2006;316(2):875–80.
55. Longhurst PA, Leggett RE, Briscoe JA. Characterization of the functional muscarinic receptors in the rat urinary bladder. Br J Pharmacol. 1995;116(4):2279–85.
56. Boberg L, Poljakovic M, Rahman A, Eccles R, Arner A. Role of Rho-kinase and protein kinase C during contraction of hypertrophic detrusor in mice with partial urinary bladder outlet obstruction. BJU Int. 2012;109(1):132–40.
57. Eto M, Ohmori T, Suzuki M, Furuya K, Morita F. A novel protein phosphatase-1 inhibitory protein potentiated by protein kinase C. Isolation from porcine aorta media and characterization. J Biochem. 1995;118(6):1104–7.
58. Eto M, Senba S, Morita F, Yazawa M. Molecular cloning of a novel phosphorylation-dependent inhibitory protein of protein phosphatase-1 (CPI17) in smooth muscle: its specific localization in smooth muscle. FEBS Lett. 1997;410(2–3):356–60.
59. Adelstein RS, Eisenberg E. Regulation and kinetics of the actin-myosin-ATP interaction. Annu Rev Biochem. 1980;49:921–56.
60. Ng YK, de Groat WC, Wu HY. Muscarinic regulation of neonatal rat bladder spontaneous contractions. Am J Physiol Regul Integr Comp Physiol. 2006;291(4):R1049–1059.
61. Hristov KL, Parajuli SP, Soder RP, Cheng Q, Rovner ES, Petkov GV. Suppression of human detrusor smooth muscle excitability and contractility via pharmacological activation of large conductance Ca2 + –activated K+ channels. Am J Physiol Cell Physiol. 2012;302(11):C1632–1641.
62. Brading AF. Ion channels and control of contractile activity in urinary bladder smooth muscle. Jpn J Pharmacol. 1992;58 Suppl 2:120P–7P.
63. Rivera L, Brading AF. The role of Ca2+ influx and intracellular Ca2+ release in the muscarinic-mediated contraction of mammalian urinary bladder smooth muscle. BJU Int. 2006;98(4):868–75.
64. Klockner U, Isenberg G. Action potentials and net membrane currents of isolated smooth muscle cells (urinary bladder of the guinea-pig). Pflugers Arch. 1985;405(4):329–39.
65. Nakamura Y, Ishiura Y, Yokoyama O, Namiki M, De Groat WC. Role of protein kinase C in central muscarinic inhibitory mechanisms regulating voiding in rats. Neuroscience. 2003;116(2):477–84.
66. Hristov KL, Chen M, Kellett WF, Rovner ES, Petkov GV. Large-conductance voltage- and Ca2 + –activated K+ channels regulate human detrusor smooth muscle function. Am J Physiol Cell Physiol. 2011;301(4):C903–912.
67. Nobe K, Fujii A, Saito K, Negoro T, Ogawa Y, Nakano Y, et al. Adiponectin enhances calcium dependency of mouse bladder contraction mediated by protein kinase Calpha expression. J Pharmacol Exp Ther. 2013;345(1):62–8.

68. Takahashi R, Nishimura J, Hirano K, Seki N, Naito S, Kanaide H. Ca2+ sensitization in contraction of human bladder smooth muscle. J Urol. 2004;172(2):748–52.
69. Yoshimura Y, Yamaguchi O. Calcium independent contraction of bladder smooth muscle. Int J Urol. 1997;4(1):62–7.
70. Boopathi E, Gomes C, Zderic SA, Malkowicz B, Chakrabarti R, Patel DP, et al. Mechanical stretch upregulates proteins involved in Ca2+ sensitization in urinary bladder smooth muscle hypertrophy. Am J Physiol Cell Physiol. 2014;307(6):C542–553.
71. Ji G, Barsotti RJ, Feldman ME, Kotlikoff MI. Stretch-induced calcium release in smooth muscle. J Gen Physiol. 2002;119(6):533–44.
72. Downing JE, Role LW. Activators of protein kinase C enhance acetylcholine receptor desensitization in sympathetic ganglion neurons. Proc Natl Acad Sci U S A. 1987;84(21):7739–43.
73. Sculptoreanu A, de Groat WC, Buffington CA, Birder LA. Protein kinase C contributes to abnormal capsaicin responses in DRG neurons from cats with feline interstitial cystitis. Neurosci Lett. 2005;381(1–2):42–6.
74. Zhou Y, Zhou ZS, Zhao ZQ. PKC regulates capsaicin-induced currents of dorsal root ganglion neurons in rats. Neuropharmacology. 2001;41(5):601–8.
75. Parajuli SP, Hristov KL, Cheng Q, Malysz J, Rovner ES, Petkov GV. Functional link between muscarinic receptors and large-conductance Ca-activated K channels in freshly isolated human detrusor smooth muscle cells. *Pflugers Archiv.* 2015;467(4):665-75. doi:10.1007/s00424-014-1537-8. Epub 2014 May 28.
76. Parajuli SP, Hristov KL, Cheng Q, Malysz J, Rovner ES, Petkov GV. Functional link between muscarinic receptors and large-conductance Ca2 + – activated K+ channels in freshly isolated human detrusor smooth muscle cells. Pflugers Arch. 2015;467(4):665–75.
77. Levin RM, Haugaard N, Hypolite JA, Wein AJ, Buttyan R. Metabolic factors influencing lower urinary tract function. Exp Physiol. 1999;84(1):171–94.
78. Levin RM, Monson FC, Haugaard N, Buttyan R, Hudson A, Roelofs M, et al. Genetic and cellular characteristics of bladder outlet obstruction. Urol Clin North Am. 1995;22(2):263–83.
79. Shahab N, Kajioka S, Takahashi-Yanaga F, Onimaru M, Matsuda M, Seki N, et al. Obstruction enhances rho-kinase pathway and diminishes protein kinase C pathway in carbachol-induced calcium sensitization in contraction of alpha-toxin permeabilized guinea pig detrusor smooth muscle. Neurourol Urodyn. 2012;31(4):593–9.
80. Zhang EY, Stein R, Chang S, Zheng Y, Zderic SA, Wein AJ, et al. Smooth muscle hypertrophy following partial bladder outlet obstruction is associated with overexpression of non-muscle caldesmon. Am J Pathol. 2004;164(2):601–12.
81. Choi BH, Jin LH, Kim KH, Kang SA, Kang JH, Yoon SM, et al. Cystometric parameters and the activity of signaling proteins in association with the compensation or decompensation of bladder function in an animal experimental model of partial bladder outlet obstruction. Int J Mol Med. 2013;32(6):1435–41.
82. Levin RM, Longhurst PA, Monson FC, Kato K, Wein AJ. Effect of bladder outlet obstruction on the morphology, physiology, and pharmacology of the bladder. Prostate Suppl. 1990;3:9–26.
83. Stein R, Gong C, Hutcheson JC, Canning DA, Zderic SA. The decompensated detrusor III: impact of bladder outlet obstruction on sarcoplasmic endoplasmic reticulum protein and gene expression. J Urol. 2000;164(3 Pt 2):1026–30.
84. DiSanto ME, Stein R, Chang S, Hypolite JA, Zheng Y, Zderic S, et al. Alteration in expression of myosin isoforms in detrusor smooth muscle following bladder outlet obstruction. Am J Physiol Cell Physiol. 2003;285(6):C1397–1410.
85. Macarak EJ, Schulz J, Zderic SA, Sado Y, Ninomiya Y, Polyak E, et al. Smooth muscle trans-membrane sarcoglycan complex in partial bladder outlet obstruction. Histochem Cell Biol. 2006;126(1):71–82.
86. Sjuve R, Haase H, Ekblad E, Malmqvist U, Morano I, Arner A. Increased expression of non-muscle myosin heavy chain-B in connective tissue cells of hypertrophic rat urinary bladder. Cell Tissue Res. 2001;304(2):271–8.
87. Iguchi N, Hou A, Koul HK, Wilcox DT. Partial bladder outlet obstruction in mice may cause E-cadherin repression through hypoxia induced pathway. J Urol. 2014;192(3):964–72.
88. Chacko S, Chang S, Hypolite J, Disanto M, Wein A. Alteration of contractile and regulatory proteins following partial bladder outlet obstruction. Scand J Urol Nephrol Suppl. 2004;215:26–36.
89. Chang S, Gomes CM, Hypolite JA, Marx J, Alanzi J, Zderic SA, et al. Detrusor overactivity is associated with downregulation of large-conductance calcium- and voltage-activated potassium channel protein. Am J Physiol Renal Physiol. 2010;298(6):F1416–1423.
90. Malykhina A, Hanno P. How are we going to make progress treating bladder pain syndrome? ICI-RS 2013. Neurourol Urodyn. 2014;33(5):625–9.
91. Sadler KE, Stratton JM, Kolber BJ. Urinary bladder distention evoked visceromotor responses as a model for bladder pain in mice. *J Vis Exp.* 2014:(86).

18

Anticholinergic burden and comorbidities in patients attending treatment with trospium chloride for overactive bladder in a real-life setting

A. Ivchenko[1], R.-H. Bödeker[2], C. Neumeister[3*] and A. Wiedemann[1]

Abstract

Background: Elderly people are representative for the patients most likely to be treated with anticholinergics for overactive bladder (OAB). They often receive further drugs with anticholinergic properties for concomitant conditions. This increases the risk for side effects, including central nervous system disorders. Data on comorbidities and baseline anticholinergic burden of OAB patients seen in urological practice is scarce. Therefore, we included an epidemiological survey on these issues in our study which assessed the effectiveness and tolerability of trospium chloride (TC) in established dosages under routine conditions.

Methods: Outpatients (≥ 65 years of age), for whom treatment with TC was indicated, were eligible to participate in this non-interventional, prospective study performed in 162 urological practices in Germany. Epidemiological questions were evaluated by the Anticholinergic Burden (ACB) scale and the Cumulative Illness Rating Scale for Geriatrics (CIRS-G) at baseline. Efficacy was assessed by changes in symptom-related variables of OAB after treatment. Dosage regimen, duration of treatment, adverse events, withdrawals, and ease of subdivision of the prescribed SNAP-TAB tablet were documented. Patients and physicians rated efficacy and tolerability of treatment. Statistics were descriptive.

Results: Four hundred fourty-five out of 986 (47.54%) patients in the epidemiological population had a baseline ACB scale score > 0, 100 (24.72%) of whom a score ≥ 3. The median CIRS-G comorbidity index score for all patients was 5. 78.55% (608/774) of patients in the efficacy population received a daily dose of 45 mg TC. 60.03% (365/608) of them took this dose by dividing the SNAP-TAB tablet in three equal parts. Before-after-comparisons of the core symptoms of OAB showed clear improvements. An influence of the dosage scheme (1 × 45 mg TC/d vs 3 × 15 mg TC/d) on clinical outcome could not be observed. Most urologists and patients rated TC treatment as effective and well tolerated. 44 (4.37%) out of 1007 patients in the safety collective ended their treatment prematurely, while 75 patients (7.45%) experienced adverse events.

Conclusions: Anticholinergic burden and comorbidities in elderly OAB patients are frequent. The acceptance of the SNAP-TAB tablet, which facilitates flexible dosing with TC, was high, which is supportive in ensuring adherence in therapy.

(Continued on next page)

* Correspondence: claudia.neumeister@dr-pfleger.de
[3]Department of Medical Science/Clinical Research, Dr. R. Pfleger GmbH, Dr.-Robert-Pfleger-Strasse 12, 96052 Bamberg, Germany
Full list of author information is available at the end of the article

(Continued from previous page)

Keywords: Anticholinergic burden, Comorbidity index, CIRS-G, Overactive bladder, Elderly patients, Trospium chloride, Non-interventional study

Background

Trospium chloride, a synthetic quaternary antimuscarinic, is intended for symptomatic treatment of the overactive bladder syndrome, providing patients with a fast, reliable and considerable improvement or cure of the stressful symptoms: urinary incontinence, urgency and frequency [1–6]. The recommended daily dose is 45 mg TC (3 × 15 mg).[1] It is adequate for most patients with OAB. Flexible dosing up to daily doses of 90 mg TC is safe and well tolerated, permitting treatment to be tailored to the patient's optimal individual balance between efficacy and side effects [1, 7–9].

Increasing attention is paid to safety and compliance concerns, as older people show an increased prevalence of gradually declining human organ and body functions, resulting in physical, physiological and/or cognitive impairments, multi- and co-morbidities, and/or frailty [10]. They are exposed to an increasing number of medications (polypharmacy), often with known or unknown anticholinergic activity, including prescriptions and over-the-counter products [10, 11]. Estimates suggest that one third to half of commonly prescribed drugs for the elderly have anticholinergic properties [12]. Due to the pattern of receptor distribution and their mechanisms of action, anticholinergic drugs as well as many other drugs not usually denoted as anticholinergics, show their anticholinergic activity throughout the human body. This is often associated with a variety of adverse effects (AEs). The most common are peripheral AEs, such as dry mouth, blurred vision, constipation, and tachycardia, as well as central nervous system (CNS) AEs, including dizziness, sedation, falls, confusion, delirium and cognitive impairment [12–20]. These can, in turn, further worsen patient's mental and physical health status, often leading to dependence [21]. On the other hand, OAB is a common yet disabling condition with a considerably negative impact on the patient's quality of life, sleep, sexual function, work productivity and general mental health [11, 22–24]. Therefore, it is often associated with a significant increase in troublesome symptoms and comorbidities in those patients, such as falls, urinary tract infections, hypertension, diabetes [25–27], as well as higher odds for loneliness and depression [26, 28–30]. The causal relationship between many of these comorbid conditions as well as the question whether treatment of one condition improves or exacerbates the other have thus far largely remained unclear [26]. Nevertheless, muscarinic receptor antagonists are universally accepted to be the first-line pharmacotherapy of OAB [31, 32].

Physicians prescribe drugs with primary or secondary anticholinergic properties based on their anticipated therapeutic benefits. Herein, they sometimes overlook that the concurrent use of several drugs with anticholinergic properties likely results in cumulating effects in the vulnerable elderly patients [12, 15, 21, 33]. This so-called anticholinergic burden (or anticholinergic load) can adversely impact both cognitive and functional status of patients further. Moreover, elderly individuals are thought to be particularly vulnerable to central nervous system AEs of anticholinergics due to age-associated morphological, biochemical, physiological and pathological changes in the brain [12, 34, 35]. A comprehensive systematic review examining associations between drugs with anticholinergic properties and adverse outcomes in older adults concluded that exposure to certain individual drugs with anticholinergic effects or increased overall anticholinergic exposure may increase the risk of falls, cognitive impairment and all-cause-mortality in these patients [36]. Therefore, physicians should carefully consider medical history and concomitant medications when initiating antimuscarinic treatment of OAB in elderly patients.

Generally, however, on the comorbidities and the baseline anticholinergic burden of OAB patients seen in daily urological practice very little information exists. To address this gap of knowledge, we included an epidemiological survey on these two issues in a non-interventional study (NIS) assessing treatment responses and tolerability to TC administered according to current routine treatment schemes in a diverse population of OAB outpatients. Evaluating the ease of subdivision of the SNAP-TAB tablet preparation, containing 45 mg of TC, by the elderly participants was a further objective of this study.

Methods

Study design

This open, prospective, observational study was conducted in 162 urology practices in Germany between November 2014 and October 2015. The number of patients that could be recruited by a single centre was limited to 10 to ensure that the data was not predominantly generated by few large practices, which could jeopardize the representativeness of the sample. The selection and number of study centres was set as is to reflect the most representative picture of "medical practice" in Germany possible. Regarding the data to be gathered in the epidemiological part of the study, 1250 patients were to be recruited into this study to obtain a final sample size of approximately 1000 patients for the analysis of epidemiological research questions. The TC therapy was prescribed by the participating urologists in the course of normal outpatient care, was commercially available and funded according to local practice in usual routine care. The study protocol, therefore, did not contain any specifications regarding dosing of TC or duration of treatment. Instead, the advising urologists were asked to follow the recommendations defined in the licensed approval by the national regulatory authorities. The contraindications, special warnings, precautions for use, interactions, information on use during pregnancy and lactation, effects on ability to drive and use machines, as well as undesirable effects specified in the Summary of Product Characteristics (SmPC) had to be observed.

Compliance with ethics

This post-registration trial conforms with § 67(6) of the German Drug Law. All procedures were carried out in accordance with the official recommendations regarding the conduct of non-interventional studies by the Federal Institute for Drugs and Medical Devices (BfArM) and the Paul-Ehrlich-Institute [37], and the recommendations for assuring Good Epidemiological Practice [38]. Accordingly, the study was notified to the federal authority and the relevant associations. Approval of an ethical committee was not required for such a non-interventional trial in Germany [§67(6) of the German Drug Law]. Nevertheless, the study protocol was submitted to the Ethics Committee of the Medical Chamber Westphalia-Lippe and the Westphalian Wilhelm University Münster, Germany, which gave a favourable recommendation prior to the start of the study (September 2014). All data and information collected in the scope of this study was gathered in accordance with the recommendations for baseline diagnosis specified in the AWMF Guideline No. 084/001 *Urinary Incontinence*, published by the German Geriatric Society [39]. The study was performed within the indication approved in the marketing authorization and under consideration of the contraindications and precautions defined therein [40]. Each physician had to decide on the OAB-therapy independently from the assignment of a patient's inclusion into the study. Patients were admitted only after they had given their written consent to the data protection policy at the first visit. Participants were free to withdraw at will at any time without giving reasons and without incurring disadvantages. Documentation of study-related data of each patient was performed solely in accordance with routine urological assessments.

Patients and treatment

Elderly men and women (≥ 65 years of age) with symptoms of OAB for whom the attending urologist had decided to prescribe a TC preparation containing 45 mg active agent per tablet (Spasmex® 45 mg film-coated tablets) were included in this trial. Consistent with the non-interventional nature of the study, no further restrictions were applied in respect to the inclusion of patients or to the dose and duration of treatment. The preparation Spasmex® 45 mg is a modern SNAP-TAB tablet designed for easy and precise subdivision [41, 42].

Assessments

Participation in this trial included three visits per patient, defined as first, interim and last visit (= Visit 1, 2, 3), with a recommended minimum interval between visits of 10 days. The minimum duration of treatment was recommended to be no less than 6 weeks.

At Visit 1, patients were questioned regarding their comorbidities and their anticholinergic burden, using established scales and questionnaires. The Anticholinergic Cognitive Burden Scale, adapted to the German market, was selected to measure anticholinergic burden [19, 43, 44]. The level of burden caused by chronic illnesses was assessed using the German version of the Cumulative Illness Rating Scale for Geriatrics, which rates the severity of chronic diseases in 14 organ-specific categories on a five-point scale of 0 to 4 [45]. The illness ratings across all organ categories are subsequently summed up to create the comorbidity index (CMI).

The attending urologists entered the patient's data online via an encrypted website, using a validated German Internet-based input system (portal of MedSurv GmbH, Nidderau, Germany). They collected the following information at the specified time points and/or, if applicable, at the time of premature discontinuation of treatment: demography, medical history, pre-treatment of OAB, anticholinergic burden-related medications contributing to the ACB scale score, concomitant diseases contributing to the baseline CIRS-G score, further relevant comedication, OAB symptoms (number of voids/24 h, number of nocturnal voids/hour sleeping time, severity of urgency symptoms, occurrence and number of incontinence episodes, usual amount of urine leakage), prescribed dose and timing of administration of TC 45 mg, any adverse events as well as premature treatment termination. At Visits 2 and 3, physicians and patients were asked to assess effectiveness and tolerability of therapy using the following four categories: very good, good, poor, very poor. Additionally, at Visit 3 or time of premature discontinuation of treatment the investigator queried the patient to rate the ease of subdivision of the SNAP-TAB tablets on a four-point scale with the categories: very easy, easy, somewhat difficult, very difficult.

Data management and statistics

The validity of the anonymized submission data was checked for plausibility and completeness. Missing data on patient and physician assessments of treatment efficacy and tolerability and variables describing OAB symptoms at the last visit was replaced by the corresponding data collected at the interim visit in cases where the time difference between the first and the interim visit was at least 10 days. Adverse events were classified using the MedDRA coding system V19.1.

Transformation, preparation and exploratory analyses of data were carried out using the statistical software package SAS® V9.3 and 9.4, respectively. Since direct calculation of the exact confidence interval of the median was not possible with SAS, it was done using the DescTools package in R-version 3.3.1. The IML module was used to call R from SAS.

Data was analysed using descriptive statistical methods. The distributions of the qualitative and discrete quantitative variables were described in terms of absolute and relative frequencies based on sample size of the respective collective and were presented by three age classes and gender separately, and globally for all patients. The distributions of the continuous variables and quantitative discrete variables with a lot of values were described by sample size, number of missing values, minimum, 1. quartile (Q1), median, 3. quartile (Q3), maximum, and confidence interval (CI) of the median.

To answer the epidemiological research questions, we used logistic regression methods. Since the target variable, the ACB scale score, was extremely skewed to the right, we divided the variable "ACB score" into two classes (ACB = 0 and ACB > 0) before evaluating the data. Since a linear influence of age and CIRS-G score-derived comorbidity index on the probability of the presence of an anticholinergic burden could also not be assumed, the explanatory variable "age" was divided into three classes (65 years to < 75 years, 75 years to < 85 years, and ≥ 85 years), and the explanatory variable "comorbidity index" was divided into four quartile classes (0–2, 3–4, 5–7, and ≥ 8). Effects of the potential effect modifiers age, gender and CIRS-G derived comorbidity index as a measure of the number of health problems were then studied using logistic regression. Because the comorbidity index was also extremely right-skewed, we also transformed this index into a dichotomous variable (≤ 4 versus > 4) when handling the age–/gender-related question to the presence of comorbidity burden.

Efficacy outcomes were evaluated by change in the quantitative variables describing OAB symptoms which was defined as the score difference between the respective variable at Visit 1 and by using a new target variable constructed using the combined data from Visits 3 and 2 (last evaluable Visit minus Visit 1).

Post hoc subgroup analysis

After the statistical analysis was finished as laid down in the study protocol, a subgroup of the efficacy analysis set (n = 385 patients) consisting of two treatment groups according to the dosage regime "1 times a day 45 mg of TC" (n = 90 patients) or "3 times a day 15 mg of TC" (n = 295 patients) documented over the whole treatment period, was used to compare treatment outcomes in relation to the two administration schemes (Fig. 1). All analyses were descriptive and explorative in nature.

For between-group comparisons relating the main variables, we used effect size measures for evaluating the strength of the observed result. We calculated *Cohen's r* for the median *change of average number of voids/24 h between Visit 1 and the last evaluable visit*; and *Cramér's V* for the *combination in the occurrence of incontinence episodes at Visit 1 to the last evaluable visit*, as well as for the assessments of efficacy and tolerability by physicians and patients. For facilitating the interpretation of effect sizes, we used the defined reference values by Cohen [46] and Ellis [47].

Results

Participants

All 1007 recruited participants, including one patient who had been treated before the start of the study and whose data had been submitted retroactively, were included in the safety analysis. In accordance with the study protocol, data sets from 986 patients were available for the epidemiological analysis, and 774 were available for the efficacy analysis (Fig. 1).

Epidemiological population and research-related characteristics

Out of the 986 patients, 564 (57.2%) were women and 422 (42.8%) were men (Table 1). The median age in this population was 75.0 years (range: 65–97; Q1: 70.0, Q3: 79.0) with equal distributions by gender (Hodges-Lehmann estimator: 1 year, 95% CI: [0 years, 2 years]).

At Visit 1, data of 936 patients was analysed and scored on the ACB scale. Overall, 491 (52.46%) patients in the epidemiological population were not taking any drugs with potential anticholinergic effects, as reflected by an ACB scale score of 0; while 445 patients (47.54%; 95% CI [44.30%; 50.80%]) of all patients with evaluable ACB score data at Visit 1 had a baseline anticholinergic burden, as defined as an ACB scale score of > 0 (Fig. 2).

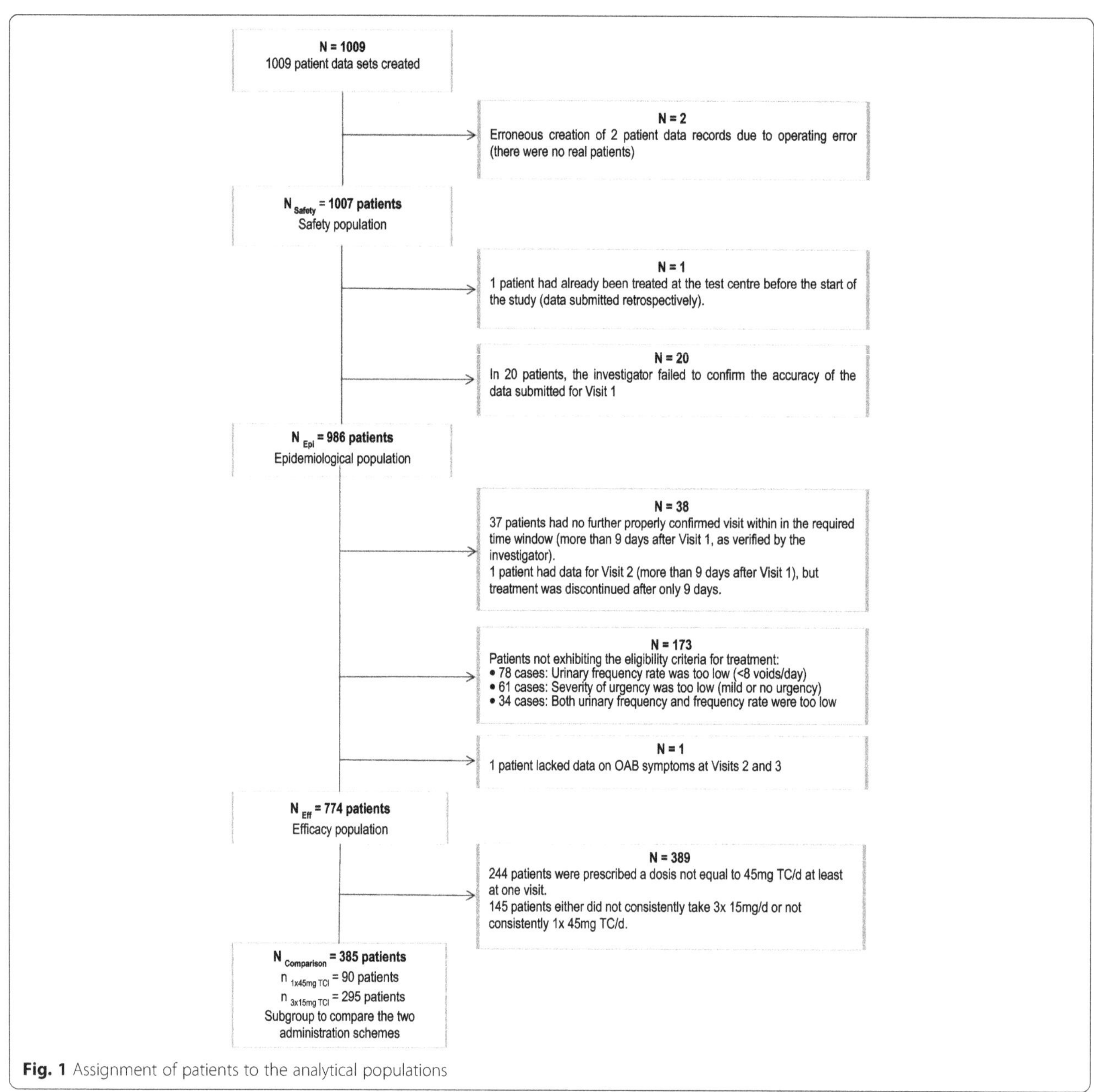

Fig. 1 Assignment of patients to the analytical populations

Table 1 Epidemiological population: Frequency distribution of age classes at the first visit, by sex, and globally

Sex	Patient age at Visit 1 (3 classes)						Total
	65 years to < 75 years		75 years to < 85 years		≥ 85 years		
	n	%	n	%	n	%	N
Female	281	49.82	239	42.38	44	7.80	564
Male	184	43.60	192	45.50	46	10.90	422
All patients	465	47.16	431	43.71	90	9.13	986

The total number of ACB-related drugs taken by the participants was 657. Of them, 479 (72.91%) had an ACB score of 1, 115 (17.50%) had a score of 2, and 63 (9.59%) were anticholinergics with an ACB score of 3. The most commonly used anticholinergic medication was metoprolol ($n = 159$), followed by TC ($n = 101$) and furosemide ($n = 66$).

The median comorbidity index, as calculated from the CIRS-G data for all patients of the epidemiological population, was 5 (exact 95% CI [4.0%; 5.0%]; sum of items 1–14, observed range 0–33), with 52.03% (513/986) of patients observed with a CMI of > 4. Most patients (837/986, 84.89%) did not have any relevant

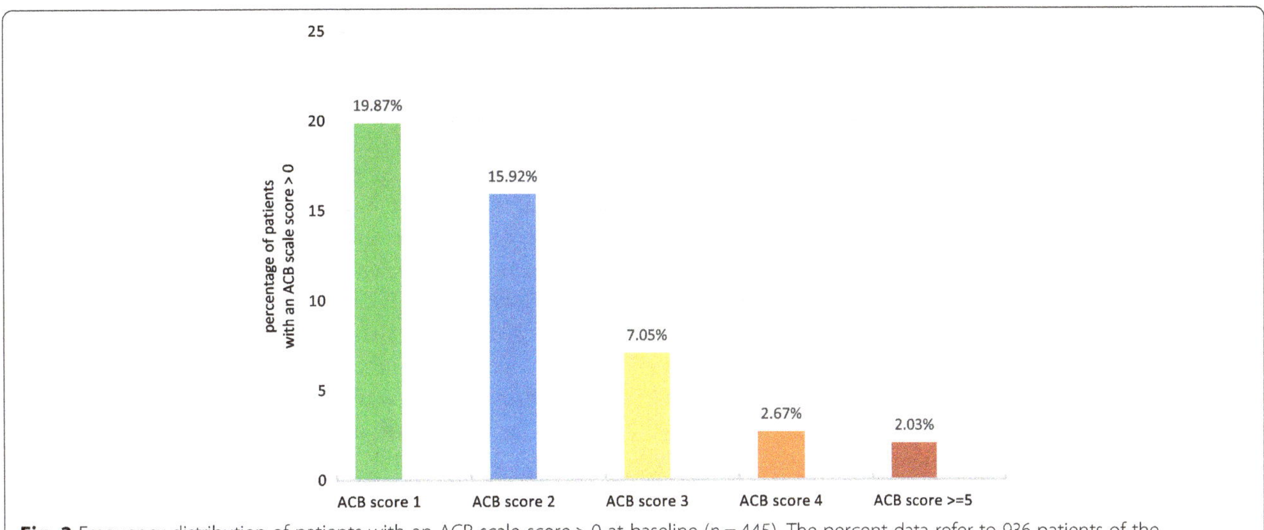

Fig. 2 Frequency distribution of patients with an ACB scale score > 0 at baseline (*n* = 445). The percent data refer to 936 patients of the epidemiological population. An ACB scale score of ≥3 was considered clinically relevant [19]

somatic morbidity (RSM, number of items with a rating of 3 or 4, except for psychiatric disorders = 0), 11.16% of patients (110/986) had a RSM of 1, 3.25% (32/986) a RSM of 2, and 0.71% (7/986) a RSM score between 3 and, at maximum, 5.

The data analysis of possible effect modifiers for the ACB score indicated that the chances of having an anticholinergic burden (ACB > 0) might be higher in patients aged ≥85 years and seemed to be higher in men than in women; additionally, the odds of having an anticholinergic burden seemed to increase with an increasing CMI (Table 2). Similarly, regarding the CIRS-G score-related comorbidity index in this population, the occurrence of having a CMI of > 4 seemed to increase with increasing age and women might have a lower likelihood than men.

Evaluation of efficacy

The population of the efficacy analysis set comprised 774 patients, 456 women and 318 men, with a median age of 75.0 years (range: 65–97; Q1: 70.0, Q3: 79.0) and equal distributions by sex (Hodges-Lehmann estimator for the difference between the location: 1 year, 95% CI: [0 years, 2 years]).

At study entry, 256 out of 764 patients (33.51%) suffered from OAB symptoms for years, 408 patients (53.40%) for months, and 100 patients (13.09%) reported symptoms occurring during the last weeks or days. 34.37% (266/774) of patients had received medical pre-treatment for their OAB syndrome; most frequently used drugs were anticholinergics (62.41%) and herbal drugs for urological disorders (11.28%). The reasons for switching of medication were "insufficient efficacy" in

Table 2 Epidemiological population: Effects of age and sex on ACB score and CMI

Effect	Category of interest versus reference category	Point estimate of the odds ratio	95% confidence interval (Wald's type)
A. Effects of age, gender and/or CIRS-G score-related comorbidity index on ACB score			
Sex	Female vs. male	0.72	[0.55; 0.94]
Age class	75 years to < 85 years vs. 65 years to < 75 years	1.13	[0.85; 1.50]
	≥ 85 years vs. 65 years to < 75 years	1.79	[1.08; 2.94]
CMI (4 classes)	Quartile 2 CMI 3–4 vs. Quartile 1 CMI 0–2	1.69	[1.13; 2.52]
	Quartile 3 CMI 5–7 vs. Quartile 1 CMI 0–2	2.03	[1.38; 2.99]
	Quartile 4 CMI ≥ 8 vs. Quartile 1 CMI 0–2	3.29	[2.23; 4.86]
B. Effects of age and/or gender on the comorbidity index			
Sex	Female vs. male	0.57	[0.44; 0.74]
Age class	75 years to < 85 years vs. 65 years to < 75 years	2.28	[1.74; 2.99]
	≥ 85 years vs. 65 years to < 75 years	2.79	[1.73; 4.51]

Odds ratio point estimates and confidence intervals calculated by comparing the respective category of interest with the reference category for the possible explanatory variables included in the model for the likelihood of having an anticholinergic burden (A) or a comorbidity index of > 4 (B)

221 out of 267 cases (82.77%) and "lack of tolerance" in 31 cases (11.61%).

At Visit 1, 78.55% (608/774) of patients were instructed to take a daily dose of 45 mg TC (Fig. 3). Of them, 60.03% (365/608) took the prescribed dose by dividing the SNAP-TAB tablet in three equal parts corresponding to 15 mg of TC each, to be taken in the morning, noon and night; 19.41% (118/608) took the whole 45 mg tablet as a single daily dose, and 20.56% (125/608) divided the tablet in two doses, one of 30 mg and one of 15 mg of TC.

At Visit 2, the physician decided on the patient's individual response to treatment whether a dose adjustment and/or a change in dosage regimen was necessary or not. In 81.61% (630/772) of patients, the prescribed daily dose remained unchanged (Fig. 4).

The median treatment period documented at the last evaluable visit ($n = 774$) was 64 days (min = 10 (predefined), max = 325; Q1: 46, Q3: 98). Treatment with TC improved symptoms of OAB as evaluated by before-and-after comparisons of different variables. The median change in the average *number of voids per 24 h*, as calculated by subtracting the outcome for Visit 1 from that for the last evaluable Visit, was – 4 (Q1: -6, Q3: -2; exact 95% CI [– 4 voids/24 h; – 4 voids/24 h]) for all patients included in the efficacy population (n = 774). The data analysis by logistic regression indicated that women were more likely to have a ≥ 4-void reduction in the average number of voids per 24 h than men (female vs. men: point estimate of the odds ratio (OR) 1.41, 95% $CI_{Wald's\ type}$ [1.05; 1.91]). Moreover, patients aged ≥75 years to < 85 years seemed to have a lower chance to experience this improvement than patients aged ≥65 years to < 75 years: OR 0.71 (95% $CI_{Wald's\ type}$ [0.52; 0.97]). The median change in the average *number of nocturnal voids/hour sleeping time in the last 7 days* was – 0.3 (Q1: -0.4, Q3: -0.1; $n = 769$). Under treatment, the *severity of urgency symptoms* decreased in 655 (84.63%, 95% CI [81.89%; 87.10%]) out of 774 patients.

38.50% (298/774) of the patients included in the efficacy analysis did not have any incontinence episodes by the time of the first and the last visit. Improvement in the *occurrence of incontinence episodes* was observed in 231 (29.84%, 95% CI [26.64%; 33.21%]) out of 774 individuals, 528 (68.22%) showed no change, and 15 (1.94%) reported worsening of accident occurrence. The *number of incontinence episodes* in this population ($n = 470$) decreased by a median of 5 incontinence episodes (Q1: -10, Q3: -2; 95% CI [– 5.0; – 4.0]). Six further patients confirmed the occurrence of incontinence episodes in the last 7 days before the respective visit but did not provide valid data describing the number of incontinence episodes or the amount of urine leakage. In 349 cases (74.26%) the *amount of urine leakage* decreased from Visit 1 to the last evaluable visit.

The post hoc subgroup analysis did not indicate a difference in treatment outcome between the two dosage regimens "1 x 45 mg TC/day" and "3 x 15 mg TC/day" for any of the efficacy variables. This was also obvious from the effect size measures relating to the variables, with *Cohen's* $r = 0.103$ for the median *change in the number of voids/24 h between Visit 1 and the last evaluable visit*, and *Cramér's* $V = 0.050$ for the *combination in the occurrence of incontinence episodes at Visit 1 to the last evaluable visit*. As the effect size of any variable was < 0.1 or only marginally greater than 0.1, this had to be considered a trivial effect in accordance with the conventions by Cohen [46] and Ellis [47].

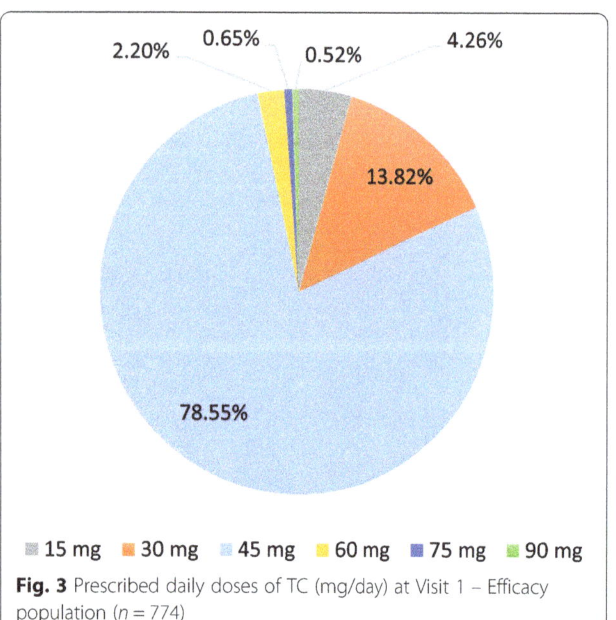

Fig. 3 Prescribed daily doses of TC (mg/day) at Visit 1 – Efficacy population ($n = 774$)

Global assessment of effectiveness and tolerability

At the last evaluable visit, 91.21% of the physicians (706/774) assessed the effectiveness of the OAB treatment with TC 45 mg tablet as either "very good" or "good", as did 89.53% of patients (693/774). The question relating to therapy continuation with 45 mg of TC was answered affirmatively for 672 patients (89.36%); 57 patients (7.58%) required no further treatment and 23 (3.06%) were switched to another treatment modality.

Tolerability was assessed predominantly "very good" or "good" by 94.32% (730/774) of the physicians and by 90.96% (704/774) of the patients.

This trend was also observed in the post hoc analysis regarding the global assessment of effectiveness and tolerability across the two analysed dosage regimens; effectiveness: physicians – *Cramér's* $V = 0.122$, patients – *Cramér's* $V = 0.161$; tolerability: physicians – *Cramér's* $V = 0.075$, patients – *Cramér's* $V = 0.107$. Based on the reference values for effect size measures by Ellis [47], this

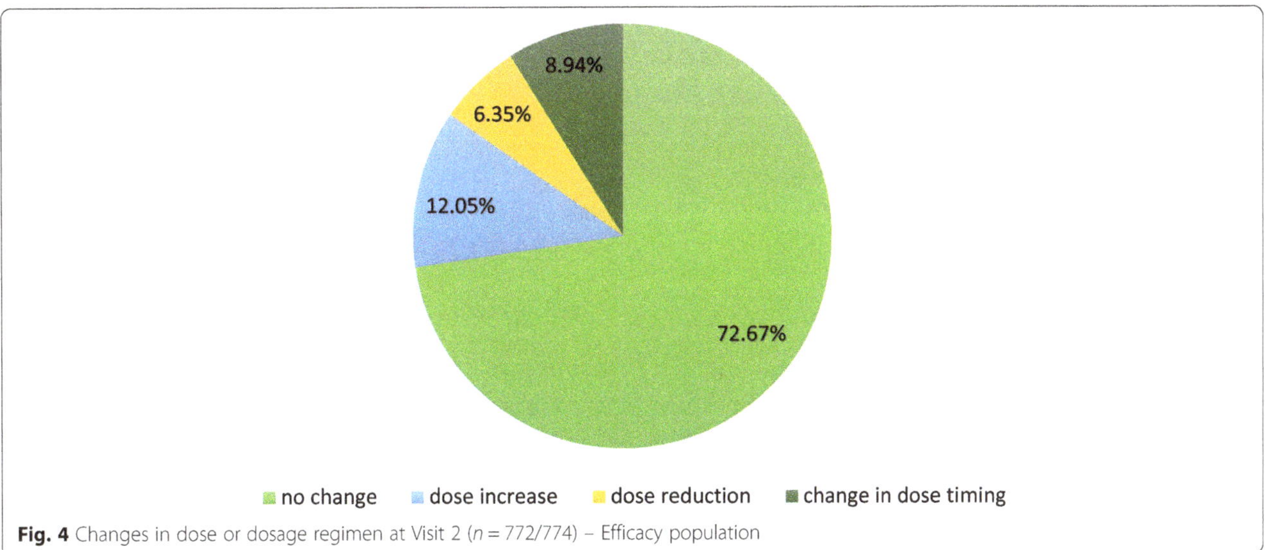

Fig. 4 Changes in dose or dosage regimen at Visit 2 (n = 772/774) – Efficacy population

indicated that the observed effect differences between the two treatment regimens were either irrelevant or very small at maximum.

Ease of subdivision analysis

The distribution of this variable is shown by age classes in Fig. 5. Since only 12.01% (91/758) of the patients rated the ease of subdivision as "difficult to divide" or "very difficult to divide", we constructed a new variable for the analysis by combining these two categories into one category and the other two categories ("very easy to divide" and "easy to divide") into a second. 87.99% (667/758; 95% CI [85.47%; 90.22%]) of the study participants (≥ 65 years of age) rated the ease of subdivision of the SNAP-TAB tablet into three equal parts as "very easy or easy to divide". An influence of age or gender of patients on the relative frequency at which the ease of subdivision was rated like this could not be observed ($p_{\text{Likelihood ratio}} = 0.127$).

Therapy withdrawals and adverse events

Treatment with TC was prematurely terminated in 44 (4.37%) out of 1007 patients recruited. The most common reason for withdrawal was "adverse event" (43.18%) followed by "lack of efficacy" (22.73%).

Overall, the attending physicians documented a total of 110 adverse events in 75 (7.45%) patients of the safety population; 82.72% of these were well-known side effects of TC listed in the SmPC. The most frequently reported AEs were dry mouth (4.87%) and constipation (1.49%). All other documented AEs occurred at a frequency of ≤0.5%. One serious AE was reported (postrenal failure), of which the causality to the study drug was assessed by the physician as unlikely. An at least possible causal

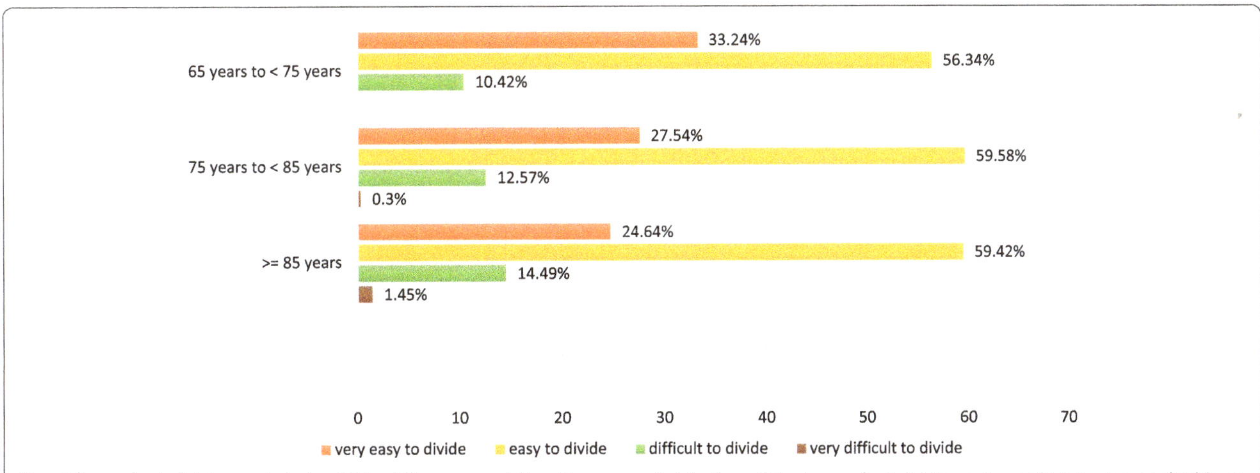

Fig. 5 Ease of subdivision analysis (n = 758) – Efficacy population. Frequency distribution of the "ease of subdivision rating at Visit 3 or, as applicable, at the time of premature discontinuation of treatment" by age classes

relationship between an AE and TC treatment was considered in 97 cases (88.18%) by the investigator, and in 91 cases (82.27%) by the marketing authorization holder. Treatment with the study drug was discontinued in 32 (29.09%) patients, the dosage was reduced in 16 (14.55%) patients, and no measures were taken to treat the AE in 49 (44.55%) cases.

Discussion

This non-interventional study examined the importance of real-life anticholinergic treatment of elderly outpatients with idiopathic OAB in view of their anticholinergic load and comorbidities, which to our knowledge was not done in any trial before it. The median age of the participants was 75 years; therefore, this population represents the group of adults most frequently affected by the OAB syndrome [13, 27, 48, 49]. 47.54% (445/936) of the elderly in our study were exposed to at least one anticholinergic medication at baseline, as indicated by an ACB scale score of > 0. Thereof 24.72% had an ACB score of ≥3, which is considered by Boustani et al. [19] as clinically relevant. Relating this to the total number of patients in the epidemiological group for which valuable information was available, the percentage of patients with an ACB scale score ≥ 3 was 11.75% (110/936). In a retrospective study of anticholinergic burden in a large cohort of hospitalized geriatric patients (89,579 analysed individuals with a median age of 82 years), 41,456 (46.3%) patients took at least one prescribed anticholinergic drug [50]. Of them, 24,569 (59.3%) had an ACB total score of 1, 5765 (13.9%) a score of 2, and 11,122 (26.8%) a score of 3 or more. Although we observed a population of outpatients in urological practice which is not directly comparable with the hospitalized population in the cohort study, and there is a difference in the median age of the patients in both studies, the magnitude of anticholinergic burden is broadly in line. The observed rate of prescriptions for drugs with anticholinergic properties in our study is also comparable with data from other previous studies, wherein rates vary between 25% in community-dwelling patients to up to 80% in nursing-home residents with cognitive impairments [14, 43, 51].

Several ranked lists have been compiled to assess anticholinergic burden of drugs. The ACB scale identifies the severity of anticholinergic AEs on cognition for many prescribed and over-the-counter medications in a single list [19]. Drugs are rated regarding their anticholinergic burden either through serum anticholinergicactivity or in vitro affinity to muscarinic receptors, and then scored according to their clinical relevance [36]. The study by Pasina et al. [21] found that the ACB scale might help to rapidly identify drugs potentially associated with cognitive impairment in a dose-response pattern.

The epidemiological survey in our study additionally showed a median CIRS-G score-based CMI for all patients of 5 at baseline, and a CMI of > 4 in 52.03% of all patients. The occurrence of a higher comorbidity index, which was found to increase with increasing age, was identified as a potential effect modifier for the ACB scale score, as was age of ≥85 years. These results are supported by an analysis of a large representative primary care dataset (1,751,841 patients) which showed that the prevalence of multimorbidity, defined in this study as the concomitant presence of ≥2 illnesses, increased substantially with age and was present in most people aged 65 years or older [52]. The percentage of subjects with multimorbidity was 64.9% (95% CI [64.7%, 65.1%]) in the group of 65–84 years olds compared to 81.5% (95% CI [81.1%, 81.9%]) in the group of ≥85 years olds. Laux et al. [53] observed a strong correlation between age, gender, multimorbidity (co-occurrence of ≥2 chronic diseases) and health care utilization in the context of the German CONTENT project, analysing the data from 39,699 patients. They discovered that the number of patients' chronic conditions have a significant impact on the number of different prescriptions ($ß = 0.226$, $P < 0.0001$) as well as on the number of referrals ($ß = 0.3$, $P < 0.0001$). In the 60–69 years age group, the average number (± SE) of different prescriptions per patient was 4.45 ± 0.19 in men and 4.55 ± 0.16 in female, whereas the average number of prescriptions rose to 6.51 ± 0.69 and 6.57 ± 0.24, respectively, in the age group ≥80 years.

Currently, there are no CIRS-G based cut-offs for the illness severity and CMI established [54], making the classification of the observed results difficult. Miller et al. [55] identified a mean (± SD) CMI of 4.5 ± 2.5 for a healthy elderly individual with a mean age of 71.1 ± 5.3 years ($n = 35$). In contrast, the total CIRS-G score (± SD) was 12.7 ± 4.7 ($n = 76$) for people with Parkinson's disease [56]. A CIRS score of ≤6 is used to differentiate between patients who are eligible for intensive chemoimmunotherapy and those who are not [57]. If we apply the cut-off from Miller et al. [55] to our results, then slightly less than half (47.97%) of the study participants in the epidemiological group (473/986) had a CMI score of ≤4, corresponding with that of a healthy elderly subject.

Since anticholinergic activity affects both central and peripheral systems, these drugs are indicated in a wide spectrum of conditions. Multimorbidity and polypharmacy increase the cumulative anticholinergic burden and thus the risk for side effects, including the well-known risk for neurodegenerative disorders [12, 13, 19, 20, 35, 58, 59]. Apart from age-associated changes in pharmacokinetic and pharmacodynamic properties, elderly people may also be more sensitive to anticholinergic effects in the central nervous system because of age-related physiological and pathological changes at the brain [20, 34, 35]. An American population-based study in 12,423 men and women even showed that, comparable to the percentage of anticholinergic users in our study, 47% of the elders (≥ 65 years) used a medication with possible anticholinergic properties, which increased the cumulative risk of cognitive decline and mortality over 2 years in participants with normal or mildly impaired cognition at baseline [18]. Risacher et al. [60] observed that cognitively normal older adults ($n = 402$) taking medications with medium or high anticholinergic activity showed poorer memory and executive function, reduced cerebral glucose metabolism, whole-brain and temporal lobe atrophy, and increased clinical decline compared with non-users; these symptoms were most severe in those with the highest total anticholinergic burden scores. Using data from a well-established prospective cohort study, Chuang et al. [61] discovered that exposure to medications with mild anticholinergic activity in midlife is associated with greater risk of Alzheimer's disease and accelerated brain atrophy before cognitive impairment. In a population-based, longitudinal study of individuals 65 years or older, higher cumulative use of anticholinergics was associated with an increased risk for all-cause dementia and Alzheimer's disease [14]. In the cohort study by Pfistermeister et al. [50], anticholinergic drugs with an ACB score of 3 clearly contributed most to the patients' overall anticholinergic load for all patients having ACB total scores of ≥3. They further found a high anticholinergic burden to be associated with patients with severe cognitive impairment.

In contrast to all tertiary amines indicated in OAB, brain penetration of TC is highly restricted by the molecule's polar structure and its low lipophilicity, as well as by a P-glycoprotein mediated efflux in the endothelial cells of the blood-brain-barrier (BBB) [62, 63]; in a mouse model, TC permeation across the BBB was not increased with ageing [64]. A recent randomized placebo-controlled clinical study in 59 women aged 50 years and older being treated for OAB with 60 mg of TC per day for 4 weeks, measured no changes in cognitive function between the TC group and the placebo group [65]. Previous clinical studies investigating different indicators for cognitive function and neuropsychological effects, including electroencephalogram and sleep studies, have proven that TC is largely free of CNS effects [66–74]. The drug may therefore provide an effective approach to treating OAB without increasing the patient's central nervous anticholinergic burden.

This is also supported by the nature and the low frequency of AEs in our study. All documented AEs with an at least causal relationship are well-known side effects of oral TC. In general, TC was well tolerated which is reflected by the subjective assessments of physicians and patients. An observational study of TC 30 mg film-coated tablets in 4092 patients with OAB symptoms achieved comparable results: its tolerability was rated as "very good" or "good" by physicians in 90.2% of cases, and by patients in 87.1% [9].

The relevant changes in characteristic OAB symptoms, observed in the present trial after a median treatment period of 64 days and determined by before-after-comparisons of different variables, indicated that an oral dose of 45 mg TC per day is a potent treatment strategy, providing patients pronounced improvement or cure of the most bothersome symptoms of OAB. This has previously been proven in a previous 12-week, randomised, double-blind, phase IIIb study in 1658 patients with urinary urge incontinence evaluating the efficacy and tolerability of TC which demonstrated that urinary frequency and urge incontinence can be reduced significantly through a flexible dosing strategy [1, 7]. It has further been shown that these clinical effects are associated with improvements in several areas of health-related quality of life of those patients, suggesting a real clinically and personally relevant treatment success [1].

The majority of the patients in our trial (78.55%) - as in the preceding clinical study – were using the approved dose of 45 mg (3 × 15 mg) TC daily, which is defined in the current SmPC [75]. The flexible dosing strategy in our study allowed the physician together with the patient to decide at Visit 2 whether to increase, decrease or maintain the starting dose, or switch to another dosage regimen, until the end of the treatment period. 81.61% (630/772) of patients did not change their initial prescribed daily dose, and only 8.94% (69/772) of patients switched to another dosage regimen. This confirmed that a daily dose of 45 mg of TC is adequate for most patients with idiopathic OAB. This conclusion is supported further by the favourable assessment of efficacy by both the urologists and the patients, as well as the fact that the physicians answered the question relating to therapy continuation affirmatively for 672 out of 752 patients (89.36%) after the observational period. Pooled data from three non-interventional studies in a total of 9366 patients showed that flexible dosing of TC is commonly used in urological practice in Germany [76].

The post hoc analysis in our study, regarding the two dosage schemes "1 x 45 mg TC/day" and "3 x 15 mg TC/day", did not indicate a difference in clinical outcome for any of the variables. As was further shown in the present study, the SNAP-TAB tablet can be easily divided in three equal units, thereby providing a patient-friendly option in flexible drug dosing. This way of administration simplifies the optimal treatment with TC which should be individualised considering the patient's comorbidities and comedications, especially in the elderly, and based on the patient's individual responses to treatment, to ensure an optimal balance between efficacy and tolerability [1, 7–10]. Thus, in turn, it supports close patient adherence and persistence to treatment [76].

Due to its non-interventional and observational character the current trial has distinct advantages and disadvantages associated with it. Limitations are the heterogeneity of participants, the variable dosage regimen and the lack of a comparator group, such as tertiary amines. It must be noted that the epidemiological population in our NIS consisted only of elderly patients (although they account for most patients). While the urologists that attended asked follow-up questions (queries), the possibility that the ACB score data reported by the physicians may have been partly incomplete cannot be ruled out. Missing data for the efficacy analysis was handled by replacing missing values with the corresponding values documented at the last evaluable visit (Last-Observation-Carried-Forward method). Only those patients with evaluable data for the first and last visit and minimum of ≥10 days between the two visits were included in the sensitivity analysis for the variable of interest. This decreased the sample size by approximately 3%. Furthermore, the analysis of the data collected in this NIS and the interpretation of the results could solely be carried out in a descriptive manner.

On the plus side, our study follows national and international recommendations dealing with quality aspects of NIS. With its safety population of 1007 elderly patients and 162 attended urologists nationwide, it comprises a cross-section of the typical population of patients treated for symptoms of idiopathic OAB in daily practice. The open observational scenario highly reflects common use of the study drug. Moreover, the validated instruments, the ACB score and the German version of the CIRS-G scale, used in this NIS cover relevant epidemiological aspects related to the representative patient population. The NIS can therefore be a scientific instrument that completes the results of randomized controlled studies by contributing important data on the use of the drug in real-life practice, for example on medical prescription, dosage recommendations, patients' compliance, and on safety aspects [77]. The evaluation and demonstration of the adequate patient acceptability of a medicinal product is also presented as a major issue in the EMA Reflection Paper on the Pharmaceutical Development of Medicines for Use in the Older Population [10].

Conclusions

This NIS focussed on less-known epidemiological issues relating to comorbid conditions and anticholinergic burden from concomitant medications when treating idiopathic OAB. It adds evidence from daily therapeutically practice supporting the favourable benefit-risk profile of TC as reported from the randomized controlled trials. The use of the SNAP-TAB tablet containing 45 mg of TC was shown to be an effective, safe and easy to manage new type of drug administration that facilitates flexible dosing of TC to achieve the optimal patient-related balance between efficacy and tolerability in real-life practice.

Endnotes

[1]Trademark: *Spasmex*® 45 mg film-coated immediate -release tablets (Dr. R. Pfleger GmbH, Bamberg, Germany)

Abbreviations

ACB: Anticholinergic burden; AE(s): Adverse event(s); AWMF: Arbeitsgemeinschaft der Wissenschaftlichen Medizinischen Fachgesellschaften (Association of the Scientific Medical); BBB: Blood-brain-barrier; BfArM: Federal Institute for Drugs and Medical Devices; CI: Confidence interval; CIRS-G: Cumulative Illness Rating Scale for Geriatrics; CMI: Comorbidity index; CNS: Central nervous system; DRKS: German Register of Clinical Studies; EMA: European Medicines Agency; MedDRA: Medical Dictionary for Regulatory Activities; NIS: Non-interventional study; OAB: Overactive bladder; OR: Odds ratio; Q1/Q3: 1. quartile / 3. quartile; RSM: Relevant somatic morbidity; SmPc: Summary of Product characteristics; TC: Trospium chloride

Acknowledgements

Medical writing support was provided by Petra Schwantes, BioMedical Services, Germany.

Funding

This study was designed by Dr. R. Pfleger GmbH. Data entry, statistical analysis and medical writing support was funded by Dr. R. Pfleger GmbH.

Authors' contributions

All authors were involved in the study conception and project coordination. RHB was responsible for the statistical analysis. RHB, AI and AW were involved in the interpretation of data. CN and RHB wrote the study protocol and the study report. All authors read and approved the final manuscript.

Ethics approval and consent to participate

All procedures performed in this study were in accordance with the German Drug Law, with the joint recommendations of the Federal Institute for Drugs and Medical Devices (BfArM) and the Paul-Ehrlich-Institute relating to the conduct of non-interventional trials [37], and with the recommendations for assuring Good Epidemiological Practice [38]. Written informed consent regarding data protection was obtained from all patients before being included in the study. The Ethics Committee of the Medical Chamber Westphalia-Lippe and the Westphalian Wilhelm University Münster, Germany, approved the study protocol. This decision was provided to each urologist within the regulatory jurisdiction of the Ethics Committee. No further Ethics Committee was involved as ethics approval in general was not mandatory and all participating urologists were satisfied with the vote of the Ethics Committee of the Medical Chamber Westphalia-Lippe and Westphalian Wilhelm University Münster.This NIS was registered with the number DRKS00007109 at the German Register of Clinical Studies (DRKS) on October 29, 2014.

Competing interests

Alexander Ivchenko received cost reimbursement of travel expenses by Dr. R. Pfleger GmbH. Rolf-Hasso Bödeker is paid-consultant (statistical planning and analysing) to Dr. R. Pfleger GmbH, Andreas Wiedemann is a consultant of Dr. R. Pfleger GmbH, Claudia Neumeister is employee (Senior Project Manager Clinical Research) of Dr. R. Pfleger GmbH.

Author details

[1]Department of Urology, Evangelisches KrankenhausWitten gGmbH, UniversityWitten/Herdecke, Pferdebachstrasse 27, 58455 Witten, Germany. [2]Department of Statistics, Institute of Medical Informatics, University Clinic Giessen, Rudolf-Buchheim-Strasse 6, 35392 Gießen, Germany. [3]Department of Medical Science/Clinical Research, Dr. R. Pfleger GmbH, Dr.-Robert-Pfleger-Strasse 12, 96052 Bamberg, Germany.

References

1. Zellner M, Madersbacher H, Palmtag H, et al, and the P195 Study Group. Trospium chloride and oxybutynin hydrochloride in a German study of adults with urinary urge incontinence: results of a 12-week, multicenter, randomized, double-blind, parallel-group, flexible-dose noninferiority trial. Clin Ther 2009; 31: 2519–2539.
2. Ulshöfer B, Bihr AM, Bödeker RH, et al. Randomised, double-blind, placebo-controlled study on the efficacy and tolerance of trospium chloride in patients with motor urge incontinence. Clin Drug Invest. 2001;21(8):563–9.
3. Cardozo L, Chapple CR, Toozs-Hobson P, et al. Efficacy of trospium chloride in patients with detrusor instability: a placebo-controlled, randomised, double-blind, multicentre clinical trial. BJU. 2000;85:659–64.
4. Alloussi S, Laval KU, Eckert R, et al. Trospium chloride (Spasmo-lyt®) in patients with motor urge syndrome (detrusor instability): a double-blind, randomised, multicentre, placebo-controlled study. J. Clin Res. 1998;1:439–51.
5. Jünemann KP, Füsgen I, Svetlana T. Trospium chloride 40 mg – a placebo-controlled, randomised, double-blind clinical trial on the efficacy and tolerability for 3 weeks in patients with urge-syndrome. Eur Urol. 2000;37:84.
6. Jünemann KP, Füsgen I. Placebo-controlled, randomised, double-blind, multicentre clinical trial on the efficacy and tolerability of 1x40 mg and 2x40 mg trospium chloride (Spasmo-lyt®) daily for 3 weeks in patients with urge-syndrome. Neurourol Urodynam. 1999;18:375_6.
7. Bödeker RH, Madersbacher H, Neumeister C, Zellner M. Dose escalation improves therapeutic outcome: post hoc analysis of data from a 12-week, multicentre, double-blind, parallel-group trial of trospium chloride in patients with urinary urge incontinence. BMC Urol. 2010;10:15.
8. Wiedemann A, Neumann G, Neumeister C, et al. Efficacy and tolerability of add-on trospium chloride in patients with benign prostate syndrome and overactive bladder: a non-interventional trial showing use of flexible dosing. UroToday Int J. 2009;2(2) https://doi.org/10.3834/uij.1944-5784.2009.04.02.
9. Wiedemann A, Kusche W, Neumeister C. Flexible dosing of trospium chloride for the treatment of OAB – results of a non-interventional study in 4,092 patients. The Open Clinical Trials Journal. 2011;3:1–5.
10. EMA/CHMP/QWP/292439/2017 Rev.: 4.0. Reflection paper on the pharmaceutical development of medicines for use in the older population. EMA 18 May 2017. www.ema.europa.eu/docs/en_GB/document_library/Scientific_guideline/2017/08/WC500232782.pdf. Accessed 09-12-2017.
11. Wiedemann A, Füsgen I. Harninkontinenz bei Älteren. © pharma-aktuell Verlagsgruppe GmbH/Geriatrie-Report, Varel. Bamberg, Germany; 2017. (German)
12. Wagg A. The cognitive burden of anticholinergics in the elderly – implications for the treatment of overactive bladder. Eur Urol Rev. 2012; 7(1):42_9.
13. Lenherr SM, Cox L. Cognitive effects of anticholinergics in the geriatric patient population: safety and treatment considerations. Cur Bladder Dysfunct Rep. 2017;12:104–11.
14. Gray SL, Anderson ML, Dublin S, et al. Cumulative use of strong anticholinergics and incident dementia. A prospective cohort study. JAMA Intern Med. 2015;175(3):401–7.
15. Salahudeen MS, Duffull SB, Nishtala PS. Anticholinergic burden quantified by anticholinergic risk scales and adverse outcomes in older people: a systematic review. BMC Geriatr. 2015;15:31.
16. Marcum ZA, Wirtz HS, Pettinger M, et al. Anticholinergic medication use and falls in postmenopausal women: findings from the women's health initiative cohort study. BMC Geriatr. 2016;16:76.
17. Zia A, Kamaruzzaman S, Myint PK, Tan MP. Anticholinergic burden is associated with recurrent and injurious falls in older individuals. Maturitas. 2015; https://doi.org/10.1016/j.maturitas.2015.10.009. Accessed 10-05-2017
18. Fox C, Richardson K, Maidment ID, et al. Anticholinergic medication use and cognitive impairment in the older population: the medical research council cognitive function and ageing study. J Am Geriatr Soc. 2011;59:1477–83.
19. Boustani M, Cambell N, Munger S, et al. Impact of anticholinergics on the aging brain: a review and practical application. Aging Health. 2008;4(3):311–20.
20. Campbell N, Boustani M, Limbil T, et al. The cognitive impact of anticholinergics: a clinical review. Clin Interv Aging. 2009;4:225–33.
21. Pasina L, Djade CD, Lucca U, et al. Association of anticholinergic burden with cognitive and functional status in a cohort of hospitalized elderly: comparison of the anticholinergic cognitive burden scale and anticholinergic risk scale. Drugs Aging. 2013;30:103–12.
22. Kelleher CJ. Economic and social impact of OAB. Eur Urol. 2002;1:11–6.
23. Luscombe FA. Socioeconomic burden of urinary incontinence with focus on overactive bladder and tolterodine treatment. Rev Contemp Pharmacother. 2000;11:43–62.
24. Tubaro A. Defining overactive bladder: epidemiology and burden of disease. Urology. 2004;64(Suppl 6A):2–6.
25. Lua LL, Pathak P, Dandolu V. Comparing anticholinergic persistence and adherence profiles in overactive bladder patients based on gender, obesity, and major anticholinergic agents. Neurourol Urodyn. 2017;36:2123–31.
26. Coyne KS, Wein A, Nicholson S, et al. Comorbidities and personal burden of urgency urinary incontinence: a systematic review. Int J Clin Pract. 2013; 67(10):1015–33.
27. Irwin DE, Milsom I, Hunskaar S, et al. Population-based survey of urinary incontinence, overactive bladder, and other lower urinary tract symptoms in five countries: results of the EPIC study. Eur Urol. 2006;50:1306–15.
28. Stickley A, Santini ZI, Koyanagi A. Urinary incontinence, mental health and loneliness among community-dwelling older adults in Ireland. BMC Urol. 2017;17:29.
29. Lai HH, Shen B, Rawal A, Vetter J. The relationship between depression and overactive bladder/urinary incontinence symptoms in the clinical OAB population. BMC Urol. 2016;16:60.
30. Felde G, Ebbesen MH, Hunskaar S. Anxiety and depression associated with urinary incontinence. A 10-year follow-up study from the Norwegian HUNT study (EPINCONT). Neurourol Urodynam. 2017;36:322–8.
31. Corcos J, Przydacz M, Campeau L, et al. CUA guideline on adult overactive bladder. Can Urol Assoc J. 2017;11(5):E142–73. https://doi.org/10.5489/cuaj.4586. Accessed 09-20-2017
32. Andersson KE, Chapple CR, Cardozo L, et al. Pharmacological treatment of urinary incontinence. In: Abrams P, Cardozo L, Khoury S, Wein A, editors. Incontinence. 4th international consultation on incontinence. UK, Plymouth: Plymouth, Plymbridge Contributors Ltd; 2009. p. 631–700.
33. Lechevallier-Michel N, Molimard M, Dartigues JF, et al. Drugs with anticholinergic properties and cognitive performance in the elderly: results from the PAQUID study. Br J Clin Pharmacol. 2004;59(2):143–51.
34. Erdo F, Denes L, de Lange E. Age-associated physiological and pathological changes at the blood-brain-barrier: a review. J Cereb Blood Flow Metab. 2017;37(I):4–24.
35. Gerretsen P, Pollock BG. Cognitive risks of anticholinergics in the elderly. Aging Health. 2013;9(2):159–66.
36. Ruxton K, Woodman RJ, Mangoni AA. Drugs with anticholinergic effects and cognitive impairment, falls and all-cause mortality in older adults: a systematic review and meta-analysis. Br J Clin Pharmacol. 2015;80(2):209–20.
37. BfArM. Empfehlungen des Bundesinstituts für Arzneimittel und Medizinprodukte und des Paul-Ehrlich-Instituts zur Planung, Durchführung und Auswertung von Anwendungsbeobachtungen. 2010. http://www.bfarm.de/SharedDocs/Bekanntmachungen/DE/Arzneimittel/klinPr/bm-KlinPr-20100707-NichtinterventePr-pdf.pdf?__blob=publicationFile&v=5. Accessed 09-01-2017.
38. Hoffmann W, Latza U, Terschüren C. Leitlinien und Empfehlungen zur Sicherung von Guter Epidemiologischer Praxis (GEP). German: Deutsche Gesellschaft für Epidemiologie (DGEpi); 2008.

39. AWMF. Guideline No. 084/001. Harninkontinenz. German: Leitlinien der Deutschen Gesellschaft für Geriatrie; 2010.
40. Summary of Product Characteristics (SmPC). Spasmex® 45 mg film-coated tablets. Dr. R. Pfleger GmbH. Version 09/2013. www.fachinfo.de.
41. Van Santen E, Barends DM, Frijlink HW. Breaking of scored tablets: a review. Eur J Pharma Biopharm. 2002;53:139–45.
42. Wening K, Breitkreutz J. Oral drug delivery in personalized medicine: unmet needs and novel approaches. Int J Pharm. 2011;404:1–9.
43. Kolanowski A, Fick DM, Campbell J, et al. A preliminary study of anticholinergic burden and relationship to quality of life indicator, engagement in activities, in nursing home residents with dementia. J Am Med Dir Assoc. 2009;10(4):252–7.
44. Lertxundi U, Domingo-Echaburu S, Hernandez R, et al. Expert-based drug list to measure anticholinergic burden: similar names, different results. Psychogeriatrics. 2013;13:17–24.
45. Hock G, Nosper M. Manual CIRS-G. Cumulative Illness Rating Scale. Skala zur kumulierten Bewertung von Erkrankungen. V 2.1, MDK Rheinland-Pfalz 2003. English original paper: a manual of guidelines for scoring the cumulative illness rating scale (CIRS-G), by Miller MD & Towers A. Department of Geriatric Psychiatry, University of Pittsburgh, USA, 1991.
46. Cohen J. Statistical power analysis for the behavioral sciences. 2nd ed. Hillsdale, NJ: L. Erlbaum Associates; 1988.
47. Ellis PD. The essential guide to effect sizes: statistical power, meta-analysis, and the interpretation of research results. Cambridge: Cambridge University Press; 2010.
48. Irwin DE, Kopp ZS, Agatep B, et al. Worldwide prevalence estimates of lower urinary tract symptoms, overactive bladder, urinary incontinence and bladder outlet obstruction. BJU Int. 2011;108:1132–9.
49. Milsom I, Abrams P, Cardozo L, et al. How widespread are the symptoms of an overactive bladder and how are they manages? A population-based prevalence study. BJU Int. 2001;87:760–6.
50. Pfistermeister B, Tümena T, Gaßmann K-G, et al. Anticholinergic burden and cognitive function in a large German cohort of hospitalized geriatric patients. PLoS One. 2017; https://doi.org/10.1371/hournal.pone.0171353.
51. Koyama A, Steinman M, Ensrud K, et al. Long-term cognitive and functional effects of potentially inappropriate medications in older women. J Gerontol A Biol Sci Med Sci. 2014;69(4):423–9.
52. Barnett K, Mercer SW, Norbury M, et al. Epidemiology of multimorbidity and implications for health care, research, and medical education: a cross-sectional study. Lancet. 2012;380:37–43.
53. Laux G, Kuehlein T, Rosemann T, Szecsenyi J. Co- and multimorbidity patterns in primary care based on episodes of care: results from the German CONTENT project. BMC Health Serv Res. 2008;8:14.
54. Salvi F, Miller MD, Grilli A, et al. A manual of guidelines to score the modified cumulative illness rating scale and its validation in acute hospitalized elderly patients. J Am Geriatr Soc. 2008;56:1926–31.
55. Miller MD, Paradis CF, Houck PR, et al. Rating chronic medical illness burden in geropsychiatric practice and research: application of the cumulative illness rating scale. Psychiatry Res. 1992;41:237–48.
56. King LA, Priest KC, Nutt J, et al. Comorbidity and functional mobility in persons with Parkinson's disease. Arch Phys Med Rehabil. 2014;95(11):2152–7.
57. Cramer P. The management of fit, unfit, and high-risk CLL patients. New Evid Oncol. 2014;25:52–7.
58. Ancelin ML, Artero S, Portet F, et al. Non-degenerative mild cognitive impairment in elderly people and use of anticholinergic drugs: longitudinal cohort study. BMJ. 2006;332:455–9.
59. Turnheim K. When drug therapy gets old: pharmacokinetics and pharmacodynamics in the elderly. Exp Gerontol. 2003;38:843–53.
60. Risacher SL, McDonald BC, Tallman EF, et al. Association between anticholinergic medication use and cognition, brain metabolism, and brain atrophy in cognitively normal older adults. JAMA Neurol. 2016; https://doi.org/10.1001/jamaneurol.2016.0580.
61. Chuang Y-F, Elango P, Gonzalez CE, Thambisetty M. Midlife anticholinergic drug use, risk of Alzheimer's disease, and brain atrophy in community-dwelling older adults. Alzheimers Dement Transl Res Clin Intervent. 2017;3: 471–9.
62. Geyer J, Gavrilova O, Petzinger E. The role of P-glycoprotein in limiting brain penetration of the peripherally acting anticholinergic overactive bladder drug trospium chloride. Drug Metab Dispos. 2009;37:1371–4.
63. Geyer J, Gavrilova O, Schwantes U. Differences in the brain penetration of the anticholinergic drugs trospium chloride and oxybutynin. UroToday Int J. 2010;3(1) https://doi.org/10.3834/uij.1944-5784.2010.02.12.
64. Kranz J, Petzinger E, Geyer J. Brain penetration of the OAB drug trospium chloride is not increased in aged mice. World J Urol. 2011;31(1):219–24.
65. Geller EJ, Dumond JB, Bowling JM, et al. Effect of trospium chloride on cognitive function in women aged 50 or older: a randomized trial. Female Pelvic Med Reconstr Surg. 2017;23(2):118–23.
66. Pietzko A, Dimpfel W, Schwantes U, Topfmeier P. Influences of trospium chloride and oxybutynin on quantitative EEG in healthy volunteers. Eur J Clin Pharmacol. 1994;47:337–43.
67. Todorova A, Vonderheid-Guth B, Dimpfel W. Effects of tolterodine, trospium chloride, and oxybutynin on the central nervous system. J Clin Pharmacol. 2001;41:636–44.
68. Diefenbach K, Arold G, Wollny A, et al. Effects on sleep of anticholinergics used for overactive bladder treatment in healthy volunteers aged ≥ 50 years. BJU Int. 2005;95(3):346–9.
69. Diefenbach K, Donath F, Maurer A, et al. Randomised, double-blind study of the effects of oxybutynin, tolterodine, trospium chloride and placebo on sleep in healthy young volunteers. Clin Drug Invest. 2003;23(6):395–404.
70. Staskin D, Kay G, Goldman H, et al. Central nervous system penetration and effect on memory: comparison of trospium chloride and oxybutynin in patients with overactive bladder and age-associated memory impairment. Neurourol Urodynam. 2012; https://doi.org/10.1002/nau.
71. Staskin D, Kay G, Tannenbaum C, et al. Trospium chloride has no effect on memory testing and is assay undetectable in the central nervous system of older patients with overactive bladder. Int J Clin Pract. 2010;64(9):1294–300.
72. Staskin D, Kay G, Tannenbaum C, et al. Trospium chloride is undetectable in the older human central nervous system. J Am Geriatr Soc. 2010;58(8):1618–9.
73. Staskin DR, Harnett MD. Effect of trospium chloride on somnolence and sleepiness in patients with overactive bladder. Curr Urol Rep. 2004;5:423–6.
74. Isik AT, Celik T, Bozoglu E, Doruk H. Trospium and cognition in patients with late onset Alzheimer disease. J Nutr Health Aging. 2009; https://doi.org/10.1007/s12603-009-0144-4.
75. Summary of Product Characteristics (SmPC) Spasmex® 45 mg film-coated tablets. Dr. R. Pfleger GmbH. 2017. http://www.fachinfo.de; 014933.pdf. Accessed 11-16-2017.
76. Schwantes U, Grosse J, Wiedemann A. Refractory overactive bladder: a common problem? Int Urogynecol J. 2015;26:1407–14.
77. Von Jeinsen BKJG, Sudhop T. A 1-year cross-sectional analysis of non-interventional post-marketing study protocols submitted to the German Federal Institute for Drugs and Medical Devices (BfArM). Eur J Clin Pharmacol. 2013;69:1453–66.

19

Urinary proteomics and metabolomics studies to monitor bladder health and urological diseases

Zhaohui Chen[1] and Jayoung Kim[2,3,4*]

Abstract

Background: Assays of molecular biomarkers in urine are non-invasive compared to other body fluids and can be easily repeated. Based on the hypothesis that the secreted markers from the diseased organs may locally release into the body fluid in the vicinity of the injury, urine-based assays have been considered beneficial to monitoring bladder health and urological diseases. The urine proteome is much less complex than the serum and tissues, but nevertheless can contain biomarkers for diagnosis and prognosis of diseases. The urine metabolome has a much higher number and concentration of low-molecular metabolites than the serum or tissues, with a far lower lipid concentration, yet informs directly about dietary and microbial metabolism.

Discussion: We here discuss the use of mass spectrometry-based proteomics and metabolomics for urine biomarker assays, specifically with respect to the underlying mechanisms that trigger the pathological condition.

Conclusion: Molecular biomarker profiles, based on proteomics and metabolomics studies, reliably distinguish patients from healthy controls, stratify sub-populations with respect to treatment options, and predict therapeutic response of patients with urological disease.

Keywords: Urinary biomarkers, Proteomics, Metabolomics, Bladder diseases

Background

Personalized medicine aims for a customized healthcare for each patient to match treatments with the right patients at the perfect timing. Gene-specific data (SNP genotyping as well as epigenetics) is too static to enable such timed treatments. It is therefore essential to collect variable biomarker, along with other clinical information, data to achieve accurate diagnostic assessment for individual patients [1–3]. Multi-omic readouts of cellular and organ phenotypes (RNA-Seq, proteomics and metabolomics) will be indispensible in the era of personalized medicine. Only through a combination of exact genotypic and molecular phenotypic information we will improve the development of custom and precision therapies [4–6]. Sub-grouping of patients is necessary to define the evidence-based protocol for matching treatments to the right patients with appropriate timing [5, 7]. The necessity of compiling molecular information and clinical outcomes in personalized medicine prompted us to believe that the use of multi-omic data in conjunction with clinical outcome data is ever more important not only at the time of medical intervention, but throughout patients' lives. The need for and possibilities associated with big data approach to gain insight into biological processes driving diseases and to identify novel diagnostics is enlarging. In this review, we will discuss how far metabolomic and proteomic approaches have come to aid in this long-term goal.

Urological diseases including urological cancers and benign bladder dysfunctions are complex in nature and require powerful, precise treatments. Tests to find patient candidates for a specific or combination of therapy and to identify biomarkers are incredibly challenging to determine [6, 8, 9]. Urine contains information not only from the urinary track, but also from other organs, providing biomarkers for bladder and other systemic

* Correspondence: Jayoung.Kim@cshs.org
[2]Department of Surgery, Cedars-Sinai Medical Center, 8700 Beverly Blvd, Los Angeles, CA 90048, USA
[3]Department of Biomedical Sciences, Cedars-Sinai Medical Center, 8700 Beverly Blvd, Los Angeles, CA 90048, USA
Full list of author information is available at the end of the article

diseases [10–12]. Looking at urine data in conjunction with other available patient clinical data may enable us to understand the molecular signature, which helps monitor the stages of the diseases and responses to therapies. This is particularly true in urological diseases, where urine samples provide the primary window for diagnosis and drug behavior observation [13].

A common definition of the proteome is the entire set of proteins expressed by a cell, tissue or organism at a certain time. Since proteomics is the large-scale study of proteome, it can contribute to expanding the understanding of biological systems and functions in cells or organs. Proteomes are directly responsible for cell functions, and therefore, abnormal protein expression is an indication of cellular disruption due to the pathological conditions [14, 15]. Current global proteomic technologies may provide a comprehensive understanding of urological diseases, characteristics of the disease's state, and novel approaches to relieve the clinical symptoms [16–18].

Metabolomics provides a global chemical fingerprint of the metabolism of cells and indicates physiological and pathological states of biological samples [19–21]. Thus, the power of metabolomics opens up an unparalleled opportunity to query the molecular mechanisms of the disease. Metabolites are not merely the end products of gene/protein expression, rather, they are the result of the interactions of the genome and proteome with their environment in the cells. They play as powerful mediators of cellular events both in long-distance actions (e.g. hormones), stress and physiological actors (e.g. oxylipins) [22] and as cell-internal mediators (e.g. α-ketoglutarate in pluripotency) [23]. Thus, analyzing metabolic differences between pathological and normal conditions could provide undiscovered insights into the underlying disease pathology.

In addition to the advancements in multi-omics data acquisitions, novel bioinformatics methods enable an integrated view to identify the combined action of biomarkers as well as to develop drugs [24–27]. A significant volume of data with various omics data, including genetic, epigenetic, transcriptomic, proteomic, metabolomic and clinical outcome data, provides researchers with the capability to see a broader perspective and make discoveries that couldn't previously be delivered [28–31]. Integrative approaches have become the essential part of experimental designs aimed at better understanding the biology of bladder diseases.

The main goal of this article is to provide the reader with an up-to-date summary of the main molecular variations taking place in biofluids with respect to various urological diseases including urological cancers (e.g., prostate cancer (hereafter PCa) and bladder cancer (BCa)) and benign bladder dysfunctions (e.g., benign prostatic hyperplasia (BPH), interstitial cystitis/pelvic bladder syndrome, bladder pain syndrome (IC)), as well as of the analytical strategies employed to unveil urinary biomarkers.

We here focus on mainly two omics analyses—proteomics and metabolomics—and associated data integration strategies. These approaches enable researchers to: (a) identify unknown molecular mechanisms; (b) select molecular markers that can be used for drug discovery, preclinical, and clinical drug development; (c) develop diagnostic tools. First, we present a short review on the urine-based studies. Second, we discuss analytical techniques that are used in urinary omics analyses, including computational methods for data processing. Next, we present studies that have used proteomics or metabolomics approaches to reveal the fingerprints of urological diseases. Finally, we discuss the future research directions and prospective how to apply to diagnosis and precision medicine for patients to summarize the review.

Discussion

Urine-based biomarkers for diagnosis, prognosis, or monitoring the treatment efficiency

A concerted effort bridging basic biology and clinical research is needed to identify high quality predictive biomarkers [31]. Discovery and validation of predictive biomarkers should be an integral part of clinical trials. In the clinical setting, the best diagnostic value is given by noninvasive biomarker tests that have both high sensitivity and specificity. A non- or minimally invasive diagnostic method using biofluids (e.g., urine, blood, saliva, fecal extract, and sputum specimens) may play a significant role in urological diseases with regard to early detection, diagnosis, prognosis, drug development, and sensitivity prediction to clinical treatments [12, 32–34].

So far the most attractive biofluids for biomarker discovery in bladder health and urological diseases are serum and urine [32–34]. Serum is a relatively accessible, stable and informative biofluid, making it ideal for early detection of systemic alteration in a wide range of diseases [35, 36]. Monitoring of serum has several advantages mainly due to its stability and minimum dilution effect. Proteomic and metabolic profiles of serum can be regarded as important indicators of physiological and pathological states and may aid in the understanding of the mechanism behind disease occurrence and progression [37–39]. However, blood samples pose certain disadvantages. During blood sample collection, proteases are often activated, which degrades proteins quickly and introduces a range of variability. On the other hand, 20 highly abundant proteins in the blood, which correspond to 99 % of the proteins, may hinder the identification of other less abundant, potentially important, proteins [40–43]. This feature makes it challenging to develop plasma or serum based assays and often analytes enrichment or protein depletion is needed.

Urine definitely is not a waste in regards to gaining patients' diagnostics and therapeutic information [18, 44, 45]. However, it is still in debate whether urine plays an active role in regulating bladder biology. Urine's composition is 95 % of water with small amounts of ammonia, sulfate, and other constituents. Total protein concentration in urine from healthy donor is very low (<100 mg/L) and urinary proteome contains over 100,000 different peptides [18, 32, 44, 46, 47]. Approximately 1500 proteins have been shown to constitute the urinary proteome, of which large proportions are extra cellular proteins, plasma membrane proteins, and lysosomal proteins [18, 48]. The Human Kidney and Urine Proteome Project by the Human Proteome Organization (HUPO) suggested that urine is an ultra filtration of the blood in the body, since urine and blood samples share the proteome profile [49–51]. Approximately 30 % of the proteins in normal human urine are plasma proteins, while the other 70 % are proteins derived from the kidney and genitourinary tract [49, 50].

Urine samples usually need special treatments to meet the requirements of reproducible measurements after sample collections. To obtain reliable and consistent profiles of urine, first, urine must be collected in a sterile bag or plastic container, because urinary bacteria metabolism significantly interferes on the urine proteome and metabolome. Secondly, urine samples must be properly processed (e.g., pH adjustment and/or removal of cell debris) and frozen at −80°C immediately after collection, until analysis [40, 46]. In addition, analysis of urine samples poses several analytical challenges for profiling owing to wide variations in the ionic strength, pH, and osmolality, particularly under conditions of physiological stress, diet, exercise, medication, health condition, and environmental exposure [46, 52, 53]. Furthermore, urine samples typically have a huge dynamic range of metabolite and protein concentrations. Another potential problem is the presence of proteolytic activity in the urine by urokinase and other enzymes [54]. Proteases found in stored urine degrade urinary albumin to a substantial degree. However, the extent to which proteases affect biomarkers in the urine is still unclear.

Despite all these shortcomings, urine is still an attractive source for studying bladder diseases. To monitor bladder condition, urine-based assays present the most attractive strategy, among other biofluids-based methods, given that the body fluids that are most proximal to a disease site often can provide a source of informative biomarkers. Urine is readily obtained and available with no required preparations by the patient and it is less complex than other body fluids. The ease of collection allows for serial sampling to monitor disease and therapeutic responses. Care must be taken in interpreting urine-based proteomics and metabolomics data. The main disadvantage of urine is the variation in protein concentration due to differences in fluid consumption during the day, which can be countered by normalizing with creatinine. However, although creatinine is the best possible internal standard for correcting urine volume effects, creatinine levels can vary due to dietary intake and pathological conditions. Computational approaches for data normalization methods can be applied to reduce artifacts due to sample variability using currently developed probabilistic quotient- and median-fold changes in normalization strategies [55].

Analytical techniques and databases for urine-based omics for bladder diseases

With the latest advances in high-throughput technologies, the pace of advances in the "omics" field accelerated the rate of novel biomarker discovery and therapeutic targets for various bladder diseases. Various omics technologies for personalized medicine are shown in Fig. 1, and ideal applications and workflow of urine-based biomarkers in clinical settings are shown in Fig. 2.

Proteomic technology has made a dramatic progress in the overall quality and information content over the past 5 years [56]. When computationally matching identified proteins (or metabolites) against knowledge-based databases, proteomics or metabolomics profiles today provide direct insights for biological interpretation of molecular perturbations unique in patients with urological diseases [47, 57, 58]. In this section, we review the current proteomic and metabolomic techniques and analytical tools/softwares that are used to identify signatures of urological diseases.

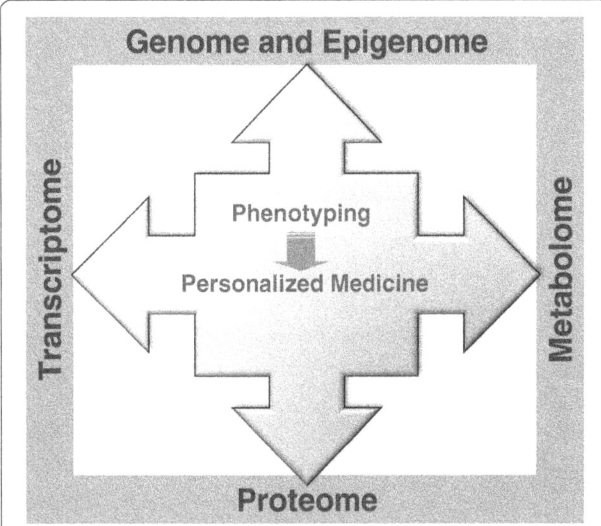

Fig. 1 Overview of multi-omics technologies, which can be applied to urine-based biomarker study

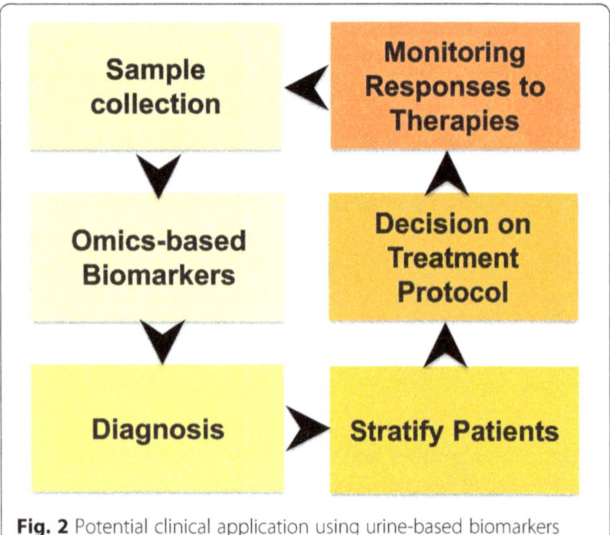

Fig. 2 Potential clinical application using urine-based biomarkers

Urinary proteomics studies

Proteins are the major players influencing a person's health, since proteins frequently have the greatest clinical significance for the diagnosis of diseases. Studies in the field of proteomics aim to elucidate proteomes and understand the identity, quantity, modification, localization, interaction, and function of all proteins in a given cell type or tissue. A number of powerful proteomic technologies were developed, demonstrating that proteomic approaches have wide utility [59, 60]. Proteomics profiling enabled the comparing of protein differences between patients suffering from a wide range of ailments and healthy controls to discover biomarkers for diagnosis and monitoring treatment response [49, 56]. Further developments to understand the post-translational modifications (PTMs) in tissues and biological fluids from patients have been achieved through the development of mass spectrometry instrumentation with increasing sensitivity [61, 62]. Established protocols for PTM enrichment and pipelines for high-throughput assays for clinical specimens may provide the potential of automated and large-scale identification and quantification of PTM-ome and its biological role in diseases [63].

For urine proteomics, many mass spectrometry techniques, such as 2D PAGE-mass spectrometry (MS), liquid chromatography-mass spectrometry (LC-MS/MS), capillary electrophoresis-mass spectrometry (CE-MS), surface-enhanced laser desorption/ionization time-of-flight mass spectrometry (SELDI-TOF MS), matrix assisted laser desorption/ionization time-of-flight (MALDI-TOF) MS and nano-liquid chromatography-tandem mass spectrometry (Nano-MALDI-MS) have been used with some advantages and limitations [64–68]. We described here only a few analytical tools that highlight the usefulness of it for urinary proteomics research. Briefly, 2D PAGE-MS is time consuming and technically challenging but very effective for large molecules. LC-MS is also time-consuming but pretty sensitive. CE-MS is cheap and good for biomarker discovery. MALDI-TOF MS is relatively simple, inexpensive, and, thus, a good option for fast screening. In general, nano-MALDI-MS is known to be much more sensitive than MALDI-TOF MS [64].

The gel-based 2-DE method enables urinary proteins to be resolved based on their molecular weight and isoelectric point. Several tools for image noise subtraction, protein spot detection, spot quantification, and spot matching can be used for 2-DE analysis including *Melanie*, *ImageMaster2D*, and *PDQuest* et al. The main steps in differential analysis of 2DE gels involve and statistical analysis. Often, the 2-DE method is coupled with MALDI-TOF MS or LC-MS/MS. Peptides from protein spots of interest are mixed with a matrix (*e.g.*, α-cyano-4-hydroxycinnamic acid) solution and are spotted onto a MALDI plate and analyzed with a MALDI-TOF MS to identify a peptide-mass fingerprint. These peptides can also be analyzed with nanoLC-MS/MS to sequence each peptide and thus identify the protein.

Besides identification and characterization, urine proteins can also be quantified. Today, label-free proteomics is the primary approach to relative quantifications of the human urinary proteome [69, 70]. A major advantage of label-free quantification is that this method is cheaper, simpler and involves less complicated data analysis than isotope-labeled approaches. Data processing is often performed by softwares such as *Decyder MS, Protein Lynx, SIEVE,* and *skyline* [71]. However, label-free quantification is limited by its lower quantification accuracy (especially for spectral counting in data dependent scan methods), and label-free data dependent acquisition quantifications are generally results in the identifications of less proteins and poor reproducibility. Currently SWATH and other data independent mass spectrometry acquisition methods and several computational algorithms are tested in their potential to overcome these limitations [59, 69, 70, 72].

The use of the most advanced proteomics mass spectrometry technologies has allowed discovering and verifying several urinary biomarkers of bladder diseases. In a large proteomics study, 407 patient urine samples were analyzed using MALDI-TOF MS. Two markers, uromodulin and semenogelin, could distinguish PCa versus BPH with 71.2 % sensitivity and 67.4 % specificity [9]. In another study on prostate cancer (PCa), capillary electrophoresis was coupled with MS detection of proteins and was able to identify and validate 12 novel urinary biomarkers for PCa [73]. This report suggested that collecting mid-stream urine samples was uninformative, but that first void urine was able to identify patients with PCa with 91 % sensitivity and 69 % specificity [73]. Due to its limited size, this study certainly requires additional validation in a larger cohort. In general, it can be assumed that a panel of biomarkers will most likely achieve an overall high level of specificity and robustness than using a single urinary protein biomarker. Further development of quantitative proteomics and selective or multiple reaction monitoring (SRM/MRM) methods [74–76] may allow the protein-quantification data to stand by their own without redundant validation using traditional protein quantification methods such as Western blot and ELISA. In many cases, there is no antibody available, and the capability of measuring multiple biomarkers in a panel for immune-based assays is very limited.

Urinary metabolomics studies

Metabolomic profiling, or metabolomics, is the systemic study of the unique small chemical fingerprints in a biological sample, and is the collection of small-molecule profiles that represent the end products of cellular processes in biological systems (e.g., cells, tissues, or organs) [20, 77]. As little as 5 ul of plasma or urine allows the characterization of hundreds of metabolites that provide a functional readout of the metabolic state. A recent effort to characterize the metabolomes of human urine has completed to identify and annotate approximately 2500 urinary metabolites using nuclear magnetic resonance spectroscopy (NMR, in most cases ^{1}H-NMR), gas chromatography mass spectrometry (GC-MS), direct flow injection mass spectrometry (DFI/LC-MS/MS), inductively coupled plasma mass spectrometry (ICP-MS) and high performance liquid chromatography (HPLC) [78]. The detailed information of metabolite structures, concentrations, related literature references and disease associations is publically available via an online database (http://www.urinemetabolome.ca) [77]. Urinary metabolite levels are usually standardized by creatinine concentrations. Endogenous substrate levels in normal healthy subjects can inform on the status of each subject's metabolizing enzyme activities. The comparison of urinary metabolite levels of patients vs. healthy controls, and responders vs. non-responders to a particular drug should facilitate the development of useful biomarkers to diagnose the disease or to predict the response, respectively. Also, understanding of urinary metabolome in healthy condition may help the titration of drug dose and monitoring drug response [18, 77].

Metabolomic studies typically begin with sample collection followed by sample analysis. A number of analytical techniques including NMR spectroscopy, GC-MS, and liquid chromatography-mass spectrometry (LC-MS) are used as methods of analysis [19]. NMR spectroscopy has proven to be particularly good for urine metabolomics analysis, because the technique is highly reproducible, requires minimal sample handling, and is straightforward to implement [79]. While the reproducibility, quantitative ability, and structure information derived from the NMR methods are big advantages, the relatively lower sensitivity and less straightforward identification methods are disadvantages of the NMR method [79]. MS-based metabolomics is considered more sensitive, providing greater coverage, and to be more cost-efficient than NMR-based applications. Given that the coverage varies with different technologies and instruments, the combination of different metabolomic approaches may provide a broad range of information that covers the metabolite profile and may maximize the capability of metabolomics analysis [19–21].

For metabolomics data processing, several statistical tools are currently used to analyze NMR and MS-based metabolomics datasets (e.g., MS-DIAL [80], XCMS, MZmine, MetAlign, MathDAMP, and LCMStats) [81, 82]. As metabolite databases, the Human Metabolome DataBase (HMDB), Madison Metabolomics Consortium Database, METLIN, and LipidMaps are generally used. To further understand the biology of the identified metabolites, HMDB (http://www.hmdb.ca/), METLIN (http://metlin.scripps.edu/), MassBank (http://www.massbank.jp), PubChem (https://pubchem.ncbi.nlm.nih.gov/) and KEGG (http://www.genome.jp/kegg/) can be used.

There is an increasing awareness of standardization or careful accounting in experimental design of urinary metabolomics study. To overcome possible limitations and pitfalls of the metabolomics approach, specific recommendations for urine collection, sample handling, storage, data acquisition, and statistical validation are also needed [78].

Urinary extracellular vesicle-derived omics studies

Most cells including cancer cells shed different types of vesicles into extracellular environment [83]. These vesicles are so-called extracellular vesicles (EV) including microvesicles, exosomes, and oncosomes, which are named based mainly on their size and characteristics [84]. EV have an increasing attention in the field of biomarker discovery. Given that EV are membrane bound structures, the components should be protected from degradation by extracellular proteases, DNAse and RNAse. A possibly selective package process during EV formation and shedding may lead to the reduced complexity of the contents [83, 84].

EV were originally considered a cleaning system to trash away the unnecessary molecules from cells. However, accumulated evidence demonstrates that EV influence their microenvironments by altering signaling pathways and delivering genetic information to other cells within close proximity [85–88]. Today, EV are accepted as potent mediators of cellular communication and as selectively packed delivery vehicle, which can provide clues to EV biogenesis, targeting, and cellular effects [87–89]. EV may also be used as a source of biomarkers for disease diagnosis, prognosis and response to treatment [89, 90]. Since EV can be readily isolated from multiple biological fluids (e.g., urine, serum, plasma, pleural effusion and saliva et al.), they have been considered to contain non-invasive biomarker candidates. In some pathological conditions including urological cancers, EV are easily secreted into the urine, and the urinary EV contain rich molecular information specific to the disease conditions such as cytoplasmic RNAs, miRNAs, metabolites and proteins [91]. Several disease-associated proteome were identified in urine from patients. Since EV-based urinary biomarkers are cell-free and do not rely on the presence of shed cells, urine provides a promise for the easy detection of bladder diseases [92, 93].

Unfortunately, there is no gold-standard technique for enriching and isolating EV in the clinical practice [94]. Nevertheless, several techniques have been developed to enrich and isolate urinary EV. This section discusses the different methods used to isolate urinary EV. Before isolating EV, it is advised to remove well-known abundant proteins in urine (e.g., uromodulin) [95]. Step-wise differential ultracentrifugation including low speed and high-speed centrifugation, and immuno-affinity and peptide-based isolation methods can be applied. The so-called Vn-96 peptide, based on surface marker of EV, was introduced to capture EV from biological fluids including urine. ExoQuick-TC™, Exospin™, and miRCURY™ EX isolation kits are based on aggregating agents followed by a low-speed centrifugation. Size-exclusion chromatography was also introduced to fractionate urine samples and isolate EV. Exochip™, a microfluidic-based method, has been recently shown to isolate EV. In particular, the hydrostatic dialysis method is efficient to enrich EV from highly diluted samples with molecular weight cut-off of 1000 kDa [94]. After omics analysis is done using EV isolated from urine samples, data can be analyzed using three major publically accessible EV-associated databases, EVpedia, ExoCarta, and Vesiclepedia [71, 96].

Because the variable results have been obtained with different isolation techniques, further discussion on the standard protocols for EV isolation, and normalization problem, which are major obstacles for the quantitative omics studies of EV, will be needed to apply this interesting biological resource into clinical practice.

Computational approaches to integrate data for better knowledge extraction

Using all information available from a wide variety of sources, including behavioral, genomic and life-style data has been coined "Big Data". In clinical research, Big Data approaches show promise to connect information for individualized therapy approaches, called Personalized Medicine, once Big Data Initiative has been shown to lead to new scientific insights to better understand the biology [4]. Omics studies generate long lists of interconnected genes, proteins and metabolites, which may be integrated in clinical settings via computational approaches [18, 21, 28, 75]. The systems approach, integrating multi-omics, data will increase the reliability of discovering biomarkers and development therapeutic strategies for bladder diseases.

Currently available tools for integrating omics data can be categorized (i) to identify parameters of disease-associated biological networks and (ii) to identify pathway-based targets. Computational methods and tools for identification of important molecular targets and biomarker candidates are summarized. The major network-based visualization tools include VANTED (https://immersive-analytics.infotech.monash.edu/vanted/), VisAnt (visant.bu.edu/), Metscape2 (metscape.ncibi.org/metscape2/), Arena3D (arena3d.org/) and MetaMapR [97]. In order to construct a disease-perturbed network, several softwares and integrative querying systems for interaction information (PSICQUIC), network modeling and analysis tools (STRING [98] and Cytoscape [99]), and pathway analysis (KEGG [100]) might be useful. Commercial tools (e.g., GeneGo and Ingenuity Pathway Analysis (IPA)) are also helpful to construct a network. For pathway visualization, various tools are available, including Pathguide (www.pathguide.org/), KEGG-based pathway visualization tool (www.genome.jp/kegg/pathway.html), Paintomics (www.pantomics.com/), ProMeTra (https://www.cebitec.uni-bielefeld.de/polyomics/index.php/comics-software/75-prometra/), KaPPa-View (kpv.kazusa.or.jp/), MapMan (mapman.gabipd.org/), MAYDAY, and PaVESy (pavesy.mpimp-golm.mpg.de/). Based on the biochemical activities extracted from experimental datasets, interactive pathways can be constructed [101].

Importantly, in order to extract biological knowledge and to perform successful data integration across multiple resources, it is always essential to understand the context of the biology. Most current approaches, maybe with the exception of the Ingenuity Pathway analysis, are ignorant of disease etiologies and common pathological information that are very well known to clinical scientists. Hence, it is critical that scientists using pathway or genomic software are aware of this pitfall and use such network analyses only as additional tool to structure data and information, but not to expect immediate understanding. Only under careful interpretation of clinical knowledge and scientific literature can Omics data and software provide new hypotheses on undiscovered biological pathways and processes, eventually allowing us to personalized care and therapies on bladder diseases.

Potential biomarkers of bladder diseases

Next, we review the current state of proteomics and metabolomics in conjunction with recent technical advances in mass spectrometry in this section. The key applications and achievements by urinary proteomics and metabolomics in clinical biomarker research are discussed. Focus will be given to PCa, BCa, BPH and IC among other urological diseases. Examples of urine-based biomarkers suggested by previous studies are shown in Fig. 3.

Urinary biomarkers for prostate cancer

As the second most prevalent cancer in men, PCa's incidence reaches 899,000 new cases and 258,000 deaths per year [102]. One of the gold standard diagnostic tools for PCa progression detection is the measurement of prostate specific antigen (PSA) in serum [102].

There have been many proteomic approaches to identify the urine-based biomarkers of PCa. For example, a large study using urine samples from 591 patients reported Annexin A3, a calcium-binding protein that plays a role in the regulation of cellular growth and in signal transduction pathways, as a novel urine-based biomarker for early PCa detection when used in conjunction with PSA [103]. Using CE-MS, 12 urinary biomarkers for PCa, including sodium/potassium-transporting ATPase γ, collagen α-1(III), collagen α-1(I), psoriasis susceptibility 1 candidate gene 2 protein, hepatocellular carcinoma associated protein TB6, histone H2B, osteopontin, polymeric Ig receptor, transmembrane secretory component, prostatic acid phosphatase, fibrinogen α chain precursor, and semenogelin 1, were identified and validated (91 % sensitivity and 69 % specificity) [104].

These findings strongly suggest that the use of a panel of biomarkers for disease diagnosis rather than a stand-alone biomarker, which may not be as specific, would benefit to diagnostic precision. However, unfortunately, currently none of these urinary protein biomarkers have been introduced into clinical practice, since current diagnostic biomarkers are suboptimal and of poor utility for low-grade disease and surveillance. To become routine tests, these biomarker candidates should be carefully tested in multicenter clinical trials and should be measured in biological fluids by robust, standardized analytical methods.

For development of metabolite markers, both LC-MS and GC-MS methods were applied to profile various clinical samples (including tissues, urine, and plasma) from PCa patients and identified 87 metabolites that distinguished PCa from normal subjects [105]. This study suggested that an interesting urinary metabolite, sarcosine (N-methylglycine), associates with PCa progression to metastasis with significant predictive value [105]. A following nested case control study showed that urinary sarcosine (and cysteine) levels were significantly higher in 54 PCa patients who had a recurrence after treatment [106]. However, another follow-up study done using an independent cohort of 106 PCa patients failed to reproduce the ability of urinary sarcosine (normalized to creatinine) as a PCa biomarker [107]. It is certainly possible that sarcosine may serve only as cell-internal signal, and not be excreted or shed into biofluids.

In addition, several cell-free and exosome-derived urinary microRNAs were suggested as PCa biomarkers [43]. The following reports provided evidence that circulating miRNAs might be a next-generation biomarker and contribute to cancer screening in non-invasive liquid biopsy. Only few studies for PCa-associated miRNA in urine were reported. Five of the miRNAs were differentially quantified in PCa patients compared to controls (miR-107, miR-574-3p, miR375, miR200b and miR-141) in urine of men with cancer, compared to that of healthy

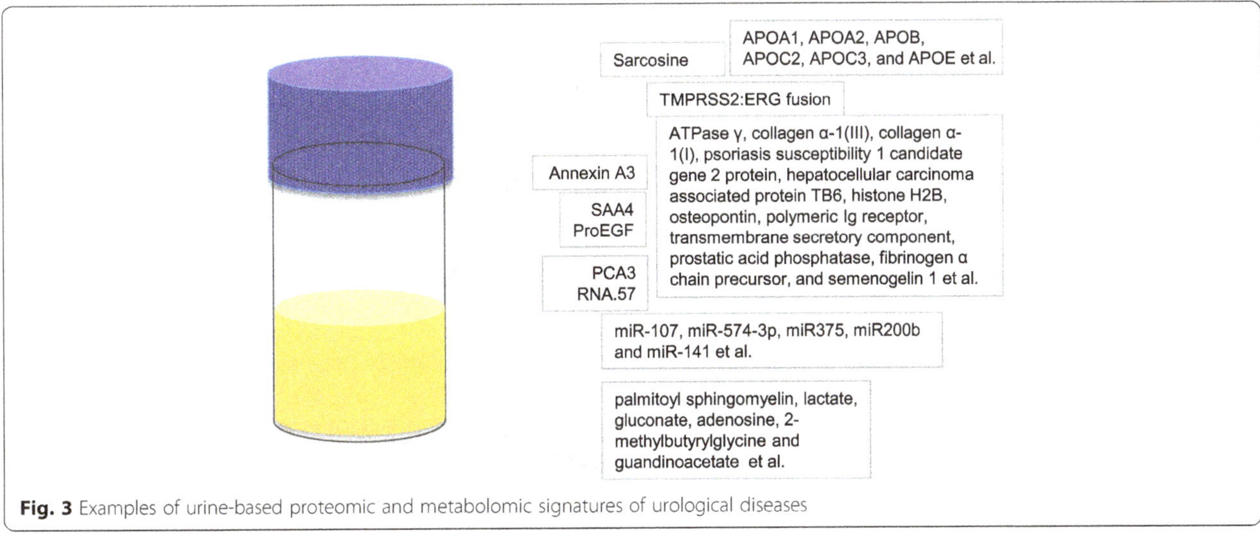

Fig. 3 Examples of urine-based proteomic and metabolomic signatures of urological diseases

volunteers [108]. Among them, two miRNAs (miR-141 and miR-375) were also found higher in the PCa patient blood [108]. In the case of miR-141, the urinary levels were approximately 50 fold higher in metastatic PCa patients, compared to the healthy controls. Nilsson et al. found that exosomes were carriers for the TMPRSS2:ERG fusion, which is an early molecular event associated with PCa invasion, and PCA3 RNA.57, which were originally found as PCa biomarkers in prostate tissues [108].

Recently we also found interesting urinary miRNAs including virus-encoded miRNAs, which are specific to PCa, suggesting that this miRNA panel can be usable for the clinical setting [88]. This miRNA panel showed much better specificity and sensitivity to PSA for the early PCa patients whose serum PSA levels are undetectable [88]. In addition to RNA detection, proteomic profiling of exosomes and EV in human urine is underway and may lead to new biomarker development for a variety of diseases, including urological cancers and other benign diseases, with a hope of the potential use of EV as reservoirs of disease biomarkers.

Urinary biomarkers for bladder cancer

Urinary bladder cancer (BCa), the fourth most common cancer worldwide, is a significant cause of morbidity and mortality with a high recurrence rate [109]. For a follow-up surveillance, the diagnostic methods have been mostly instrumental in approaches including cystoscopy and cytology, which are painful and invasive. Thus, the molecular assays in a non-invasive fashion are needed for BCa patient surveillance at an early stage. High-throughput proteomic profiling technologies will identify molecular signatures that are associated with BCa, and will provide us understanding on bladder cancer biology, eventually leading to the development of targeted therapeutics [57, 110].

The complementary techniques of high-resolution MS and Western blotting/dot blot were able to quantify the urinary proteome specific to NMIBC. 29 proteins had a significantly higher abundance ($p < 0.05$) in urine samples of NMIBC compared with matched controls [111]. Another MS analysis using a Bruker Ultraflextreme MALDI-TOF-MS revealed that the urine peptidome was associated with MIBC [57, 112]. Using hexapeptide-based library beads and an antibody-based affinity column using the iTRAQ technique, six apolipoproteins (APOA1, APOA2, APOB, APOC2, APOC3, and APOE) were suggested as BCa-associated urine proteins [112]. In this study, SAA4 and ProEGF were also significantly altered in BCa subgroups [112]. The combined signatures of SAA4 and ProEGF were demonstrated to have a good diagnostic capacity (AUC = 0.80 and $p < 0.001$) on BCa [112]. The other urine proteomic study using 2-DE MS demonstrated the increased level of urinary apolipoprotein-A1 (Apo-A1) in BCa patients compared to control subjects. Additional validation assays ($n = 379$) supported that Apo-A1 could be used as a BCa biomarker with a sensitivity and specificity of 89.2 and 84.6 %, respectively [113].

An unbiased global metabolomic profiling using high-performance liquid chromatography-quadrupole time-of-flight mass spectrometry (HPLC-QTOFMS) profiled urine metabolites of BCa patients and controls. Comprehensive data analyses suggested 12 differential metabolites that contributed to the distinction between the BCa and control groups with a great sensitivity (91.3 %) and specificity (92.5 %) (AUC = 0.937) [114]. Interestingly, BCa-associated urinary metabolomes are enriched in glycolysis and beta-oxidation [114]. Recent urine metabolic profiling was performed on two subject cohorts with and without BCa in three independent platforms, which include ultrahigh-performance liquid chromatography/tandem mass spectrometry (UHPLC-MS/MS) in the negative ion mode, UHPLC-MS/MS in the positive ion mode, and GC-MS. As a set of candidate biomarkers for bladder cancer, 6 biomarkers (palmitoyl sphingomyelin, lactate, gluconate, adenosine, 2-methylbutyrylglycine and guandinoacetate) were suggested [115].

There is no study on urine exosome-derived miRNA signature associated with BCa, however, exosome proteomics studies demonstrated exosomes were highly purified from cultured BCa cells. Using ultracentrifugation on a sucrose cushion, Western blotting and flow cytometry of exosome-coated beads, 18 urine exosome proteins (e.g., basigin, galectin-3, and trophoblast glycoprotein (5 T4) et al.) were identified and validated [116], suggesting that exosomes in urine are a highly stable resource of biomarkers for BCa.

Urinary biomarkers for BPH

Incidence of benign prostatic hyperplasia (BPH), the most common benign disease among men, is known to be associated with age. Since BPH patients have similar symptoms to those of PCa patients, there have been diagnostic challenges in clinical settings.

The urine proteome-based method for discrimination of BPH from high-grade prostatic intraepithelial neoplasia or PCa was developed through testing 407 patient samples using MALDI-TOF [73]. Recently performed urinary proteome profiling of men with BPH vs. PCa using iTRAQ LC/LC/MS/MS have identified 25 proteins that were differentially expressed in urines [73]. Three proteins, β2M, PGA3, and MUC3, were further validated by western blot analysis. The combination of these three proteins showed an AUC of 0.710 (95 % CI: 0.631–0.788, $P < 0.001$) and enhanced a diagnostic accuracy when combined with PSA (AUC = 0.812, (95 % CI:

0.740–0.885, $P < 0.001$), suggesting a useful biomarker candidate panel segregating BPH from PCa [9].

Urinary biomarkers for IC

IC is a chronic bladder syndrome with bladder pain, urinary frequency/urgency, pressure, discomfort, and nocturia, which cause the suppressed physical function and social activity and adverse impact on the quality of life [117–119]. Approximately 1 out of 77 people in the United States have been diagnosed with IC. There is no gold standard for IC diagnosis. Objective diagnostic markers are urgently needed to improve prospects for clinical care. Etiologies of IC remain unknown. Prescription of medications has not been clearly suggested in clinical settings. Thus, there is a clear clinical need for the identification of biomarkers of IC.

The urine-based omics approaches to identify IC diagnostic markers have been employed. A small glycosylated peptide, antiproliferative factor (APF) was found in urine samples derived from IC patients [120]. Urinary APF bioactivity could segregate IC patients from controls (94 % sensitivity and 95 % specificity). The following global and unbiased quantitative proteomics combined with bioinformatics analysis performed by our group has enabled us to reveal the in vitro APF signaling network [121, 122]. Additional proteomics profiles associated with IC were suggested by studies using various technologies. Using 2-DE and MALDI-TOF, urine samples from 9 IC patients and 9 asymptomatic controls were analyzed, and the proteins such as uromodulin, kininogens (precursors of kinin) and inter-α-trypsin inhibitory heavy chain H4 were significantly altered in urine samples of IC patients [123]. A study by Kuromitsu et al. suggested that neutrophil elastase is significantly higher in IC subset with bladder pain and small bladder capacity than in other IC patients and healthy controls by using the 2D-DIGE nanoLC-MS/MS [124]. Another urinary proteome identified by Goo et al. revealed that α-1B-glycoprotein, orosomucoid-1, transthyretin and hemopexin were altered in 60 % of IC patients compared to controls [125].

A few attempts to use metabolomics analysis to identify an IC signature have suggested promising metabolite signatures specific to IC. Fukui et al. used ultra-performance liquid chromatography-mass spectrometry (UPLC-MS) and found that the urinary ratio of phenylacetylglutamine to creatinine can be correlated to the clinical grade of IC (e.g. mild to severe based on symptoms) [126]. A report from Van et al. has suggested that IC patients exhibited distinct MS and NMR spectral patterns from non-IC patients [127]. With follow-up studies in a larger cohort, global metabolite profiling combined with multivariate statistical and bioinformatics analysis may validated some of these compounds as important biomarker metabolites contributing to the biological responses, such as the drug-induced toxicity, or response as metabolic biomarkers.

Conclusion: concluding remarks and perspectives

In this short review, we have provided information on the current state of 'omics' studies and available data sets relevant to bladder health and pathological condition, and presents opportunities for new research directed at understanding the pathogenesis of this complex condition. We believe that the ultimate goals of urine profiling of proteome and metabolome should be (i) to identify non-invasive diagnostic and prognostic biomarkers of bladder diseases, (ii) to better understand the biology of bladder diseases, and (iii) to determine the therapeutic strategies targeting the critical pathways of various bladder diseases. Recent efforts in the generation of large genomics, transcriptomics, proteomics, metabolomics, and other types of 'omics' data sets have provided a series of urinary biomarker candidates of bladder diseases. In spite of much efforts to identify candidate urinary biomarkers, it is still required to validate such markers in larger numbers of urine samples using targeted proteomics and metabolomics analyses in a prospective way.

Diagnostic and treatment modalities, even subjective diagnostic tools, are largely unavailable. As described here, our attempts to perform a systematic review and to build a pooled database using existing public 'omics' data associated with bladder health and various pathological conditions revealed the significant limitations and challenges facing investigators in the field. Many reports have suggested that natural diversity of patient population clearly plays a role in the difficulty of validating urine biomarkers. Expanding tests to include the general population often leads to loss or decrease in sensitivity. However, if tests are used for patients presenting specific symptoms in the clinic, and not for the general population, to inform about prognosis or treatment options, the pitfalls of general-population based urinary biomarkers may be alleviated. However, the cost of developing and validating a clinical grade assay is clearly beyond regular laboratory funding and would require concerted efforts by health agencies.

Collectively, despite these numerous pitfalls, urine is an interesting source of biomarkers for monitoring the bladder health. Rather than a single urinary molecular biomarker, a panel of biomarkers may be required to achieve the overall high level of specificity needed, so the trend is shifting towards implementing a panel of biomarkers, which may increase specificity. In order to translate potential biomarkers to clinical practice, vigorous validation must be pursued, with input from industry or large collaborative studies. Computational approaches combined with high quality 'omics' data could provide new insights in the field, essential molecular details about regulatory mechanisms and perturbations leading to bladder diseases, and essential information if we are to offer improved diagnostic capability and treatment strategies for patients.

Abbreviations

APF: antiproliferative factor; BCa: bladder cancer; BPH: benign prostatic hyperplasia; DEPs: differentially expressed proteins; DFI/LC-MS/MS: direct flow injection mass spectrometry; EV: extracellular vesicles; GC-MS: gas chromatography mass spectrometry; HMDB: human metabolome database; HPLC: high performance liquid chromatography; IC: interstitial cystitis/pelvic bladder syndrome/bladder pain syndrome; ICP-MS: inductively coupled plasma mass spectrometry; iTRAQ: isobaric tags for relative and absolute quantitation; LC-MS: liquid chromatography-mass spectrometry; MALDI-TOF: matrix assisted laser desorption/ionization time-of-flight; MIBC: muscle invasive bladder cancer; MS: mass spectrometry; nano-MALDI-MS: nano-liquid chromatography-tandem mass spectrometry; NMIBC: non-muscle invasive bladder cancer; NMR: nuclear magnetic resonance spectroscopy; PCa: prostate cancer; PTMs: posttranslational modifications; SELDI-TOF: surface-enhanced laser desorption/ionization time-of-flight; SILAC: stable-isotope labeling by amino acids; SRM/MRM: selective or multiple Reaction monitoring.

Competing interests

The authors declare that they have no competing interests.

Authors' contributions

ZC and JK participated in the design of the study and performed the analysis of references. JK led obtaining funding and drafted the manuscript. All authors read and approved the final manuscript.

Acknowledgements

The authors would like to thank Dr. Oliver Fiehn (UC Davis) for careful review and editing the manuscript.

Funding

The authors acknowledge support from National Institutes of Health grants (1U01DK103260, 1R01DK100974, U24 DK097154, NIH NCATS UCLA CTSI UL1TR000124 (to J.K.)), Department of Defense grants (PR140285 (to J.K.)), Centers for Disease Control and Prevention (1U01DP006079 (to J.K.)), IMAGINE NO IC Research Grant, the Steven Spielberg Discovery Fund in Prostate Cancer Research Career Development Award. J.K. is former recipient of Interstitial Cystitis Association Pilot Grant, a Fishbein Family IC Research Grant, New York Academy of Medicine, and Boston Children's Hospital Faculty Development.

Author details

[1]Advanced Clinical Biosystems Research Institute, Cedars-Sinai Medical Center, Los Angeles, CA, USA. [2]Department of Surgery, Cedars-Sinai Medical Center, 8700 Beverly Blvd, Los Angeles, CA 90048, USA. [3]Department of Biomedical Sciences, Cedars-Sinai Medical Center, 8700 Beverly Blvd, Los Angeles, CA 90048, USA. [4]Department of Medicine, University of California, Los Angeles, CA, USA.

References

1. Roper N, Stensland KD, Hendricks R, Galsky MD. The landscape of precision cancer medicine clinical trials in the United States. Cancer Treat Rev. 2015; 41(5):385–90.
2. Roychowdhury S, Chinnaiyan AM. Advancing precision medicine for prostate cancer through genomics. J Clin Oncol. 2013;31(15):1866–73.
3. Rubin MA. Toward a prostate cancer precision medicine. Urol Oncol. 2015; 33(2):73–4.
4. Garay JP, Gray JW. Omics and therapy - a basis for precision medicine. Mol Oncol. 2012;6(2):128–39.
5. Robinson PN. Deep phenotyping for precision medicine. Hum Mutat. 2012; 33(5):777–80.
6. Zhao Y, Polley EC, Li MC, Lih CJ, Palmisano A, Sims DJ, Rubinstein LV, Conley BA, Chen AP, Williams PM et al. GeneMed: an informatics hub for the coordination of next-generation sequencing studies that support precision oncology clinical trials. Cancer Informat. 2015;14 Suppl 2:45–55.
7. Wei WQ, Denny JC. Extracting research-quality phenotypes from electronic health records to support precision medicine. Genome Med. 2015;7(1):41.
8. Meric-Bernstam F, Johnson A, Holla V, Bailey AM, Brusco L, Chen K, Routbort M, Patel KP, Zeng J, Kopetz S et al. A decision support framework for genomically informed investigational cancer therapy. J Natl Cancer Inst 2015;107(7). doi: 10.1093/jnci/djv098.
9. Yang J, Roy R, Jedinak A, Moses MA. Mining the human proteome: biomarker discovery for human cancer and metastases. Cancer J. 2015;21(4): 327–36.
10. Antunes-Lopes T, Cruz CD, Cruz F, Sievert KD. Biomarkers in lower urinary tract symptoms/overactive bladder: a critical overview. Curr Opin Urol. 2014; 24(4):352–7.
11. Kamat AM, Vlahou A, Taylor JA, Hudson ML, Pesch B, Ingersoll MA, Todenhofer T, van Rhijn B, Kassouf W, Barton Grossman H et al. Considerations on the use of urine markers in the management of patients with high-grade non-muscle-invasive bladder cancer. Urol Oncol. 2014;32(7): 1069–77.
12. Kuo HC. Potential urine and serum biomarkers for patients with bladder pain syndrome/interstitial cystitis. Int J Urol. 2014;21 Suppl 1:34–41.
13. Pedroza-Diaz J, Rothlisberger S. Advances in urinary protein biomarkers for urogenital and non-urogenital pathologies. Biochemia Medica. 2015;25(1): 22–35.
14. Filip S, Zoidakis J, Vlahou A, Mischak H. Advances in urinary proteome analysis and applications in systems biology. Bioanalysis. 2014;6(19):2549–69.
15. Mendez O, Villanueva J. Challenges and opportunities for cell line secretomes in cancer proteomics. Proteomics Clin Appl. 2015;9(3–4):348–57.
16. Anderson L. Six decades searching for meaning in the proteome. J Proteome. 2014;107:24–30.
17. Iliuk AB, Arrington JV, Tao WA. Analytical challenges translating mass spectrometry-based phosphoproteomics from discovery to clinical applications. Electrophoresis. 2014;35(24):3430–40.
18. Zou L, Sun W. Human urine proteome: a powerful source for clinical research. Adv Exp Med Biol. 2015;845:31–42.
19. Naz S, Moreira dos Santos DC, Garcia A, Barbas C. Analytical protocols based on LC-MS, GC-MS and CE-MS for nontargeted metabolomics of biological tissues. Bioanalysis. 2014;6(12):1657–77.
20. Weckwerth W, Morgenthal K. Metabolomics: from pattern recognition to biological interpretation. Drug Discov Today. 2005;10(22):1551–8.
21. Zhang A, Sun H, Yan G, Wang P, Wang X. Metabolomics for biomarker discovery: moving to the clinic. BioMed Res Int. 2015;2015:354671.
22. Hou Q, Ufer G, Bartels D. Lipid signalling in plant responses to abiotic stress. Plant Cell Environ. 2015. doi: 10.1111/pce.12666.
23. Carey BW, Finley LW, Cross JR, Allis CD, Thompson CB. Intracellular alpha-ketoglutarate maintains the pluripotency of embryonic stem cells. Nature. 2015;518(7539):413–6.
24. Benjamin DI, Cravatt BF, Nomura DK. Global profiling strategies for mapping dysregulated metabolic pathways in cancer. Cell Metab. 2012;16(5):565–77.
25. Di Girolamo F, Del Chierico F, Caenaro G, Lante I, Muraca M, Putignani L. Human serum proteome analysis: new source of markers in metabolic disorders. Biomark Med. 2012;6(6):759–73.
26. Fischer R, Bowness P, Kessler BM. Two birds with one stone: doing metabolomics with your proteomics kit. Proteomics. 2013;13(23–24):3371–86.
27. Zhang A, Sun H, Wang P, Han Y, Wang X. Recent and potential developments of biofluid analyses in metabolomics. J Proteome. 2012;75(4):1079–88.
28. Alyass A, Turcotte M, Meyre D. From big data analysis to personalized medicine for all: challenges and opportunities. BMC Med Genet. 2015;8:33.
29. Boja ES, Rodriguez H. Proteogenomic convergence for understanding cancer pathways and networks. Clin Proteomics. 2014;11(1):22.
30. Stransky B, Barrera J, Ohno-Machado L, De Souza SJ. Modeling cancer: integration of "omics" information in dynamic systems. J Bioinforma Comput Biol. 2007;5(4):977–86.
31. Goossens N, Nakagawa S, Sun X, Hoshida Y. Cancer biomarker discovery and validation. Translat Cancer Res. 2015;4(3):256–69.

32. Dijkstra S, Mulders PF, Schalken JA. Clinical use of novel urine and blood based prostate cancer biomarkers: a review. Clin Biochem. 2014;47(10–11): 889–96.
33. Hessels D, Schalken JA. Urinary biomarkers for prostate cancer: a review. Asian J Androl. 2013;15(3):333–9.
34. Sorio C, Mauri P, Pederzoli P, Scarpa A. Non-invasive cancer detection: strategies for the identification of novel cancer markers. IUBMB Life. 2006; 58(4):193–8.
35. Kumar A, Baycin-Hizal D, Shiloach J, Bowen MA, Betenbaugh MJ. Coupling enrichment methods with proteomics for understanding and treating disease. Proteomics Clin Appl. 2015;9(1–2):33–47.
36. Stastna M, Van Eyk JE. Secreted proteins as a fundamental source for biomarker discovery. Proteomics. 2012;12(4–5):722–35.
37. Deutsch EW, Eng JK, Zhang H, King NL, Nesvizhskii AI, Lin B, Lee H, Yi EC, Ossola R, Aebersold R. Human Plasma PeptideAtlas. Proteomics. 2005;5(13): 3497–500.
38. Nanjappa V, Thomas JK, Marimuthu A, Muthusamy B, Radhakrishnan A, Sharma R, Ahmad Khan A, Balakrishnan L, Sahasrabuddhe NA, Kumar S et al. Plasma Proteome Database as a resource for proteomics research: 2014 update. Nucleic Acids Res. 2014;42(Database issue):D959–65.
39. Omenn GS. Data management and data integration in the HUPO plasma proteome project. Methods Mol Biol. 2011;696:247–57.
40. Lygirou V, Makridakis M, Vlahou A. Biological sample collection for clinical proteomics: existing SOPs. Methods Mol Biol. 2015;1243:3–27.
41. Roobol MJ, Carlsson SV. Risk stratification in prostate cancer screening. Nat Rev Urol. 2013;10(1):38–48.
42. Stovsky M, Ponsky L, Vourganti S, Stuhldreher P, Siroky MB, Kipnis V, Fedotoff O, Mikheeva L, Zaslavsky B, Chait A et al. Prostate-specific antigen/ solvent interaction analysis: a preliminary evaluation of a new assay concept for detecting prostate cancer using urinary samples. Urology. 2011;78(3): 601–5.
43. Trock BJ. Circulating biomarkers for discriminating indolent from aggressive disease in prostate cancer active surveillance. Curr Opin Urol. 2014;24(3): 293–302.
44. Emwas AH, Luchinat C, Turano P, Tenori L, Roy R, Salek RM, Ryan D, Merzaban JS, Kaddurah-Daouk R, Zeri AC et al. Standardizing the experimental conditions for using urine in NMR-based metabolomic studies with a particular focus on diagnostic studies: a review. Metabolomics. 2015; 11(4):872–94.
45. Rolfo C, Castiglia M, Hong D, Alessandro R, Mertens I, Baggerman G, Zwaenepoel K, Gil-Bazo I, Passiglia F, Carreca AP et al. Liquid biopsies in lung cancer: the new ambrosia of researchers. Biochim Biophys Acta. 2014; 1846(2):539–46.
46. Thomas CE, Sexton W, Benson K, Sutphen R, Koomen J. Urine collection and processing for protein biomarker discovery and quantification. Cancer Epidemiol Biomark Prev. 2010;19(4):953–9.
47. Wood SL, Knowles MA, Thompson D, Selby PJ, Banks RE. Proteomic studies of urinary biomarkers for prostate, bladder and kidney cancers. Nat Rev Urol. 2013;10(4):206–18.
48. Hortin GL, Sviridov D. Diagnostic potential for urinary proteomics. Pharmacogenomics. 2007;8(3):237–55.
49. Farrah T, Deutsch EW, Omenn GS, Sun Z, Watts JD, Yamamoto T, Shteynberg D, Harris MM, Moritz RL. State of the human proteome in 2013 as viewed through PeptideAtlas: comparing the kidney, urine, and plasma proteomes for the biology- and disease-driven Human Proteome Project. J Proteome Res. 2014;13(1):60–75.
50. Yamamoto T. The 4th Human Kidney and Urine Proteome Project (HKUPP) workshop. 26 September 2009, Toronto, Canada. Proteomics. 2010;10(11): 2069–70.
51. Yamamoto T, Langham RG, Ronco P, Knepper MA, Thongboonkerd V. Towards standard protocols and guidelines for urine proteomics: a report on the Human Kidney and Urine Proteome Project (HKUPP) symposium and workshop, 6 October 2007, Seoul, Korea and 1 November 2007, San Francisco, CA, USA. Proteomics. 2008;8(11):2156–9.
52. Court M, Selevsek N, Matondo M, Allory Y, Garin J, Masselon CD, Domon B. Toward a standardized urine proteome analysis methodology. Proteomics. 2011;11(6):1160–71.
53. Drake RR, White KY, Fuller TW, Igwe E, Clements MA, Nyalwidhe JO, Given RW, Lance RS, Semmes OJ. Clinical collection and protein properties of expressed prostatic secretions as a source for biomarkers of prostatic disease. J Proteome. 2009;72(6):907–17.
54. Cho YT, Chen CW, Chen MP, Hu JL, Su H, Shiea J, Wu WJ, Wu DC. Diagnosis of albuminuria by tryptic digestion and matrix-assisted laser desorption ionization/time-of-flight mass spectrometry. Clin Chim Acta. 2013;420: 76–81.
55. Dieterle F, Ross A, Schlotterbeck G, Senn H. Probabilistic quotient normalization as robust method to account for dilution of complex biological mixtures. Application in 1H NMR metabonomics. Anal Chem. 2006;78(13):4281–90.
56. Hathout Y. Proteomic methods for biomarker discovery and validation. Are we there yet? Expert Rev Proteomics. 2015;12(4):329–31.
57. Bauca JM, Martinez-Morillo E, Diamandis EP. Peptidomics of urine and other biofluids for cancer diagnostics. Clin Chem. 2014;60(8):1052–61.
58. Bechis SK, Otsetov AG, Ge R, Olumi AF. Personalized medicine for the management of benign prostatic hyperplasia. J Urol. 2014;192(1):16–23.
59. Muntel J, Xuan Y, Berger ST, Reiter L, Bachur R, Kentsis A, Steen H. Advancing urinary protein biomarker discovery by data-independent acquisition on a quadrupole-orbitrap mass spectrometer. J Proteome Res. 2015;14(11):4752–62.
60. Ovrehus MA, Zurbig P, Vikse BE, Hallan SI. Urinary proteomics in chronic kidney disease: diagnosis and risk of progression beyond albuminuria. Clin Proteomics. 2015;12(1):21.
61. Ordureau A, Munch C, Harper JW. Quantifying ubiquitin signaling. Mol Cell. 2015;58(4):660–76.
62. Weissinger EM, Mischak H. Application of proteomics to posttransplantational follow-up. Methods Mol Med. 2007;134:217–28.
63. Schwammle V, Verano-Braga T, Roepstorff P. Computational and statistical methods for high-throughput analysis of post-translational modifications of proteins. J Proteome. 2015;129:3–15.
64. Gopal J, Muthu M, Chun SC, Wu HF. State-of-the-art nanoplatform-integrated MALDI-MS impacting resolutions in urinary proteomics. Proteomics Clin Appl. 2015;9(5–6):469–81.
65. Heemskerk AA, Deelder AM, Mayboroda OA. CE-ESI-MS for bottom-up proteomics: Advances in separation, interfacing and applications. Mass Spectrom Rev. 2014. doi: 10.1002/mas.21432.
66. Hellstrom M, Jonmarker S, Lehtio J, Auer G, Egevad L. Proteomics in clinical prostate research. Proteomics Clin Appl. 2007;1(9):1058–65.
67. Robledo VR, Smyth WF. Review of the CE-MS platform as a powerful alternative to conventional couplings in bio-omics and target-based applications. Electrophoresis. 2014;35(16):2292–308.
68. Whelan LC, Power KA, McDowell DT, Kennedy J, Gallagher WM. Applications of SELDI-MS technology in oncology. J Cell Mol Med. 2008;12(5A):1535–47.
69. Collier TS, Muddiman DC. Analytical strategies for the global quantification of intact proteins. Amino Acids. 2012;43(3):1109–17.
70. Matzke MM, Brown JN, Gritsenko MA, Metz TO, Pounds JG, Rodland KD, Shukla AK, Smith RD, Waters KM, McDermott JE et al. A comparative analysis of computational approaches to relative protein quantification using peptide peak intensities in label-free LC-MS proteomics experiments. Proteomics. 2013;13(3–4):493–503.
71. Kim DK, Kang B, Kim OY, Choi DS, Lee J, Kim SR, Go G, Yoon YJ, Kim JH, Jang SC et al. EVpedia: an integrated database of high-throughput data for systemic analyses of extracellular vesicles. J Extracell Vesicles. 2013;2. doi: 10. 3402/jev.v2i0.20384.
72. Gillet LC, Navarro P, Tate S, Rost H, Selevsek N, Reiter L, Bonner R, Aebersold R. Targeted data extraction of the MS/MS spectra generated by data-independent acquisition: a new concept for consistent and accurate proteome analysis. Mol Cell Proteomics. 2012;11(6):O111.016717.
73. Jedinak A, Curatolo A, Zurakowski D, Dillon S, Bhasin MK, Libermann TA, Roy R, Sachdev M, Loughlin KR, Moses MA. Novel non-invasive biomarkers that distinguish between benign prostate hyperplasia and prostate cancer. BMC Cancer. 2015;15:259.
74. Colangelo CM, Chung L, Bruce C, Cheung KH. Review of software tools for design and analysis of large scale MRM proteomic datasets. Methods. 2013; 61(3):287–98.
75. Harlan R, Zhang H. Targeted proteomics: a bridge between discovery and validation. Expert Rev Proteomics. 2014;11(6):657–61.
76. Shi T, Su D, Liu T, Tang K, Camp 2nd DG, Qian WJ, Smith RD. Advancing the sensitivity of selected reaction monitoring-based targeted quantitative proteomics. Proteomics. 2012;12(8):1074–92.
77. Bouatra S, Aziat F, Mandal R, Guo AC, Wilson MR, Knox C, Bjorndahl TC, Krishnamurthy R, Saleem F, Liu P et al. The human urine metabolome. PLoS One. 2013;8(9):e73076.

78. Khamis MM, Adamko DJ, El-Aneed A. Mass spectrometric based approaches in urine metabolomics and biomarker discovery. Mass Spectrom Rev. 2015. doi: 10.1002/mas.21455.
79. Zheng C, Zhang S, Ragg S, Raftery D, Vitek O. Identification and quantification of metabolites in (1)H NMR spectra by Bayesian model selection. Bioinformatics. 2011;27(12):1637–44.
80. Tsugawa H, Cajka T, Kind T, Ma Y, Higgins B, Ikeda K, Kanazawa M, VanderGheynst J, Fiehn O, Arita M. MS-DIAL: data-independent MS/MS deconvolution for comprehensive metabolome analysis. Nat Methods. 2015; 12(6):523–6.
81. Krumsiek J, Suhre K, Evans AM, Mitchell MW, Mohney RP, Milburn MV, Wagele B, Romisch-Margl W, Illig T, Adamski J et al. Mining the unknown: a systems approach to metabolite identification combining genetic and metabolic information. PLoS Genet. 2012;8(10):e1003005.
82. Zhou B, Wang J, Ressom HW. MetaboSearch: tool for mass-based metabolite identification using multiple databases. PLoS One. 2012;7(6):e40096.
83. Coleman BM, Hill AF. Extracellular vesicles–Their role in the packaging and spread of misfolded proteins associated with neurodegenerative diseases. Semin Cell Dev Biol. 2015;40:89–96.
84. Yanez-Mo M, Siljander PR, Andreu Z, Zavec AB, Borras FE, Buzas EI, Buzas K, Casal E, Cappello F, Carvalho J et al. Biological properties of extracellular vesicles and their physiological functions. J Extracellular Vesicles. 2015;4: 27066.
85. Choi DY, You S, Jung JH, Lee JC, Rho JK, Lee KY, Freeman MR, Kim KP, Kim J. Extracellular vesicles shed from gefitinib-resistant nonsmall cell lung cancer regulate the tumor microenvironment. Proteomics. 2014;14(16):1845–56.
86. Jung JH, Lee MY, Choi DY, Lee JW, You S, Lee KY, Kim J, Kim KP. Phospholipids of tumor extracellular vesicles stratify gefitinib-resistant nonsmall cell lung cancer cells from gefitinib-sensitive cells. Proteomics. 2015;15(4):824–35.
87. Kim J, Morley S, Le M, Bedoret D, Umetsu DT, Di Vizio D, Freeman MR. Enhanced shedding of extracellular vesicles from amoeboid prostate cancer cells: potential effects on the tumor microenvironment. Cancer Biol Ther. 2014;15(4):409–18.
88. Yun SJ, Jeong P, Kang HW, Kim YH, Kim EA, Yan C, Choi YK, Kim D, Kim JM, Kim SK et al. Urinary MicroRNAs of prostate cancer: virus-encoded hsv1-miRH18 and hsv2-miR-H9-5p could be valuable diagnostic markers. Int Neurourol J. 2015;19(2):74–84.
89. Astro V, de Curtis I. Plasma membrane-associated platforms: dynamic scaffolds that organize membrane-associated events. Sci Signal. 2015;8(367):re1.
90. Robbins PD, Morelli AE. Regulation of immune responses by extracellular vesicles. Nat Rev Immunol. 2014;14(3):195–208.
91. Schey KL, Luther JM, Rose KL. Proteomics characterization of exosome cargo. Methods. 2015;87:75–82.
92. Gonzalez E, Falcon-Perez JM. Cell-derived extracellular vesicles as a platform to identify low-invasive disease biomarkers. Expert Rev Mol Diagn. 2015; 15(7):907–23.
93. Duijvesz D, Luider T, Bangma CH, Jenster G. Exosomes as biomarker treasure chests for prostate cancer. Eur Urol. 2011;59(5):823–31.
94. Pitto M, Corbetta S, Raimondo F. Preparation of urinary exosomes: methodological issues for clinical proteomics. Methods Mol Biol. 2015;1243: 43–53.
95. Hiemstra TF, Charles PD, Hester SS, Karet FE, Lilley KS. Uromodulin exclusion list improves urinary exosomal protein identification. J Biomol Tech. 2011; 22(4):136–45.
96. Kalra H, Simpson RJ, Ji H, Aikawa E, Altevogt P, Askenase P, Bond VC, Borras FE, Breakefield X, Budnik V et al. Vesiclepedia: a compendium for extracellular vesicles with continuous community annotation. PLoS Biol. 2012;10(12):e1001450.
97. Grapov D, Wanichthanarak K, Fiehn O. MetaMapR: pathway independent metabolomic network analysis incorporating unknowns. Bioinformatics. 2015;31(16):2757–60.
98. von Mering C, Huynen M, Jaeggi D, Schmidt S, Bork P, Snel B. STRING: a database of predicted functional associations between proteins. Nucleic Acids Res. 2003;31(1):258–61.
99. Shannon P, Markiel A, Ozier O, Baliga NS, Wang JT, Ramage D, Amin N, Schwikowski B, Ideker T. Cytoscape: a software environment for integrated models of biomolecular interaction networks. Genome Res. 2003;13(11): 2498–504.
100. Ogata H, Goto S, Sato K, Fujibuchi W, Bono H, Kanehisa M. KEGG: Kyoto Encyclopedia of Genes and Genomes. Nucleic Acids Res. 1999;27(1):29–34.
101. Fiehn O, Kim J. Metabolomics insights into pathophysiological mechanisms of interstitial cystitis. Int Neurourol J. 2014;18(3):106–14.
102. Hayes JH, Barry MJ. Screening for prostate cancer with the prostate-specific antigen test: a review of current evidence. JAMA. 2014;311(11):1143–9.
103. Schostak M, Schwall GP, Poznanovic S, Groebe K, Muller M, Messinger D, Miller K, Krause H, Pelzer A, Horninger W et al. Annexin A3 in urine: a highly specific noninvasive marker for prostate cancer early detection. J Urol. 2009; 181(1):343–53.
104. Theodorescu D, Schiffer E, Bauer HW, Douwes F, Eichhorn F, Polley R, Schmidt T, Schofer W, Zurbig P, Good DM et al. Discovery and validation of urinary biomarkers for prostate cancer. Proteomics Clin Appl. 2008;2(4): 556–70.
105. Sreekumar A, Poisson LM, Rajendiran TM, Khan AP, Cao Q, Yu J, Laxman B, Mehra R, Lonigro RJ, Li Y et al. Metabolomic profiles delineate potential role for sarcosine in prostate cancer progression. Nature. 2009;457(7231):910–4.
106. Stabler S, Koyama T, Zhao Z, Martinez-Ferrer M, Allen RH, Luka Z, Loukachevitch LV, Clark PE, Wagner C, Bhowmick NA. Serum methionine metabolites are risk factors for metastatic prostate cancer progression. PLoS One. 2011;6(8):e22486.
107. Jentzmik F, Stephan C, Miller K, Schrader M, Erbersdobler A, Kristiansen G, Lein M, Jung K. Sarcosine in urine after digital rectal examination fails as a marker in prostate cancer detection and identification of aggressive tumours. Eur Urol. 2010;58(1):12–8. discussion 20–11.
108. Bryant RJ, Pawlowski T, Catto JW, Marsden G, Vessella RL, Rhees B, Kuslich C, Visakorpi T, Hamdy FC. Changes in circulating microRNA levels associated with prostate cancer. Br J Cancer. 2012;106(4):768–74.
109. Noon AP, Catto JW. Bladder cancer in 2012: Challenging current paradigms. Nat Rev Urol. 2013;10(2):67–8.
110. Bansal N, Gupta A, Sankhwar SN. Proteometabolomics of bladder cancer: current and future prospects. Cancer Biomark. 2015;15:339–48.
111. Linden M, Lind SB, Mayrhofer C, Segersten U, Wester K, Lyutvinskiy Y, Zubarev R, Malmstrom PU, Pettersson U. Proteomic analysis of urinary biomarker candidates for nonmuscle invasive bladder cancer. Proteomics. 2012;12(1):135–44.
112. Chen CL, Lin TS, Tsai CH, Wu CC, Chung T, Chien KY, Wu M, Chang YS, Yu JS, Chen YT. Identification of potential bladder cancer markers in urine by abundant-protein depletion coupled with quantitative proteomics. J Proteome. 2013;85:28–43.
113. Li C, Li H, Zhang T, Li J, Liu L, Chang J. Discovery of Apo-A1 as a potential bladder cancer biomarker by urine proteomics and analysis. Biochem Biophys Res Commun. 2014;446(4):1047–52.
114. Jin X, Yun SJ, Jeong P, Kim IY, Kim WJ, Park S. Diagnosis of bladder cancer and prediction of survival by urinary metabolomics. Oncotarget. 2014;5(6): 1635–45.
115. Wittmann BM, Stirdivant SM, Mitchell MW, Wulff JE, McDunn JE, Li Z, Dennis-Barrie A, Neri BP, Milburn MV, Lotan Y et al. Bladder cancer biomarker discovery using global metabolomic profiling of urine. PLoS One. 2014;9(12):e115870.
116. Welton JL, Khanna S, Giles PJ, Brennan P, Brewis IA, Staffurth J, Mason MD, Clayton A. Proteomics analysis of bladder cancer exosomes. Mol Cell Proteomics. 2010;9(6):1324–38.
117. Clemens JQ, Mullins C, Kusek JW, Kirkali Z, Mayer EA, Rodriguez LV, Klumpp DJ, Schaeffer AJ, Kreder KJ, Buchwald D et al. The MAPP research network: a novel study of urologic chronic pelvic pain syndromes. BMC Urol. 2014; 14:57.
118. Lai HH, Krieger JN, Pontari MA, Buchwald D, Hou X, Landis JR, Network MR. Painful Bladder Filling and Painful Urgency Are Distinct Characteristics in Men and Women with Urologic Chronic Pelvic Pain Syndromes - A MAPP Research Network Study. J Urol. 2015;194:1634–41.
119. Landis JR, Williams DA, Lucia MS, Clauw DJ, Naliboff BD, Robinson NA, van Bokhoven A, Sutcliffe S, Schaeffer AJ, Rodriguez LV et al. The MAPP research network: design, patient characterization and operations. BMC Urol. 2014;14:58.
120. Keay SK, Szekely Z, Conrads TP, Veenstra TD, Barchi Jr JJ, Zhang CO, Koch KR, Michejda CJ. An antiproliferative factor from interstitial cystitis patients is a frizzled 8 protein-related sialoglycopeptide. Proc Natl Acad Sci U S A. 2004;101(32):11803–8.
121. Yang W, Chung YG, Kim Y, Kim TK, Keay SK, Zhang CO, Ji M, Hwang D, Kim KP, Steen H et al. Quantitative proteomics identifies a beta-catenin network as an element of the signaling response to Frizzled-8 protein-related antiproliferative factor. Mol Cell Proteomics. 2011;10(6):M110.007492.

122. Yang W, Kim Y, Kim TK, Keay SK, Kim KP, Steen H, Freeman MR, Hwang D, Kim J. Integration analysis of quantitative proteomics and transcriptomics data identifies potential targets of frizzled-8 protein-related antiproliferative factor in vivo. BJU Int. 2012;110(11 Pt C):E1138–46.
123. Canter MP, Graham CA, Heit MH, Blackwell LS, Wilkey DW, Klein JB, Merchant ML. Proteomic techniques identify urine proteins that differentiate patients with interstitial cystitis from asymptomatic control subjects. Am J Obstet Gynecol. 2008;198(5):553.e1–6.
124. Kuromitsu S, Yokota H, Hiramoto M, Morita S, Mita H, Yamada T. Increased concentration of neutrophil elastase in urine from patients with interstitial cystitis. Scand J Urol Nephrol. 2008;42(5):455–61.
125. Goo YA, Tsai YS, Liu AY, Goodlett DR, Yang CC. Urinary proteomics evaluation in interstitial cystitis/painful bladder syndrome: a pilot study. Int Brazil J Urol. 2010;36(4):464–78. discussion 478–469, 479.
126. Fukui Y, Kato M, Inoue Y, Matsubara A, Itoh K. A metabonomic approach identifies human urinary phenylacetylglutamine as a novel marker of interstitial cystitis. J Chromatogr B Anal Technol Biomed Life Sci. 2009; 877(30):3806–12.
127. Van QN, Klose JR, Lucas DA, Prieto DA, Luke B, Collins J, Burt SK, Chmurny GN, Issaq HJ, Conrads TP et al. The use of urine proteomic and metabonomic patterns for the diagnosis of interstitial cystitis and bacterial cystitis. Dis Markers. 2003;19(4–5):169–83.

Genomic case report of a low grade bladder tumor metastasis to lung

Marvin J. Van Every[1], Garrett Dancik[2], Venki Paramesh[3], Grzegorz T. Gurda[4,5], David R. Meier[5], Steven E. Cash[5], Craig S. Richmond[5] and Sunny Guin[5*]

Abstract

Background: We present a rare case where distant metastasis of a low grade bladder tumor was observed. We carried out detailed genomic analysis and cell based experiments on patient tumor samples to study tumor evolution, possible cause of disease and provide personalized treatment strategies.

Case presentation: A man with a smoking history was diagnosed with a low-grade urothelial carcinoma of the bladder and a concurrent high-grade upper urinary tract tumor. Seven years later he had a lung metastasis. We carried out exome sequencing on all the patient's tumors and peripheral blood (germline) to identify somatic variants. We constructed a phylogenetic tree to capture how the tumors are related and to identify somatic changes important for metastasis. Although distant metastasis of low-grade bladder tumor is rare, the somatic variants in the tumors and the phylogenetic tree showed that the metastasized tumor had a mutational profile most similar to the low grade urothelial carcinoma. The primary and the metastatic tumors shared several important mutations, including in the *KMT2D* and the *RXRA* genes. The metastatic tumor also had an activating *MTOR* mutation, which may be important for tumor metastasis. We developed a mutational signature to understand the biologic processes responsible for tumor development. The mutational signature suggests that the tumor mutations are associated with tobacco carcinogen exposure, which is concordant with the patient's smoking history. We cultured cells from the lung metastasis to examine proliferation and signaling mechanisms in response to treatment. The mTOR inhibitor Everolimus inhibited downstream mTOR signaling and induced cytotoxicity in the metastatic tumor cells.

Conclusion: We used genomic analysis to examine a rare case of low grade bladder tumor metastasis to distant organ (lung). Our analysis also revealed exposure to carcinogens found is tobacco as a possible cause in tumor development. We further validated that the patient might benefit from mTOR inhibition as a potential salvage therapy in an adjuvant or recurrent disease setting.

Keywords: Bladder cancer, Lung metastasis, MTOR, KMT2D, RXRA, Exome sequencing

Background

Bladder cancer is the fourth most common cancer in men, with an estimated 79,030 new cases and 16,870 deaths expected in the United States in 2017 [1]. Unlike many other cancers, bladder cancer's mortality rates and treatment options have changed very little in the last 30 years [1, 2]. Twenty-five percent of bladder cancers are muscle-invasive and life-threatening at diagnosis [3]. Non–muscle-invasive bladder cancers can recur [4], but they rarely metastasize to distant organs [4].

We present a genomic case report of a man diagnosed with low-grade bladder cancer and a separate, concurrent high-grade cancer of the upper urinary tract in 2009. The tumors were surgically removed. In 2016, the patient had a lung metastasis that, on pathology, resembled the low-grade bladder tumor that had been removed in 2009. Low-grade bladder tumors rarely metastasize to distant organs, so we used exome sequencing on the patient's three tumor biopsy specimens (from 2009 and 2016) to investigate the relationship between the metastasis and the initial low-grade and high-grade tumors, to study tumor progression, and to identify therapeutic vulnerabilities. We also carried out primary culture of the patient's lung cancer cells to study drug response.

* Correspondence: sunny.guin@gmail.com
[5]Gundersen Medical Foundation, 1300 Badger Street, La Crosse, WI 54601, USA
Full list of author information is available at the end of the article

Case presentation

In July of 2009, a 56-year-old man with a 40 pack-year smoking history presented with a low-grade papillary urothelial (transitional cell) carcinoma at the right ureteral orifice (primary bladder tumor). He also had a high-grade urothelial carcinoma of the renal pelvis with focal squamous differentiation and extensive renal parenchymal involvement. His right ureter was filled with tumor but did not show intramuscular invasion. Venous and lymphatic invasion of this tumor was absent. The patient first underwent transurethral resection of the bladder tumor (TURBT) of right ureteral orifice for the bladder carcinoma and underwent an ureteroscopic resection of the right ureter. The final pathology report characterized the bladder tumor as low-grade, non-invasive transitional cell carcinoma, and the ureteral resection demonstrated low-grade transitional cell carcinoma. In August 2009 a month later, the patient's upper urinary tract tumor was removed by hand-assisted laproscopic neproureterectomy. The final pathology on this tumor was pT3 pN0 with negative margins. The patient then underwent an intense course of 6 rounds of bacillus Calmette-Guérin (BCG) treatment in an adjuvant setting, followed by maintenance BCG treatment for 3 years.

In 2016 the patient returned with a lung tumor that, on pathologic evaluation, resembled the low grade right ureteral orifice bladder tumor (transitional cell) from July 2009. The lung tumor was surgically removed. Because low-grade bladder tumors rarely metastasize to distant organs, we consented the patient for an Institutional Review Board–approved research study to investigate the origin of the lung metastasis and also to identify genetic changes that could represent a therapeutic target for any future recurrence or metastasis.

Hematoxylin and eosin (H&E) review of the formalin-fixed paraffin-embedded

(FFPE) tumor biopsy specimens showed more than 70% tumor tissue within all the samples sent for exome sequencing (Fig. 1a). The identified variants are listed in Additional file 1: Table S1, Additional file 2: Table S2, Additional file 3: Table S3, Additional file 4: Table S4. We focused on missense and nonsense somatic mutations present in the three tumor samples. Multiple variants were shared by these three tumors, and others were unique to each individual tumor, as shown by the Venn diagram and heat map (Fig. 1b, c).

Phylogenetic analysis indicates that the lung metastasis and primary bladder tumor are most closely related, and that the upper urinary tract tumor may have developed

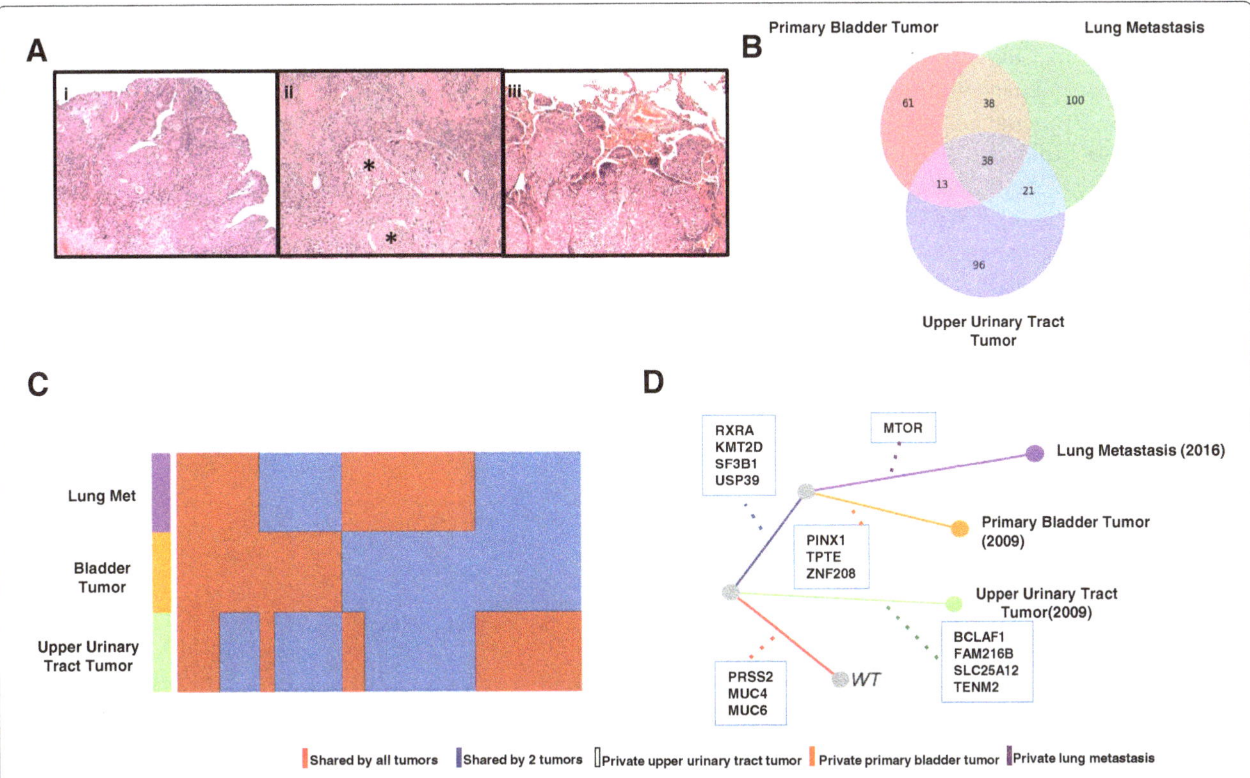

Fig. 1 a Hematoxylin and eosin stain of biopsy specimens from **i)** primary bladder tumor, **ii)** upper urinary tract tumor, and **iii)** lung metastasis. The high-grade tumor shows marked cytologic atypia and central necrosis (indicated by asterisks) not seen within the other tumors. **b, c** Venn diagram and heat map showing variant overlaps among the three tumors. **d** Phylogenetic tree showing the evolutionary relationship of the three tumors

first (the distances between normal tissue and upper urinary tract tumor and normal tissue and primary bladder tumor are very similar, 168 gain/loss of single nucleotide variants (SNVs) versus 171 (Fig. 1d, Additional file 5: Table S5). No mutations in a known oncogene or tumor suppressor gene are shared by all three tumors; however, the primary bladder tumor and the lung metastasis share known oncogenic mutations frequently found in bladder tumors, such as mutations in the *KMT2D* and *RXRA* genes. The mutational signatures, histomorphology, and distinct anatomic sites indicate that the upper urinary tract tumor and the primary bladder tumor likely are unrelated. Conversely, based on mutational profile and our model of tumor evolution, the primary bladder tumor and the lung metastasis may be related.

With evidence that the lung metastasis may be derived from the primary bladder tumor, we analyzed the somatic variants present in the primary bladder tumor and the lung metastasis that might be responsible for tumor initiation and progression. Table 1 lists some of the important variants shared between the primary bladder tumor and the lung metastasis and also variants that are unique to the lung metastasis. The primary and the metastatic tumor have mutations in the *KMT2D* and *RXRA* genes. *KMT2D* encodes the protein histone-lysine N-methyltransferase 2D which is a tumor suppressor [5, 6]. *KMT2D* is mutated in 28% of bladder tumors [7]. *RXRA*, which encodes retinoid X receptor alpha (RXR-alpha), is mutated in 10% of bladder tumors [7]. The RXRA S427F mutation present in these patient tumors is a hotspot mutation that predominantly occurs in urothelial tumors [7–10]. Initial studies show that this particular *RXRA* mutation regulates lipid metabolism via peroxisome proliferator-activated receptor gamma (PPARG) activation [8]. Among the mutations unique to the lung metastasis, a clinically actionable, activating mutation in mTOR (C1483F) was identified. This particular *MTOR* mutation is also present in the primary bladder tumor (Table 1), but at a very low frequency (1%). This C1483F mTOR mutation has been shown to activate mTOR downstream signaling via phosphorylation of p70-S6K and 4E-BP1 [11]. Development or selection of a subpopulation of cells with this activating *MTOR* mutation may be the driving event for lung metastasis within the primary bladder tumor.

We carefully examined the mutations present in the patient tumors based on the base substitutions C > A, C > G, C > T, T > A, T > C, T > G to identify how the patient tumors correlate with known mutational signatures representative of various biological processes. Figure 2a shows the mutational landscape in all the three tumors. More C > T and T > C mutations were found in the three tumors. Next we developed a mutational signature for the patient by combining all the mutations present in these three tumors (Fig. 2b). This mutational signature is characterized by predominantly C > T and T > C mutations (Fig. 2c). This patient's mutational signature resembles published mutational Signature 1A/B and Signature 5 [12]. Mutational signature 1A/B is related to the relatively elevated rate of spontaneous deamination of 5-methyl-cytosine, which results in C > T transitions and which predominantly occurs at NpCpG trinucleotides [12]. Signature 1A/B exhibits strong positive correlations with age in majority of cancers [12]. Signature 5, characterized by C > T and T > C mutations, is caused by tobacco carcinogens [12]. Our patient had a 40 pack-year smoking history, which suggests that tobacco use played a role in initiation of his tumors.

Using the Drug Gene Interaction Database [13], we identified candidate drugs targeting 12 of the 100 genes

Table 1 List of a Few Important Variants Shared Between Primary Bladder Tumor And Lung Metastasis And Variants Unique to the Lung Metastasis

							Primary Bladder Tumor		Lung Metastasis		
	Chromosome	Position	Gene	AA Change	Ref	Alt	VAF	Read Depth	VAF	Read Depth	Altered in Bladder Cancer
Shared Between Primary Bladder Tumor and Lung Metastasis	12	49,420,607	*KMT2D*	R5048C	G	A	37%	169	30%	245	28%
	9	137,328,351	*RXRA*	S427F	C	T	48%	136	28%	184	10%
	2	198,267,350	*SF3B1*	Q669H	T	A	43%	212	41%	153	6%
	2	85,868,233	*USP39*	F473 L	C	A	27%	112	34%	108	4%
	12	2,566,842	*CACNA1C*	R243C	C	T	29%	69	30%	204	6%
	X	41,204,468	*DDX3X*	D354G	A	G	79%	179	53%	104	4%
	4	183,676,006	*TENM3*	R1496W	C	T	46%	108	26%	172	8%
Unique to Lung Metastasis	1	11,217,230	*MTOR*	C1483F	C	A	1%	160	19%	172	2.4%
	6	89,616,132	*RNGTT*	R132H	C	T	0%	128	22%	82	2.4%
	8	77,761,863	*ZFHX4*	V1254A	T	C	0%	187	22%	154	18%

Ref reference sequence, *Alt* alternate sequence, *VAF* variant allele frequency

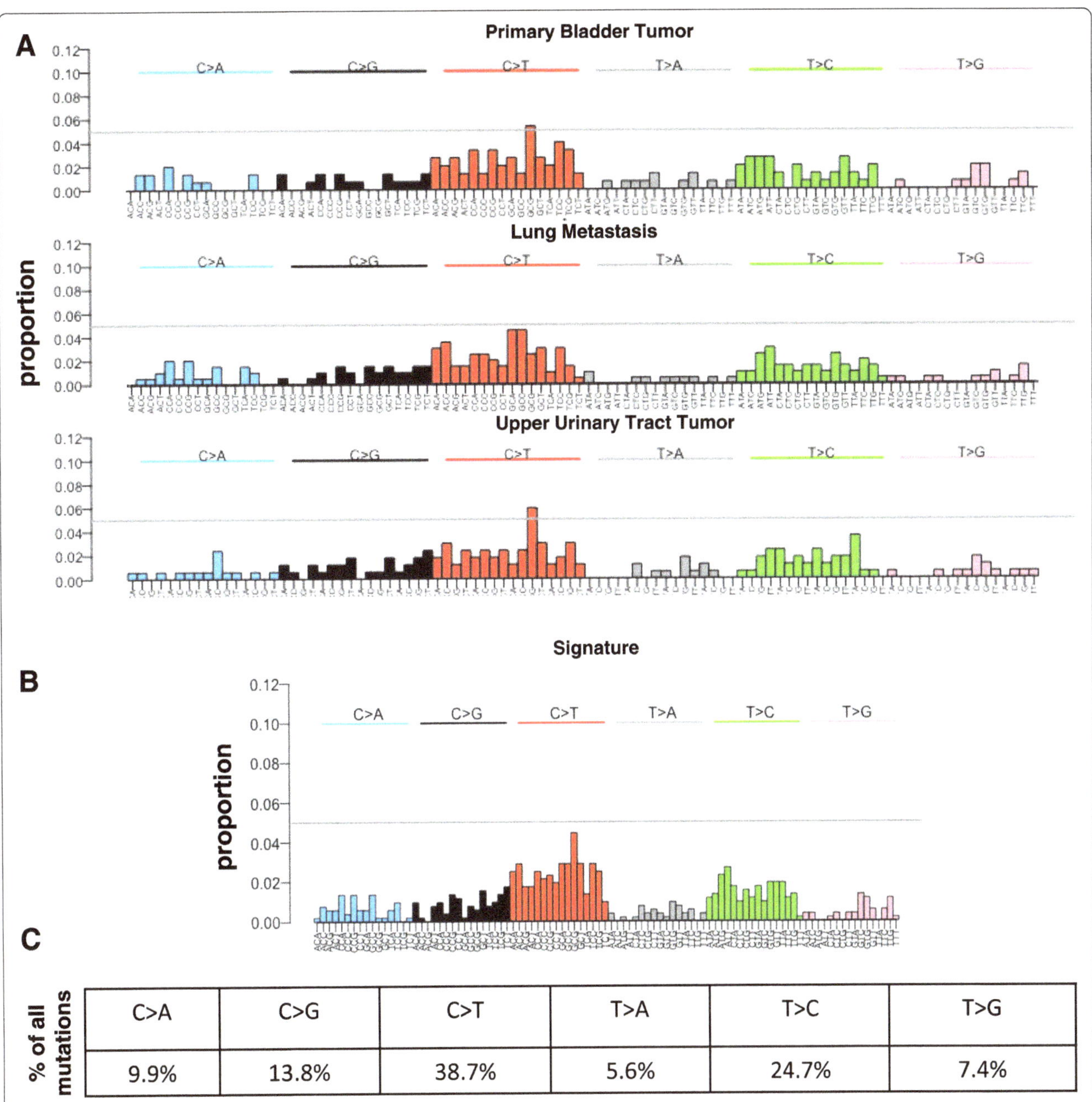

C>A	C>G	C>T	T>A	T>C	T>G
9.9%	13.8%	38.7%	5.6%	24.7%	7.4%

Fig. 2 a Substitution patterns in the upper urinary tract tumor, primary bladder tumor, and lung metastasis isolated from the same patient. Substitutions are categorized according to the pyrimidine of the mutated base pair, for all possible trinucleotides that include the mutated base along with each neighboring base on the 5′ and 3′ ends. **b** Substitution signature for upper urinary tract tumor, primary bladder tumor, and lung metastasis isolated from the same patient. Proportion of substitutions as categorized according to the pyrimidine of the mutated base pair, for all possible trinucleotides that include the mutated base along with each neighboring base on the 5′ and 3′ ends. **c** Relative frequency table showing the percentages of each substitution across all samples (516 substitutions)

with SNVs in the lung tumor (Additional file 6: Table S6). Several FDA-approved anti-cancer therapies were identified, including the *RXRA* agonist bexarotene and mTOR inhibitors, such as everolimus. We note that this analysis does not consider whether the variant is activating or deleterious, and all candidate therapies need to be evaluated. Primary culture of the lung metastasis was established in the laboratory. Since the lung metastasis has an activating *MTOR* mutation, we treated these cells with mTOR inhibitor everolimus at two concentrations (10 and 50 nM). The treatment showed a marked inhibition of mTOR activity and downstream signaling via two of its effectors, p70 S6K and 4E-BP1, at both concentrations (Fig. 3a); however, AKT activity increased with everolimus treatment (Fig. 3a). AKT can function both upstream and downstream of mTOR, but an increase in AKT activity

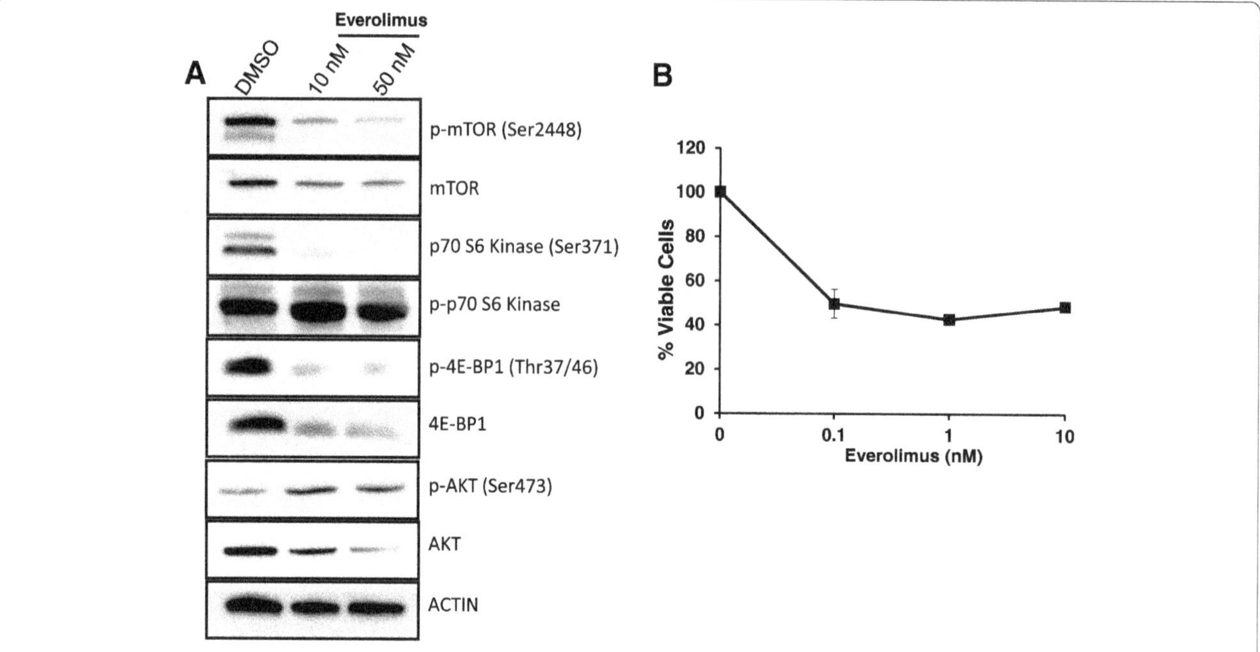

Fig. 3 a Cells from the lung metastasis were treated with Everolimus at 10 and 50 nM concentrations for 24 h. The cells were lysed, and Western blots were carried out for proteins involved in mammalian target of rapamycin (mTOR) signaling. **b** 10^3 cells were plated in triplicates in 96-well plate followed by treatment with increasing concentrations of everolimus. Cytotoxicity assay was carried out after 72-h drug treatment as described in Materials and Methods

could be a mechanism of resistance to the mTOR inhibitor.

Cytotoxicity study showed that at very low concentration (0.1 nM) everolimus reduces viability of these cells by about 60% (Fig. 3b), but even at a high concentration 40% of cells remain viable, indicating a cell population resistant to the drug.

Discussion

We present a genomic case report of rare distant metastasis of a low grade bladder tumor. Phylogenetic analysis revealed that the primary low grade bladder tumor and the lung tumor are more closely related, and shared several known oncogenic mutations frequently observed in bladder tumors. Both these tumors presented with *KMT2D* and *RXRA* gene mutations. *KMT2D* is a known tumor suppressor that is mutated in a quarter of bladder tumors [5–7] and also regulates gene transcription [6]. We speculate that the loss of function of this tumor suppressor (*KMT2D* mutation seen here is likely inactivating) is an important driver for these tumors. Another important variant present in both these tumors is a mutation in the *RXRA* gene. The S427F RXRA mutation predominantly occurs in bladder tumors [9, 10]. Preliminary studies have shown that this particular *RXRA* mutation regulates *RXRA* and PPARG interaction [8]. There is increased activation of PPARG in tumors carrying this particular *RXRA* mutation, which drives lipid metabolism [7, 8]. We believe that RXRA S427F mutation may play an important role in tumor initiation and progression. Although outside the scope of this study, the role of this *RXRA* mutation in bladder cancer should be characterized in detail as another potential therapeutic avenue for patients with advanced bladder cancer.

The lung metastasis has an activating mutation in the *MTOR* gene (C1483F). This particular C1483F mutation was presented with a variant allele frequency (VAF) of 19% (of 172 reads) in the metastatic tumor and has a VAF of 1% (of 160 reads) in the primary bladder tumor. This indicates that a small population of cells in the primary tumor probably developed this particular *MTOR* mutation and this clonal population likely migrated and was able to seed in the lung. Thus, we think that the activating *MTOR* mutation could be one of the important drivers that lead to distant metastasis, perhaps thru evolution of a subclone of the low-grade bladder tumor. Treating the lung metastasis with everolimus showed a marked decrease in p70 S6K and 4E-BP1 activity, but a concurrent increase in activated AKT. Cytotoxicity assay showed that 60% of these cells are sensitive to everolimus treatment.t. We speculate that increase in AKT activity with the drug treatment could be a mechanism of resistance to mTOR inhibition and could explain the 40% viable cells post-treatment.

Finally, we tried to understand whether the mutations present in these tumors represent a known oncogenic process. The mutational signature in this patient was dominated by predominantly C > T and T > C mutations—the hallmark of a mutational signature caused by tobacco carcinogens [12]—suggesting that our patient's tobacco use was perhaps responsible for his tumors.

We also tested whether the lung metastasis had any therapeutic vulnerability. We show that the metastasized tumor is vulnerable to mTOR inhibition because it carries an activating *MTOR* mutation. However if the patient has a recurrence of the lung metastasis and physicians choose to treat him with an mTOR inhibitor, they should take into account a possible mechanism of resistance driven by activated AKT. Thus, we believe that in case of another metastasis or a local recurrence, this patient may benefit from a combination of mTOR inhibitor and a conventional standard-of-care chemotherapy.

Conclusion

Here we used genomic analysis to study cancer evolution and present a rare case where a low grade bladder tumor metastasis to the lung. We used phylogenetic analysis to prove that the low grade bladder tumor and the lung metastasis are closely related. We also conclude that this patient may benefit from an mTOR inhibitor in case of disease recurrence since his metastatic disease carries an activating mTOR mutation and cancer cells cultured from his lung tumor showed vulnerability to mTOR inhibition. This case report points to the importance of genomic analysis of patient tumors to understand tumor biology, evolution and for personalized patient care.

Materials and methods

Sample preparation for exome sequencing

Formalin-fixed paraffin-embedded (FFPE) tumor biopsy blocks from the primary bladder tumor (2009), high-grade upper urinary tract tumor (2009), and the lung metastasis (2016) were cut and stained with hematoxylin and eosin (H&E) staining using standard protocol [14] to identify the tumor-rich regions. gDNA was isolated from the tumor-rich regions of the biopsies using Qiagen QIAamp® DNA FFPE Tissue kit, per standard manufacturer instruction. gDNA was also isolated from patient blood to detect germline genetic changes using Qiagen QIAamp® DNA Blood Mini kit. Exome sequencing and variant calling was carried out at BGI Sequencing Services.

Data analysis (exome sequencing, phylogenetic tree, substitution patterns and mutational signature, and druggable genes)

Somatic variants were identified by removing those present in the patient's blood, and then filtered to remove those observed $\geq$0.1% in the 1000 Genomes and Exome Sequencing Projects. Downstream analyses were limited to non-silent variants and indels in the coding region of the gene.

Phylogenetic trees were constructed based on the presence or absence of somatic coding variants, using the parsimony ratchet method [15] as implemented in the Bioconductor package *phangorn* [16], version 2.2.0. Branch lengths were calculated using the ACCelerated TRANsformation criteria (*acctran* function).

Substitution patterns are categorized based on the mutated pyrimidine (C or T) or the complementary pyrimidine partner of the mutated base (for substitutions involving A or G), yielding the following mutations: C > A, C > G, C > T, T > A, T > C, T > G. The immediate 5′ and 3′ bases are included, for example, ACA > AAA, to yield 96 possible trinucleotide substitutions. The identification of mutation signatures was carried out using a previously published computational framework implemented in MATLAB [17]. This approach identifies mutation patterns (i.e., mutation signatures) that explain observed mutations across samples.

Druggable genes were identified by querying genes of interest against the Drug Gene Interaction Database [13] with the results "summarized by gene." If > 3 drugs were identified for a specific gene, the top 3 drugs were reported.

Primary culture of lung metastasized tumor

Tumor tissue from the surgically removed lung metastasis was collected using an IRB-approved protocol. This tissue was first digested with collagenase/hyaluronidase (Stemcell Technologies) at 37 °C for 3 h. This was followed by Accutase (Stemcell Technologies) digestion for 30 min at 37 °C. After Accutase digestion cells were filtered using a 40 μm cell strainer. The cells were suspended in HBSS (Thermo Fisher Scientific) with 2%FBS (Stemcell Technologies), 10 μM ROCK inhibitor Y-27632 (Stemcell Technologies). Epithelial cells were isolated using Human EpCAM Positive Selection Kit (Stemcell Technologies) using standard manufacturer protocol. The isolated epithelial cells were cultured in Hepatocyte Medium (Stemcell Technologies) with 10 ng/ml EGF (Stemcell Technologies), 5% heat-inactivated charcoal stripped FBS (Stemcell Technologies), Glutamax (Thermo Fisher Scientific), 5% Matrigel (Thermo Fisher Scientific), and 10 μM ROCK inhibitor Y-27632 [18].

Western blot

Primary cells were treated with mTOR inhibitor everolimus (Cell Signaling) at 10 and 50 nM concentration for 24 h. The cells were lysed, followed by Western blot analysis for phosphorylated and total mTOR, p70 S6K, 4E-BP1, and AKT. Actin was used as housekeeping control. All primary antibodies were from Cell Signaling. HRP (Cell Signaling) labeled mouse or rabbit secondary antibodies were used, followed by chemiluminescence using ECL (Pierce, Rockford, IL).

Cytotoxicity study

Cells were plated in 96 well plates (10^3 cells/well) in triplicates and treated with different concentrations of everolimus or vehicle control. After 72 h of drug treatment, cell viability was measured using CyQUANT® Cell Proliferation Assay (Thermo Fisher Scientific) according to manufacturer instructions.

Additional files

Additional file 1: Table S1. Single nucleotide variants detected in primary bladder tumor.

Additional file 2: Table S2. Single nucleotide variants detected in upper urinary tract tumor.

Additional file 3: Table S3. Single nucleotide variants detected in lung metastasis.

Additional file 4: Table S4. Single nucleotide variants detected in peripheral blood.

Additional file 5: Table S5. Single nucleotide variants shared between and unique to the three tumors.

Additional file 6: Table S6. Candidate drug targets of genes with SNVs in the lung tumor.

Abbreviations

BCG: bacillus Calmette-Guerin; FFPE: Formalin-fixed paraffin-embedded; H&E: Hematoxylin and eosin

Acknowledgements

We thank Dr. Paraic Kenny at Gundersen Medical Foundation for his input on the project.

Funding

This study was funded by Gundersen Medical Foundation.

Authors' contributions

The study was conceived by SG and MV. The patient was seen and operated on by MV and VP. The case detail was provided by MV. The pathology was analyzed by GG. H&E was carried out by SC. DM and CR established the primary culture and carried out the cytotoxicity study. SG carried out the Western blot. SG and GD analyzed the genomic data and wrote the manuscript. All authors have read and approved the final manuscript.

Competing interests

The authors declare that they have no competing interests.

Author details

[1]Department of Urology, Gundersen Health System, 1900 South Ave, La Crosse, WI 54601, USA. [2]Department of Mathematics and Computer Science, Eastern Connecticut State University, 83 Windham Street, Willimantic, CT 06226, USA. [3]Department of Cardiothoracic Surgery, Gundersen Health System, 1900 South Ave, La Crosse, WI 54601, USA. [4]Department of Pathology, Gundersen Health System, 1900 South Ave, La Crosse, WI 54601, USA. [5]Gundersen Medical Foundation, 1300 Badger Street, La Crosse, WI 54601, USA.

References

1. Siegel RL, Miller KD, Jemal A. Cancer statistics, 2017. CA Cancer J Clin. 2017; 67(1):7–30.
2. Smith ND, Prasad SM, Patel AR, Weiner AB, Pariser JJ, Razmaria A, Maene C, Schuble T, Pierce B, Steinberg GD. Bladder Cancer mortality in the United States: a geographic and temporal analysis of socioeconomic and environmental factors. J Urol. 2016;195(2):290–6.
3. Nieder AM, Mackinnon JA, Huang Y, Fleming LE, Koniaris LG, Lee DJ. Florida bladder cancer trends 1981 to 2004: minimal progress in decreasing advanced disease. J Urol. 2008;179(2):491–5. discussion 495
4. Miyamoto H, Brimo F, Schultz L, Ye H, Miller JS, Fajardo DA, Lee TK, Epstein JI, Netto GJ. Low-grade papillary urothelial carcinoma of the urinary bladder: a clinicopathologic analysis of a post-World Health Organization/International Society of Urological Pathology classification cohort from a single academic center. Arch Pathol Lab Med. 2010;134(8):1160–3.
5. Toska E, Osmanbeyoglu HU, Castel P, Chan C, Hendrickson RC, Elkabets M, Dickler MN, Scaltriti M, Leslie CS, Armstrong SA, et al. PI3K pathway regulates ER-dependent transcription in breast cancer through the epigenetic regulator KMT2D. Science. 2017;355(6331):1324–30.
6. Ortega-Molina A, Boss IW, Canela A, Pan H, Jiang Y, Zhao C, Jiang M, Hu D, Agirre X, Niesvizky I, et al. The histone lysine methyltransferase KMT2D sustains a gene expression program that represses B cell lymphoma development. Nat Med. 2015;21(10):1199–208.
7. Cancer Genome Atlas Research N. Comprehensive molecular characterization of urothelial bladder carcinoma. Nature. 2014;507(7492):315–22.
8. Jonathan T, Goldstein CS, Duke F, Shih J, Meyerson M. Validation of PPARG and RXRA as drivers of bladder cancer. In: American association of Cancer research annual meeting. Washington DC: AACR; 2017.
9. Cerami E, Gao J, Dogrusoz U, Gross BE, Sumer SO, Aksoy BA, Jacobsen A, Byrne CJ, Heuer ML, Larsson E, et al. The cBio cancer genomics portal: an open platform for exploring multidimensional cancer genomics data. Cancer Discov. 2012;2(5):401–4.
10. Gao J, Aksoy BA, Dogrusoz U, Dresdner G, Gross B, Sumer SO, Sun Y, Jacobsen A, Sinha R, Larsson E, et al. Integrative analysis of complex cancer genomics and clinical profiles using the cBioPortal. Sci Signal. 2013;6(269):pl1.
11. Grabiner BC, Nardi V, Birsoy K, Possemato R, Shen K, Sinha S, Jordan A, Beck AH, Sabatini DM. A diverse array of cancer-associated MTOR mutations are hyperactivating and can predict rapamycin sensitivity. Cancer Discov. 2014;4(5):554–63.
12. Alexandrov LB, Nik-Zainal S, Wedge DC, Aparicio SA, Behjati S, Biankin AV, Bignell GR, Bolli N, Borg A, Borresen-Dale AL, et al. Signatures of mutational processes in human cancer. Nature. 2013;500(7463):415–21.
13. Wagner AH, Coffman AC, Ainscough BJ, Spies NC, Skidmore ZL, Campbell KM, Krysiak K, Pan D, McMichael JF, Eldred JM, et al. DGIdb 2. 0: mining clinically relevant drug-gene interactions. Nucleic Acids Res. 2016;44(D1):D1036–44.
14. Fischer AH, Jacobson KA, Rose J, Zeller R. Hematoxylin and eosin staining of tissue and cell sections. CSH Protoc. 2008;2008:pdb prot4986.
15. KC N. The parsimony ratchet, a new method for rapid parsimony analysis. Cladistics. 1999;15:407–14.
16. Schliep KP. Phangorn: phylogenetic analysis in R. Bioinformatics. 2011;27(4):592–3.
17. Alexandrov LB, Nik-Zainal S, Wedge DC, Campbell PJ, Stratton MR. Deciphering signatures of mutational processes operative in human cancer. Cell Rep. 2013;3(1):246–59.
18. Barlow LMCC, Lei M, DeCastro GJ, Badani K, Benson M, McKiernan J, Shen M. An individualized approach to bladder cancer treatment using patient-derived cell lines to predict response to chemotherapeutic agents. San Diego: American Association for Cancer Research Annual Meeting; 2014.

Uni-axial stretch induces actin stress fiber reorganization and activates c-Jun NH_2 terminal kinase via RhoA and Rho kinase in human bladder smooth muscle cells

Nobuhiro Kushida[1*], Osamu Yamaguchi[2], Yohei Kawashima[1], Hidenori Akaihata[1], Junya Hata[1], Kei Ishibashi[1], Ken Aikawa[1] and Yoshiyuki Kojima[1]

Abstract

Background: Excessive mechanical overload may be involved in bladder wall remodelling. Since the activity of Rho kinase is known to be upregulated in the obstructed bladder, we investigate the roles of the RhoA/Rho kinase pathway in mechanical overloaded bladder smooth muscle cells.

Methods: Human bladder smooth muscle cells were stimulated on silicon culture plates by 15 % elongated uni-axial cyclic stretch at 1 Hz. The activity of c-Jun NH_2-terminal kinase was measured by western blotting and actin stress fibers were observed by stained with phallotoxin conjugated with Alexa-Fluor 594.

Results: The activity of c-Jun NH_2-terminal kinase 1 peaked at 30 min (4.7-fold increase vs. before stretch) and this activity was partially abrogated by the RhoA inhibitor, C3 exoenzoyme or by the Rho kinase inhibitor, Y-27632. Stretch induced the strong formation of actin stress fibers and these fibers re-orientated in a direction that was perpendicular to the stretch direction. The average angle of the fibers from the perpendicular to the direction of stretch was significantly different between before, and 4 h after, stretch. Actin stress fibers reorganization was also suppressed by the C3 exoenzyme or Y-27632.

Conclusions: Bladder smooth muscle cells appear to have elaborate mechanisms for sensing mechanical stress and for adapting to mechanical stress overload by cytoskeletal remodeling and by activating cell growth signals such as c-Jun NH_2-terminal kinase via RhoA/Rho kinase pathways.

Keywords: Bladder smooth muscle, C-Jun NH_2 terminal kinase, Mechanical stretch, RhoA, Rho kinase

Background

Bladder wall remodeling such as smooth muscle hypertrophy/hyperplasia occurs under conditions of bladder outlet obstruction including benign prostate hyperplasia. Although these etiologies are not well understood, an excessive mechanical overload might be a prior factor. In the human obstructed bladder, sustained stretch stress is believed to cause bladder wall remodeling such as a change in the ratio of extracellular matrix and smooth muscle cells [1, 2]. In vivo animal models with a partial urethral ligature have revealed smooth muscle hypertrophy in the bladder wall, which are quite similar to the obstructed bladder in humans [3]. Although *in vitro* devices do not completely mimic the bladder wall overload, stretch devices that enable the stimulation of cultured bladder smooth muscle cells were used to reveal the pathological mechanisms under condition of mechanical overload. Park et al. indicated that angiotensin release induced by mechanical stretch acts as mitogen in bladder smooth muscle cells [4, 5].

Some studies have identified intracellular signaling pathways that mediate the biological effects evoked by mechanical stimuli and ultimately lead to nuclear events [5]. Of these pathways, the mitogen activated protein kinases

* Correspondence: no7744@fmu.ac.jp
[1]Department of Urology, Fukushima Medical University School of Medicine, 1, Hikarigaoka, Fukushima 960-1295, Japan
Full list of author information is available at the end of the article

(MAPKs), which constitute a family of serine/threonine kinases, are known to mediate signals that are activated by external stimuli and that regulate cell growth and differentiation. One MAPK family member, c-Jun NH_2-terminal kinase (JNK), has been reported to be activated by mechanical stretch in vascular smooth muscle cells [6] and cardiac myocytes [7]. In addition, Nguyen et al. indicated that cyclic stretch activates JNK in bladder smooth muscle cells [8]. We also showed that stretch stimulation activated JNK in rat bladder smooth muscle cells by the influx of Ca^{2+} through a stretch activated ion channel [9].

RhoA is a member of the Rho family of 20 to 30 kDa GTPase proteins that cycle between an active GTP-bound form and an inactive GDP-bound form. One of the important roles of RhoA is to act as a regulator of actin stress fibers [10]. RhoA is involved in cell division, movement, polarization and morphological changes via reorganization of actin stress fibers. The Rho-associated coiled-coil forming protein kinase (ROCK) is a molecule of RhoA that acts as a serine/threonine kinase and phosphorylates various substrates. Actin stress fiber reorganization was recently reported to be mediated by the ROCK pathway [11]. The physical deformation of cells appears to be caused by reorganization of actin stress fibers in order to adapt to their extracellular environments.

Previous evidence suggested that the RhoA/ROCK pathway is involved in the pathogenesis of obstructed bladder [12] and in the change in Ca^{2+} sensitization due to agonist stimulation [13]. Poley et al. indicated that quick stretch of rabbit bladder smooth muscle sufficient to induce calcium entry and stimulate a myogenic contraction does not activate the ROCK, and that basally active ROCK is necessary for stretch induced myogenic contraction [14]. We undertook to identify the roles of the RhoA/ROCK pathway in the early signalling events evoked by mechanical stimuli in human bladder smooth muscle cells (HBSMCs).

Methods

Cultured HBSMCs

Commercially established HBSMCs (Cambrex Bio Science, Walkersville, USA) were used for all experiments. Cultured cells were identified by immunostaining with anti-α smooth muscle actin (Sigma, Saint Louis, USA). Cells were maintained in the growth medium: SmBM-2 with BulletKit containing 5 % fetal bovine serum (Cambrex) in a humidified 5 % CO_2-95 % air atmosphere at 37 °C. All experiments were performed on cells between passages 2 and 4.

Application of uni-axial mechanical cyclic stretch

HBSMCs were seeded on 35-mm square silicon elastomer bottomed culture plates that had been coated with 1 µg/ml fibronectin (Wako, Osaka, Japan) dissolved in phosphate buffer saline (PBS). After achieving 90 % confluency, the cells were subjected to uni-axial cyclic stretch using a controlled motor unit; ST-140 (Strex, Kyoto, Japan). The intensity of stretch was 15 % elongation and the stretch cycle frequency was 1 Hz. These procedures were carried out in a humidified incubator with 5 % CO_2-95 % air at 37 °C.

Protein extraction and Western blotting

Stimulated HBSMCs were harvested with a cell scraper and were solubilized in a lysis buffer consisting of 20 mM Tris–HCl (pH 7.5), 1 % Nonidet P-40, 1 mM EDTA, 50 mM NaF, 50 mM sodium β-glycerophosphate, 0.05 mM Na_3VO_4, 10 µg/ml leupeptin, and 100 µM phenylmethylsulfonyl fluoride. Following centrifugation at 5000*g* for 5 min, the resultant supernatant was used as the lysate after protein concentration determination using the Bradford assay (Bio-Rad, Hercules, USA). The lysates were resolved in a 10 % SDS polyacrylamide gel and were electrotransferred to Hybond-P Polyvinylidene difluoride membrane (GE healthcare, Amersham Place, UK). Immunodetection of JNK1 and phosphorylated JNK1 was performed using anti-JNK1 (1:1000 dilution; Cell Signaling, Massachusetts, USA), and anti-phosphorylated JNK1 (Thr183/Tyr185) antibodies (1:1000; Cell Signaling), respectively. The signal was detected by incubation with an anti-rabbit secondary antibody conjugated to horseradish peroxidase (1:10,000; Promega, Tokyo, Japan), followed by chemiluminescence detection using the SuperSignal kit (Pierce Chemical Company, Rockford, USA) and Kodak BioMax light film (Kodak, Tokyo, Japan). The densities of the bands were quantified using the computer software, ImageJ (developed at the U.S. National Institutes of Health).

Labeling of actin stress fibers and nuclei

Following stretch stimulation, the cells were fixed in 3.7 % formaldehyde solution for 10 min and were permeabilized in a 0.1 % Triton X-100 solution for 5 min at room temperature. After incubation with PBS containing 1 % BSA for 30 min, the cells were stained with phallotoxin conjugated with Alexa-Fluor 594 (Molecular Probes, Eugene, USA) at 1:200 dilution for 20 min. Subsequently the cell nuclei were stained using 300 nM DAPI (Molecular Probes).

Measurement of actin stress fiber angles

Actin-stained cell images were captured and digitized using the Olympus IX71 fluorescence microscopy system (Olympus, Tokyo Japan). The angles of formed actin stress fibers were measured by using ImageJ. Stretch fibers that were perpendicular to the stretch direction were defined as having an angle of 0° and stress fibers that were parallel to the stretch direction were defined as having an angle of 90°.

Other chemicals

The *Clostridium botulinum* C3 exoenzyme and SP600125 were purchased from Sigma (Saint Louis, USA). Lipofectamine was from Invitrogen (Paisley, UK). Y-27632 was from Tocris Cookson Ltd (Bristol, UK).

Statistics

Statistical analysis between groups was performed using the Kruskal-Wallis test and Dunn's multiple comparison test for post-hoc comparison using the GraphPad Prism 6 software (GraphPad software, San Diego, USA). The null hypothesis was rejected at $p < 0.05$.

Results

The activation of JNK1 in HBSMCs exposed to uni-axial mechanical stretch

We first measured the activation of JNK1 following exposure of HBSMCs to 15 % elongation, 1 Hz cyclical uni-axial mechanical stretch over a period of 60 min. The activity of JNK1 was measured at each time point. The activity of JNK1 was enhanced from 5 min after stretching and peaked at 30 min, at which time a 4.7-fold increase in activation was detected (Fig. 1).

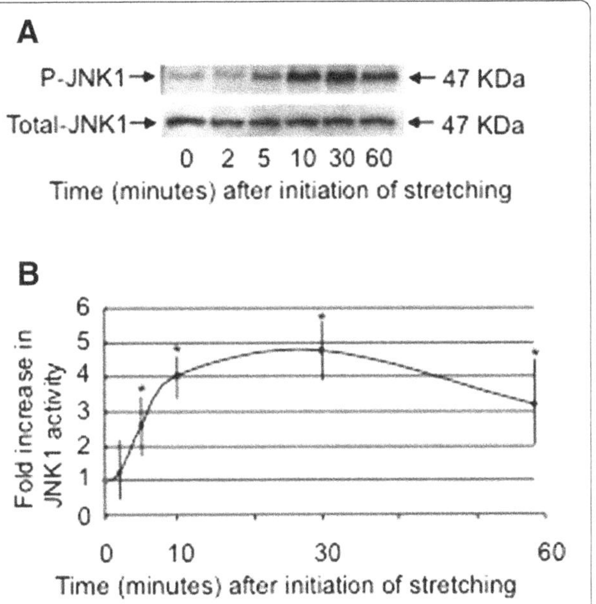

Fig. 1 Time-dependent JNK1 activation by uni-axial cyclic mechanical stretching of HBSMCs. **a** HBSMCs were exposed to uni-axial stretch (15 % elongation) for the indicated periods. The activity of JNK1 was measured by Western blotting using an anti-phosphorylated JNK1 (Thr183/Tyr185) antibody, which recognizes the active form of JNK1 (phosphorylated JNK1; P-JNK). The same filter was immunoblotted with each of the specific antibodies to demonstrate the total amount of JNK1 (Total-JNK1). **b** Quantification of the activity of JNK1 at each time point after stretch application. JNK1 activity was quantified using densitometry. The results are shown as means ± SEM ($n = 6$). The data are normalized by the total protein amount, and the intensity at 0 min was set at 1.0. An * indicates $p < 0.05$ compared to the value at time 0

Dependency of JNK1 activation on the RhoA/ROCK pathway

Based on this result, 15 % elongation and a 1 Hz cyclic stretch for 30 min were employed as the stretch conditions for analysis of the role of the RhoA/ROCK pathway in JNK1 activation by uni-axial stretch. We first analyzed the effect of inhibition of RhoA using the *botulinum* C3 exoenzyme, which is a RhoA inhibitor that specifically ADP-ribosylates RhoA at asparagine 41. As described in a previous paper [15], HBSMCs were pre-incubated with 10 μg/ml lipofectamine in order to increase the permeability of the cell membrane before C3 exoenzyme treatment. Pre-incubation of the HBSMCs with the C3 exoenzyme for 30 min before stretch inhibited JNK1 activation by uni-axial stretch in a C3 dose-dependent manner (Fig. 2a-upper blot). In a similar manner, uni-axial stretch-induced JNK1 activation was also suppressed by 30 min pre-incubation with the ROCK inhibitor, Y-27632, in a dose dependent manner (Fig. 2a-middle blot). The JNK specific inhibitor; SP600125 also inhibited JNK1 activation (Fig. 2a-lower blot). JNK1 activity was decreased to approximately 66.2, 55.9 and 39.0 % of that of the control activity by C3, Y-27632 and SP600125, respectively (Fig. 2b). As RhoA and ROCK inhibitors suppressed JNK1 phosphorylation, it is possible that RhoA/ROCK signaling may have some effect on JNK1 activation evoked by uni-axial stretch.

Actin stress fiber reorganization by uni-axial stretch

We next determined the effect of exposure of HBSMCs to uni-axial stretch with 15 % elongation on the organization of actin stress fibers by staining of cellular actin with phalloidin. Compared with non-stretched cells, cells that had been stretched for 4 h showed stronger staining of actin stress fibers. The fibers had also re-orientated so as to be more perpendicular to the stretch direction. Typical pictures of phalloidin stained cells that were not exposed, or were exposed to uni-axial stretch are shown in Fig. 3a (*a* and *b*, respectively). The angle of the stress fibers in relation to the direction of stretch was measured. For this measurement, stress fibers that were perpendicular to the direction of the stretch were defined as having an angle of 0° and fibers that were parallel to the stress fibers were defined as having an angle of 90°. The measurement of these angles is shown in Fig. 3a*c*. The angle of the actin fibers in each cell was determined by taking the average value of 5 distinct fibers, and 50 cells were counted for each time point (Fig. 3b). The graph of these values indicated that the actin

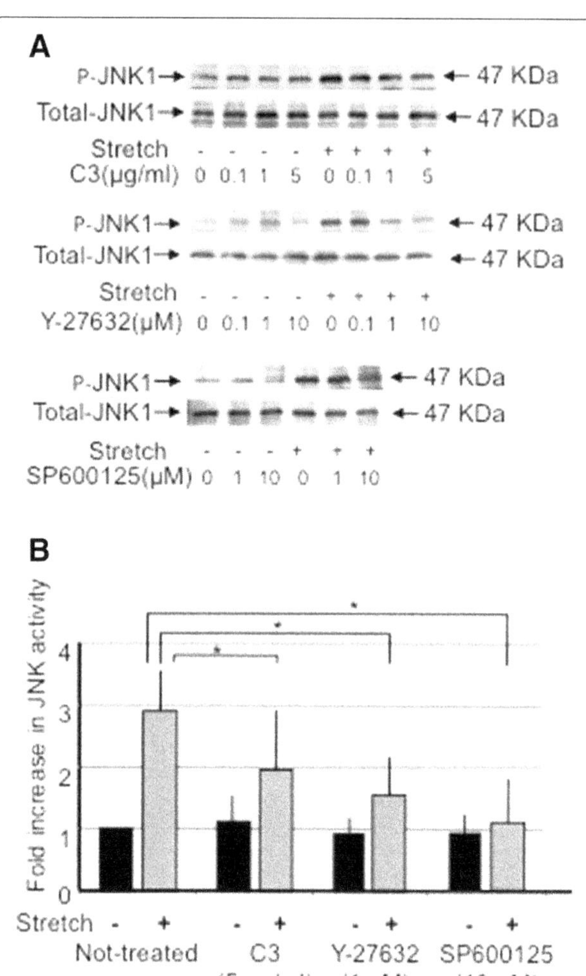

Fig. 2 The effect of signaling inhibitors on stretch-induced JNK1 activation. **a** HBSMCs were pre-incubated with 10 μg/ml lipofectamine and the RhoA inhibitor C3 exoenzyme (upper blots), the Rho kinase inhibitor Y-27632 (middle blots), or the JNK1 inhibitor SP600125 (bottom blots) at the indicated concentrations and the cells were then subjected (+), or not (–), to uni-axial stretch with 15 % elongation for 30 min. The activity of JNK1 was measured in the same manner as in Fig. 1. **b** Quantification of the effect of the inhibitors on JNK1 activation. Stretch induced JNK1 activity was quantified by densitometry. JNK1 activity under the conditions of pre-incubation with 5 μg/ml C3 exoenzyme, 1 μM Y-27632 or 10 μM SP600125 are indicated in the figure. Data were normalized by the total amount of JNK1 protein and the intensity of non-stretched, non-treated cells was defined as 1.0. Data are indicated as means ± SEM ($n = 6$). An * indicates $p < 0.05$

stress fibers in the cells moved in a direction that was perpendicular to the direction of stretch. The average angle of the actin stress fiber direction after 4 h of stretch was statistically different compared with that of non-stretched cells (41.9° [19.5, 71.6] before stretch vs. 21.7° [14.3, 43.8] [16] after 4 h of stretch. Median and interquartile values respectively are indicated in square brackets.).

Inhibitor effects on stress fiber reorganization

The effect of RhoA/ROCK pathway signaling on actin stress fiber reorganization was then investigated using the same concentration of inhibitors as those used for analysis of JNK activation above. HBSMCs were thus pre-incubated with 5 μg/ml of the C3 exoenzyme together with 10 μg/ml lipofectamine, with 1 μM Y-27632 or with 10 μM SP600125, and were then subjected to uni-axial stretch with 15 % elongation for 4 h. Actin stress fibers were then stained with phalloidin. Typical pictures of the phalloidin-stained cells are shown in Fig. 4a*a-e*. The angle of the stress fibers relative to the stretch direction was then measured and a summary graph of the effects of the inhibitors is presented in Fig. 4b. Actin stress fiber reorganization was suppressed by the C3 exoenzyme (Fig. 4a*c*) and by Y-27632 (Fig. 4a*d*) but not by the JNK1 specific inhibitor SP600125 (Fig. 4a*e*.) These results indicated that the RhoA/ROCK pathway may play a significant role in actin stress fiber reorganization, although JNK1 activation had no effect on actin stress fiber reorganization induced by uni-axial stretch.

Discussion

Mechanical overload is possibly involved in remodeling of the bladder wall, and such mechanical stress may cause morphological changes in HBSMCs. To understand the intracellular events caused by mechanical stretch, we focused on the RhoA/ROCK signaling pathway. The results demonstrated the following: 1) Uni-axial stretch activated JNK1 in HBSMCs. 2) Uni-axial stretch strongly evoked the reorganization of actin stress fibers and coordinated their orientation so that they became more perpendicular to the stretch direction. 3) The inhibitor experiments showed that the RhoA/ROCK pathway had pivotal roles in transduction of the intracellular signals induced by mechanical stretch. The stretch parameters used in this experiment were chosen to better emphasize the reaction of actin stress fiber reorganization. It should be noted that the stretch cycle used differs from the physiological condition and further assessment is needed to reflect the actual in vivo status.

RhoA mediates various extracellular signals that are induced by stimulation with agonists such as noradrenaline [17] and acetylcholine [16] in smooth muscle. RhoA was also shown to play significant roles in the signal transduction induced by mechanical stretch in endothelial cells [18] and cardiac myocytes [19]. Similarly, our data showed that RhoA appeared to have critical roles in the signaling induced by mechanical stretch in HBSMCs. However, the molecules that lead to RhoA activation by mechanical stimuli remain unclear. It is possible that scaffold proteins such as integrins or mechanosensitive ion channels [9, 20] may participate in

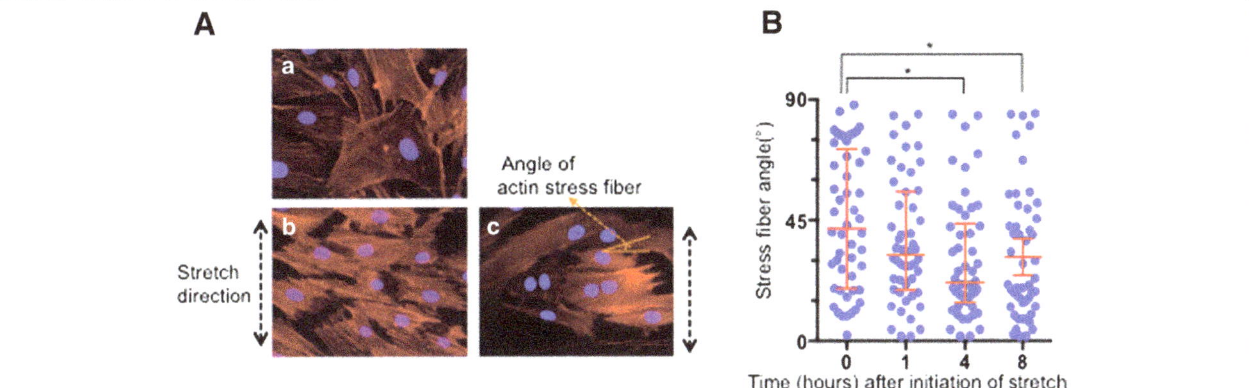

Fig. 3 Actin stress fiber re-organization induced by mechanical stretch. **a** HBSMCs were exposed to uni-axial stretch (15 % elongation) for 1, 4 or 8 h and cellular actin was then stained with phalloidin conjugated with Alexa-Fluor 594 at 1:200 dilution (red). Nuclei were dyed blue using 300 nM DAPI. Representative staining of cells (*a*) before stretch and (*b, c*) after stretching for 4 h. (*c*) The scheme of the measurement of stretch fiber angles; Actin fibers at right angles to the stretch direction were defined as having an angle of 0° and those parallel with the stretch direction were defined as having an angle of 90°. The scale bar in pictures indicates 20 μm. **b** Quantification of the angles of actin stress fibers at each time point. The direction of the actin stress fibers in each cell was determined by averaging the angles of 5 obvious fibers within a cell ($n = 50$ cells per time point). Data are expressed as the median ± interquartile. An * indicates $p < 0.05$

the activation of RhoA by sensing physical stimuli via the extracellular matrix. However, further experiments are required to clarify this mechanism.

Our results suggested the existence of signal cross-linkage between RhoA/ROCK and JNK pathways in HBSMCs. Previous papers have also reported that RhoA induces JNK activation in cardiac myocytes by mechanical stretching [15]. Furthermore, stimulation of NIH 3T3 cells with an agonist such as lysophosphatidic acid (LPA) [21] or of vascular smooth muscle cells with Angiotensin II [22] causes signaling cross-talk between the ROCK pathway and JNK. There was no clear indication as to which molecules in JNK cascades are stimulated by mechanical stretch activation of RhoA/ROCK. However, some previous reports showed that ROCK activation by LPA in NIH3T3 cells induced activation of mitogen-activated protein kinase kinase 4 (MKK4), which is an upstream kinase of JNK and leads to the

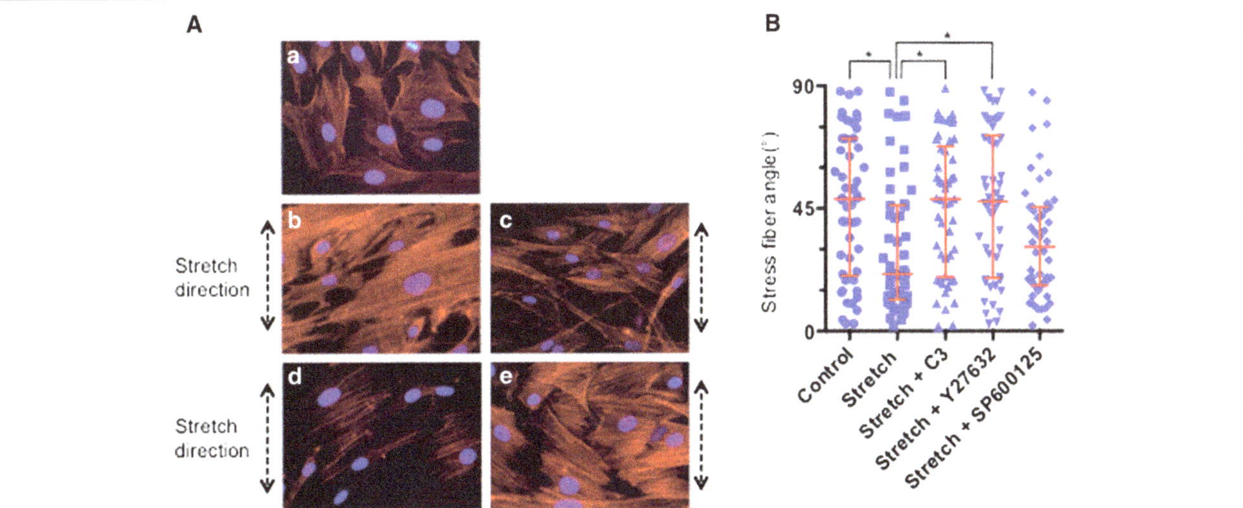

Fig. 4 The effect of signal inhibitors on stress fiber re-organization. **a** HBSMCs were not treated with inhibitor and (*a*) not-stretched or (*b*) stretched for 4 h, or were pre-incubated with 10 μM lipofectamine and 5 μg/ml of the C3 exoenzyme (*c*), 1 μM of Y-27632 (*d*) or 10 μM SP600125 (*e*) for 30 min followed by uni-axial stretching of the cells with 15 % elongation for 4 h. Actin stress fibers and nuclei were then stained and actin stress fiber angles relative to the direction of stretching were determined as in Fig. 3. The scale bar in pictures indicates 20 μm. **b** Quantification of the effect of the inhibitors on stress fiber reorganization induced by uni-axial stretch. The angles of an average of 5 actin stress fibers in a cell were counted ($n = 50$ cells for each condition). Data are expressed as the median ± interquartile. The effects of inhibitors were compared with cells not treated with inhibitors. An * indicates $p < 0.05$

phosphorylation of JNK [21]. In addition, ROCK activation by activin in keratinocytes induced activation of mitogen-activated protein kinase kinase kinase 1 (MEKK1), which is an upstream kinase of MKK4, and subsequently leads to JNK activation [23]. The activation of JNK by mechanical stretch was previously shown to promote the expression of immediate early genes in vascular smooth muscle cells [6] and cardiomyocytes [7]. Although our data indicated that the JNK inhibitor SP600125 inhibited JNK activation by mechanical stretch, it should be noted that a recent paper suggested a limitation to the specificity of SP600125 and suggested the possibility that SP600125 might also inhibit other kinases (e.g., phosphatidylinositol 3-kinase) [24].

Actin stress fibers are composed of from 20 to 30 parallel actin filaments that are bundled by a bridge protein, α-actinin [10]. Actin filaments are temporally connected to bundles of polymerized type II myosin and generate tension by utilizing the actomyosin bond. The ends of actin stress fibers connect to focal adhesions where cell membranes attach to the extra-cellular matrix [10]. Under static conditions, actin stress fibers generate an isometric contraction in order to maintain a constant length with scaffolding at both ends. Cells are thought to sense extracellular physical signals using this isometric contraction.

In the stretch experiments of the present study, actin stress fibers were reorganized by mechanical stretch, such that stronger actin stress fibers were formed as a result of the stretch stimuli and the stress fibers were organized so that their orientation came close to being perpendicular to the stretch direction. It is unclear whether actin stress fiber angle change induces alteration of cell contractility in BSMCs. Moreover, there is little evidence that actin fiber orientation change enhances smooth muscle contractility in other types of muscle cells. Many of the cells formed projections such as filopodia in the lateral side of their cell membrane, where actin stress fibers are bound. Reorganized fibers may cause isometric tension in order to maintain the cell area. These morphological changes appear to be an adaptation response for the conservation of intracellular configurations because the formation of actin stress fibers perpendicular to the direction of stretch may restrict the movement of cell organelles. In addition, the shape of some cells was also elongated perpendicular to the direction of stretch. We also conjecture that cells may try to change their polarity by using actin stress fibers as a frame in order to reduce mechanical stress. However, there was no significant difference in the overall horizontal-vertical ratio of the cell length of stretched cells vs. unstretched cells due to their wide variety of cell shapes. The morphological changes of the stress fibers may be induced via the RhoA/ROCK pathway because the C3 exoenzyme and Y-27632 inhibited their reorganization. ROCK has been reported to participate in the induction of prominent actin stress fiber formation [11]. One of the mechanisms underlying the induction of stress fiber formation by ROCK is the phosphorylation of LIM-kinase, which is an effector of cofilin. It is considered that phosphorylated cofilin is subsequently rendered inactive and that thereby actin polymerization is ultimately stabilized [25]. Moreover, Na^+/H^+ exchanger 1, which is another substrate of ROCK, is activated by ROCK and subsequently induces the connection between actin filaments and cell surface proteins [26, 27]. Furthermore, mDia, which is an effector of RhoA, is reported to induce actin stress fiber reorganization together with ROCK [28]. It is reported that stress fiber orientation change due to mechanical stretch needs mDia activation in endothelial cells [18]. ROCK has also been reported to induce actinomyosin contraction via phosphorylation of at least four substrates including myosin light chain, all of which lead to increased myosin phosphorylation and increased actomyosin contractility [10].

Our results indicated that the JNK inhibitor SP600125 did not suppress actin stress fiber reorganization, therefore the JNK pathway may not participate in this reorganization. An interesting finding was reported by Kaunas et al. that a 90° change in the direction of stretch caused re-activation of JNK, when JNK activity had disappeared after the initial stretch. In addition, JNK activity was prolonged by cytochalasin D which also suppresses actin stress fiber reorganization [29]. Hence, actin cytoskeleton contraction appears to act as some sort of trigger for JNK activation. Their concept was that deformation of the actin cytoskeleton could induce biochemical signals since the stretch-induced JNK activation subsides if stress fibers are able to organize in a configuration that minimizes the perturbation by stretch.

Since the bladder wall may be subject to mechanical stress in bladder outlet obstructive disease such as benign prostatic hyperplasia, it is important to understand how cells transduce mechanical signals and adapt themselves to them. In *our in vitro* research study, activation of RhoA/ROCK pathways by mechanical stretch induced both structural and biochemical adaptations. It is possible that the consequence of actin fibers reorganization is to lead to the preservation of the cell environment by reducing mechanical stress. Since the roles of actin stress fibers in the bladder wall in vivo have been unclear to date, further investigation is required to better understand their roles.

Conclusions

Bladder smooth muscle cells appear to have elaborate mechanisms for sensing mechanical stress and for adapting to mechanical stress overload by cytoskeletal remodeling and by activating cell growth signals such as JNK via RhoA/ROCK pathways.

Abbreviations

HBSMCs: human bladder smooth muscle cells; JNK: c-Jun NH_2 terminal kinase; LPA: lysophosphatidic acid; MAPK: mitogen activated protein kinase; MEKK1: mitogen-activated protein kinase kinase kinase 1; MKK4: mitogen-activated protein kinase kinase 4; PBS: phosphate buffer saline; ROCK: Rho-associated coiled-coil forming protein kinase.

Competing interests

The authors declare that they have no competing interests.

Authors' contributions

NK participated in the design of the study and performed the analysis, and drafted the manuscript. OY conceived of the study. YKA performed cell culture. HA and JH performed statistical analysis. KI carried out the immunohistochemical study. KA helped to draft the manuscript. YKO supervised the study design. All authors read and approved the final manuscript.

Acknowledgement

We thank Mr Jun Furasha, who kindly provided language revision.

Author details

[1]Department of Urology, Fukushima Medical University School of Medicine, 1, Hikarigaoka, Fukushima 960-1295, Japan. [2]Division of Bioengineering and LUTD Research, Nihon University School of Engineering, Nihon University, 1, Nakagawara, Tokusada, Tamura, Koriyama 963-8642, Japan.

References

1. Gilpin SA, Gosling JA, Barnard RJ. Morphological and morphometric studies of the human obstructed, trabeculated urinary bladder. Br J Urol. 1985;57(5):525–9.
2. Kim KM, Kogan BA, Massad CA, Huang YC. Collagen and elastin in the obstructed fetal bladder. J Urol. 1991;146(2 (Pt 2)):528–31.
3. Lindner P, Mattiasson A, Persson L, Uvelius B. Reversibility of detrusor hypertrophy and hyperplasia after removal of infravesical outflow obstruction in the rat. J Urol. 1988;140(3):642–6.
4. Park JM, Borer JG, Freeman MR, Peters CA. Stretch activates heparin-binding EGF-like growth factor expression in bladder smooth muscle cells. Am J Physiol. 1998;275(5 Pt 1):C1247–54.
5. Park JM, Adam RM, Peters CA, Guthrie PD, Sun Z, Klagsbrun M, et al. AP-1 mediates stretch-induced expression of HB-EGF in bladder smooth muscle cells. Am J Physiol. 1999;277(2 Pt 1):C294–301.
6. Hamada K, Takuwa N, Yokoyama K, Takuwa Y. Stretch activates Jun N-terminal kinase/stress-activated protein kinase in vascular smooth muscle cells through mechanisms involving autocrine ATP stimulation of purinoceptors. J Biol Chem. 1998;273(11):6334–40.
7. Komuro I, Kudo S, Yamazaki T, Zou Y, Shiojima I, Yazaki Y. Mechanical stretch activates the stress-activated protein kinases in cardiac myocytes. FASEB J. 1996;10(5):631–6.
8. Nguyen HT, Adam RM, Bride SH, Park JM, Peters CA, Freeman MR. Cyclic stretch activates p38 SAPK2-, ErbB2-, and AT1-dependent signaling in bladder smooth muscle cells. Am J Physiol Cell Physiol. 2000;279(4):C1155–67.
9. Kushida N, Kabuyama Y, Yamaguchi O, Homma Y. Essential role for extracellular Ca(2+) in JNK activation by mechanical stretch in bladder smooth muscle cells. Am J Physiol Cell Physiol. 2001;281(4):C1165–72.
10. Pellegrin S, Mellor H. Actin stress fibres. J Cell Sci. 2007;120(Pt 20):3491–9.
11. Fukata Y, Amano M, Kaibuchi K. Rho-Rho-kinase pathway in smooth muscle contraction and cytoskeletal reorganization of non-muscle cells. Trends Pharmacol Sci. 2001;22(1):32–9.
12. Boopathi E, Gomes C, Zderic SA, Malkowicz B, Chakrabarti R, Patel DP, et al. Mechanical stretch upregulates proteins involved in Ca2+ sensitization in urinary bladder smooth muscle hypertrophy. Am J Physiol Cell Physiol. 2014;307(6):C542–53.
13. Takahashi N, Shiomi H, Kushida N, Liu F, Ishibashi K, Yanagida T, et al. Obstruction alters muscarinic receptor-coupled RhoA/Rho-kinase pathway in the urinary bladder of the rat. Neurourol Urodyn. 2009;28(3):257–62.
14. Poley RN, Dosier CR, Speich JE, Miner AS, Ratz PH. Stimulated calcium entry and constitutive RhoA kinase activity cause stretch-induced detrusor contraction. Eur J Pharmacol. 2008;599(1–3):137–45.
15. Pan J, Singh US, Takahashi T, Oka Y, Palm-Leis A, Herbelin BS, et al. PKC mediates cyclic stretch-induced cardiac hypertrophy through Rho family GTPases and mitogen-activated protein kinases in cardiomyocytes. J Cell Physiol. 2005;202(2):536–53.
16. Patil SB, Bitar KN. RhoA- and PKC-alpha-mediated phosphorylation of MYPT and its association with HSP27 in colonic smooth muscle cells. Am J Physiol Gastrointest Liver Physiol. 2006;290(1):G83–95.
17. Sakurada S, Okamoto H, Takuwa N, Sugimoto N, Takuwa Y. Rho activation in excitatory agonist-stimulated vascular smooth muscle. Am J Physiol Cell Physiol. 2001;281(2):C571–8.
18. Kaunas R, Nguyen P, Usami S, Chien S. Cooperative effects of Rho and mechanical stretch on stress fiber organization. Proc Natl Acad Sci U S A. 2005;102(44):15895–900.
19. Torsoni AS, Marin TM, Velloso LA, Franchini KG. RhoA/ROCK signaling is critical to FAK activation by cyclic stretch in cardiac myocytes. Am J Physiol Heart Circ Physiol. 2005;289(4):H1488–96.
20. Naruse K, Yamada T, Sai XR, Hamaguchi M, Sokabe M. Pp125FAK is required for stretch dependent morphological response of endothelial cells. Oncogene. 1998;17(4):455–63.
21. Marinissen MJ, Chiariello M, Tanos T, Bernard O, Narumiya S, Gutkind JS. The small GTP-binding protein RhoA regulates c-jun by a ROCK-JNK signaling axis. Mol Cell. 2004;14(1):29–41.
22. Ohtsu H, Mifune M, Frank GD, Saito S, Inagami T, Kim-Mitsuyama S, et al. Signal-crosstalk between Rho/ROCK and c-Jun NH2-terminal kinase mediates migration of vascular smooth muscle cells stimulated by angiotensin II. Arterioscler Thromb Vasc Biol. 2005;25(9):1831–6.
23. Zhang L, Deng M, Parthasarathy R, Wang L, Mongan M, Molkentin JD, et al. MEKK1 transduces activin signals in keratinocytes to induce actin stress fiber formation and migration. Mol Cell Biol. 2005;25(1):60–5.
24. Tanemura S, Yamasaki T, Katada T, Nishina H. Limitations of SP600125, an Inhibitor of Stress-Responsive c-Jun N-Terminal Kinase. Curr Enzym Inhib. 2010;6(1):26–33.
25. Maekawa M, Ishizaki T, Boku S, Watanabe N, Fujita A, Iwamatsu A, et al. Signaling from Rho to the actin cytoskeleton through protein kinases ROCK and LIM-kinase. Science. 1999;285(5429):895–8.
26. Tominaga T, Ishizaki T, Narumiya S, Barber DL. p160ROCK mediates RhoA activation of Na-H exchange. EMBO J. 1998;17(16):4712–22.
27. Denker SP, Huang DC, Orlowski J, Furthmayr H, Barber DL. Direct binding of the Na–H exchanger NHE1 to ERM proteins regulates the cortical cytoskeleton and cell shape independently of H(+) translocation. Mol Cell. 2000;6(6):1425–36.
28. Watanabe N, Kato T, Fujita A, Ishizaki T, Narumiya S. Cooperation between mDia1 and ROCK in Rho-induced actin reorganization. Nat Cell Biol. 1999;1(3):136–43.
29. Kaunas R, Usami S, Chien S. Regulation of stretch-induced JNK activation by stress fiber orientation. Cell Signal. 2006;18(11):1924–31.

Preoperative neutrophil to lymphocyte ratio improves recurrence prediction of non-muscle invasive bladder cancer

Itamar Getzler[1*†], Zaher Bahouth[1†], Ofer Nativ[1], Jacob Rubinstein[2] and Sarel Halachmi[1]

Abstract

Background: This study aims to prospectively evaluate the ability of Neutrophil-to-Lymphocyte ratio (NLR) to forecast recurrence in patients with non-muscle invasive bladder cancer (NMIBC). This is a continuation of our two previous retrospective studies that indicated the NLR > 2.5 criterion as a predictor of recurrence in patients with NMIBC.

Methods: Since December 2013, all patients admitted to our department for TUR-BT and agreed to participate, had a blood drawn for cell count and differential 24 h prior to surgery. Patients with pathological NMIBC were followed prospectively for disease recurrence. The end-point of the follow up was either a cancer recurrence or the termination of the study. Univariate and multivariate Cox regressions were performed to assess the NLR > 2.5 predictive capability for recurrence, versus and in conjunction to the pathologically based EORTC score, among additional statistical analyses.

Results: The study cohort included 96 men and 17 women with a median age of 72 years. Sixty-four patients (56.6%) have had a recurrence during the study occurring at the median time of 9 months (IQR 6, 13), while the median follow-up time for patients without recurrence was 18 months (IQR 10, 29). Univariate Cox regressions for recurrence demonstrated significance for NLR > 2.5 for the whole cohort ($p = 0.011$, HR 2.015, CI 1.175–3.454) and for the BCG sub-group ($p = 0.023$, HR 3.7, CI 1.2–11.9), while the EORTC score demonstrated significance for the 'No Treatment' subgroup ($p = 0.024$, HR 1.278, CI 1.03–1.58). When analyzed together as a multivariate Cox model, the NLR > 2.5 and EORTC score retained their significance for the aforementioned groups, while also improving the EORTC score significance for the whole cohort.

Conclusion: NLR > 2.5 was found to be a significant predictor of disease recurrence and demonstrated high hazard ratio and worse recurrence-free survival in patients with NMIBC, especially in those treated with BCG. Additionally, our data demonstrated statistical evidence that NLR > 2.5 might have an improving effect on the EORTC score's prediction when analyzed together.

Keywords: Neutrophil-lymphocyte ratio, NLR, NMIBC, urothelial carcinoma, Recurrence, Bladder cancer

Background

Bladder cancer is the most common malignancy of the urinary tract, and the 4th most common cancer in males in developed countries [1]. Upon diagnosis, the majority (~ 75%) of patients with bladder cancer present with non-muscle invasive disease (NMIBC), which by definition includes the Tis, Ta and T1 pathologic stages [2]. As such, NMIBC represents a heterogeneous group of tumors with different rates of recurrence, progression and disease-related mortality. Consequently, each subgroup of NMIBC should be followed up and treated differently [3]. The main concern during treatment of NMIBC is progression to a muscle invasive stage (T2), which dramatically worsens prognosis [4]. To prevent this scenario, clinical and pathological factors are commonly used to categorize patients into different risk groups. These methods, such as the EORTC (European Organization for Research and Treatment of Cancer)

* Correspondence: itamargetzler@gmail.com
†Itamar Getzler and Zaher Bahouth contributed equally to this work.
[1]Department of Urology, Bnai Zion Medical Center, Faculty of Medicine, Technion - Israel Institute of Technology, Golomb 47, 31048 Haifa, Israel
Full list of author information is available at the end of the article

Risk Tables, help physicians predict the probability of progression and recurrence, and ultimately – help decide the most appropriate treatment [3, 5].

However, these grouping systems are far from optimal: would a probability of recurrence of 35% per year justify an aggressive treatment? Is a 15% chance of progression per 1 year a sufficient reason to perform a cystectomy? [5]. Thus, we still lack a strong prognostic factor that could help predict patient-specific risk rather than group-specific risk of recurrence and progression.

According to recent studies cited below, the systemic inflammatory response state triggered by the tumor microenvironment alters acute phase reactants and hematologic components - including changes in serum neutrophil and lymphocyte counts that leads to relative neutrophilia and lymphocytopenia. This state of elevated Neutrophil-Lymphocyte ratio (NLR) is associated with worse disease-free and overall survival in a variety of different malignancies [6–8].

Among patients with bladder cancer, an elevated NLR was associated with advanced stage, increased mortality, and decreased overall survival in patients with muscle-invasive disease [9–11], along with higher risk of recurrence and progression in non-muscle invasive disease [12, 13]. Specifically, in both our retrospective studies which employed different methods of analysis, NLR > 2.5 was found to be a significant predictor of recurrence [12, 13]. Following these results, and in addition to the fact that prospective data regarding the role of NLR in predicting disease recurrence and progression in NMIBC have never been published, the aim of the current study was to prospectively evaluate the role of NLR > 2.5 as a predictor of disease recurrence in patients with primary NMIBC.

Methods

Study design & procedures

This was a single center, prospective cohort study. Recruited patients were pathologically confirmed to have non-invasive BC stages – Ta, T1 and Tis, after undergoing trans-urethral resection of bladder tumor (TUR-BT). Tumors were graded and staged according to the 2004 WHO grading system [14]. Pre-operative NLR was recorded using the admission's (usually 24 h prior to surgery) complete blood count (CBC) with differential. Follow up invitations were sent out every 3 months for urine cytology, upper tract imaging, cystoscopy and treatment based on the American Urological Association (AUA) guidelines [15]. We point out that given the nature of a prospective study design, an intervention that might affect the variables is not desirable, and hence the treatment was chosen according to best practice guidelines and not according to our assumption that NLR may play a role. The end-point of the follow up was either a cancer recurrence or the termination of the study. Some degree of non-compliance to the follow up and treatment was expected, and so the last date of follow-up was recorded for missing and deceased patients. This study was based on the principles of Helsinki and was approved by the institutional review board.

Objectives

A primary objective of the study was to evaluate the effect of NLR > 2.5 on NMIBC recurrence after trans-urethral resection of bladder tumor (TUR-BT). This effect on recurrence was to be evaluated against the current standard means to predict recurrence, which is the EORTC's prediction table. Secondary objectives were to evaluate the effect of NLR > 2.5 on recurrence, when stratified by different variables including the pathologic grade, stage and the intra-vesical treatment. These objectives were set in advance, and were meant to test the hypothesis that a prediction of recurrence by NLR > 2.5 can be produced prospectively, and not only retrospectively [12, 13].

Participants

Eligible Patients were ≥ 18 years with pathologically confirmed NMIBC who underwent trans-urethral resection of bladder tumor (TUR-BT) since December 2013. An Inclusive approach was taken in order to examine broad and general effect of NLR, not only on some naïve or carefully chosen groups. Key exclusion criteria were: T2 Stage, hematologic malignancies, acute infections, and patients without preoperative NLR. All pathological grades were included.

Statistical analysis

Clinical features between groups were evaluated using Student *t*-test or chi-square test. Recurrence-free survival was evaluated using Kaplan-Meier survival plots and Log Rank was used to compare between groups. Univariate and multivariate Cox regressions were performed to assess the NLR2.5 predictive capability for recurrence, versus and in conjunction to the EORTC score. The analysis was first performed for the whole cohort, and next stratified by the 'Treatment Type' Groups: 'No Treatment', 'Mitomycin C (MMC)' or 'Bacillus Calmette–Guérin (BCG)', as the treatment choice should affect the recurrence in a meaningful way.

The EORTC Score was calculated in accordance to Sylvester et al. [5]. The tumors' pathological variables are inherently included in the EORTC score, in a way that is already established to be statistically significant. As such, further statistical analysis of the pathological variables is redundant. The results are presented as hazard ratios along with their 95% confidence intervals. A 2-sided P value of < 0.05 was considered statistically significant. Data was analyzed using IBM SPSS v23.0.

Results

Between December 2013 and October 2016, 113 patients were recruited to the study. The cohort included 96 men and 17 women with a median age of 72 years (IQR 63, 81) with a confirmed pathological diagnosis of NMIBC. Sixty-four patients (56.6%) have had a recurrence during the study, occurring at the median time of 9 months (IQR 6, 13), while the median follow-up time for patients without recurrence was 18 months (IQR 14, 30). The median NLR was 2.69 (IQR 1.9, 4.35) including 69 patients (58%) who have had NLR > 2.5. Table 1 shows an analysis of differences in clinical features between groups divided by recurrence. Table 2 shows an analysis of differences in clinical features between groups divided by NLR-2.5.

Similar to our retrospective study, NLR (> 2.5) was correlated significantly with recurrence ($p = 0.003$) but also with age (68 vs 78 years, $P = 0.0001$) and stage ($p = 0.01$). The significant p-value correlation with CIS is irrelevant as only 3 patients had CIS.

Whole cohort Kaplan-Meier survival plot factored by NLR2.5 was then performed and showed a significant difference ($p = 0.007$) in mean recurrence-free survival - (18.6 months vs 26.7 months, Fig. 1). Mean recurrence-free survival of NLR > 2.5 stratified by stage, grade and treatment type (sub-group analysis), showed statistical significance for the Ta Stage ($p = 0.022$, 18.7 vs 27 months), G1 Grade ($p = 0.031$, 17.1 vs 23 months) and the BCG sub-group ($p = 0.013$, 21.3 vs 34.1 months) of 37 patients, Figs. 2, 3 and 4. Sub-group breakdown (i.e Ta stage and T1 stage) is presented as lettered graphs ("A", "B" etc) under each figure. A persistent trend albeit without statistical significance was seen for the other stratifications (T1 Stage, G3 Grade and the other treatment types) in that the NLR > 2.5 groups always fared worse than the NLR < 2.5 groups.

In the univariate, whole cohort NLR2.5 Cox regression for recurrence, NLR2.5 was found significant ($p = 0.01$) with Hazard ratio of 2.029 (CI 1.185–3.472), indicating

Table 1 Patient and tumor characteristics of the study cohort stratified by recurrence

		Patient Groups						*P*-Value
		No Recurrence			Recurrence			
		Count	Row *N* %	Median (IQR)	Count	Row N %	Median (IQR)	
Age		49	43.4%	70 (62, 78)	64	56.6%	75 (65, 83)	0.290
Sex	Female	6	35.3%		11	64.7%		0.466
	Male	43	44.8%		53	55.2%		
Grade	1	35	45.5%		42	54.5%		0.765
	2	1	50.0%		1	50.0%		
	3	13	38.2%		21	61.8%		
Stage	Ta	38	46.3%		44	53.7%		0.299
	T1	11	35.5%		20	64.5%		
CIS	No	47	42.7%		63	57.3%		0.409
	Yes	2	66.7%		1	33.3%		
Number Of Tumors	Single Tumor	14	40.0%		21	60.0%		0.885
	2–7 Tumors	29	44.6%		36	55.4%		
	8 or More	6	46.2%		7	53.8%		
Tumor Diameter	< 30 mm	36	47.4%		40	52.6%		0.218
	30 mm or more	13	35.1%		24	64.9%		
Past TCC	No	33	41.3%		47	58.8%		0.480
	Yes	16	48.5%		17	51.5%		
WBC		49	43.4%	7.9 (7.05, 9.66)	64	56.6%	7.71 (6.17, 10)	0.373
NLR		49	43.4%	2.35 (1.7, 3.43)	64	56.6%	2.87 (2.29, 4.65)	0.287
NLR-2.5	Below 2.5	28	59.6%		19	40.4%		0.004
	Above 2.5	21	31.8%		45	68.2%		
Treatment Type	No Treatment	15	34.1%		29	65.9%		0.053
	MMC	12	37.5%		20	62.5%		
	BCG	22	59.5%		15	40.5%		

Table 2 Patient and tumor characteristics of the study cohort stratified by neutrophil-to-lymphocyte ratio (NLR)

		Patient Groups						*P*-Value
		Below 2.5			Above 2.5			
		Count	Row *N* %	Median (IQR)	Count	Row *N* %	Median (IQR)	
Age		47	41.6%	69 (59, 75)	66	58.4%	77 (70, 83)	
Status	No Recurrence	28	57.1%		21	42.9%		0.003
	Recurrence	19	29.7%		45	70.3%		
Sex	Female	6	35.3%		11	64.7%		0.568
	Male	41	42.7%		55	57.3%		
Grade	1	35	45.5%		42	54.5%		0.293
	2	0	0.0%		2	100.0%		
	3	12	35.3%		22	64.7%		
Stage	Ta	40	48.8%		42	51.2%		0.012
	T1	7	22.6%		24	77.4%		
CIS	No	44	40.0%		66	60.0%		0.037
	Yes	3	100.0%		0	0.0%		
Number Of Tumors	Single Tumor	14	40.0%		21	60.0%		0.635
	2–7 Tumors	26	40.0%		39	60.0%		
	8 or More	7	53.8%		6	46.2%		
Tumor Diameter	< 30 mm	30	39.5%		46	60.5%		0.512
	30 mm or mo re	17	45.9%		20	54.1%		
Past TCC	No	32	40.0%		48	60.0%		0.593
	Yes	15	45.5%		18	54.5%		
WBC		47	41.6%	7.58 (6.17, 8.6)	66	58.4%	8.91 (7.05, 10.5)	0.007
Treatment Type	No Treatment	17	38.6%		27	61.4%		0.317
	MMC	11	34.4%		21	65.6%		
	BCG	19	51.4%		18	48.6%		

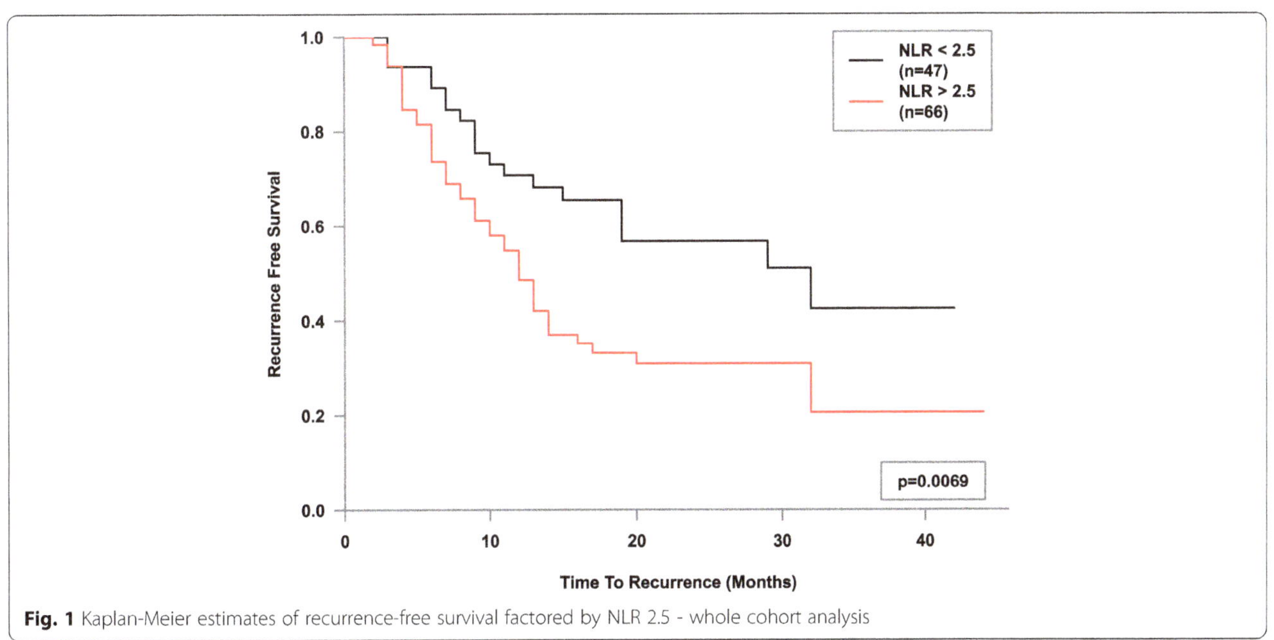

Fig. 1 Kaplan-Meier estimates of recurrence-free survival factored by NLR 2.5 - whole cohort analysis

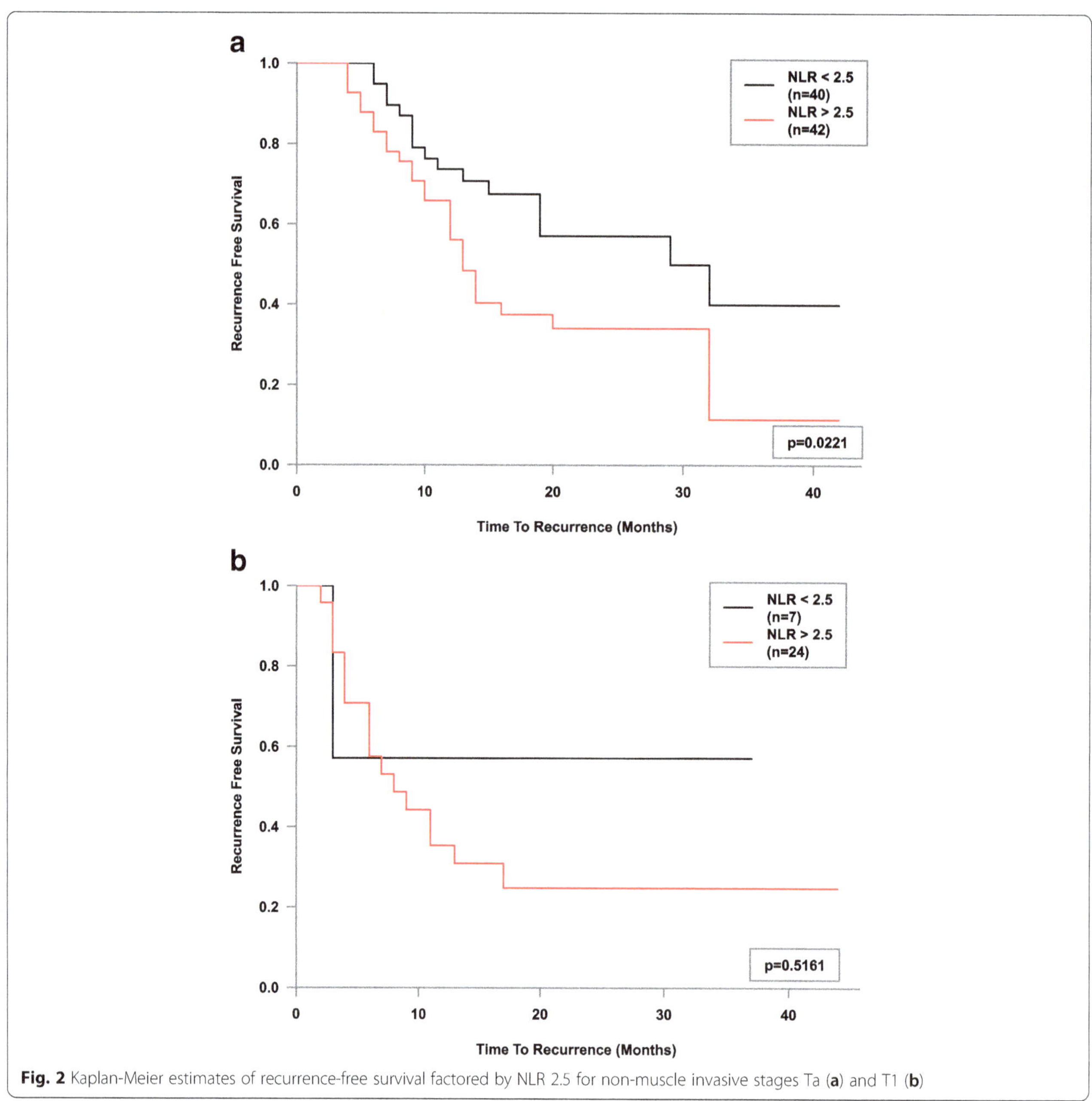

Fig. 2 Kaplan-Meier estimates of recurrence-free survival factored by NLR 2.5 for non-muscle invasive stages Ta (**a**) and T1 (**b**)

that the probability of recurrence is increased at least 2-fold for a person with NLR > 2.5 compared with NLR < 2.5 in this whole cohort analysis. After stratification by Treatment Type, NLR2.5 was only found significant for the 'BCG' subgroup ($p = 0.023$) with Hazard Ratio of 3.792 (CI 1.2–11.9) and not for the 'No Treatment' and 'MMC' subgroups ($p = 0.123$ and $p = 0.96$ respectively). (Table 3).

An identical Cox analysis was then done for the EORTC Score, which resulted in a significance only for the 'No Treatment' subgroup ($p = 0.024$) with Hazard ratio of 1.278 (CI 1.03–1.58), and interestingly not for the whole cohort ($p = 0.132$) or the other subgroups. (Table 4).

When NLR2.5 and the EORTC Score are analyzed together as a multivariate Cox model, the results per subgroups are retained: the EORTC Score is only significant for the 'No Treatment' subgroup ($p = 0.039$) and NLR2.5 is only significant for the BCG subgroup ($p = 0.025$). Although in contrast to the Univariate models, EORTC is very close to significance ($p = 0.058$, HR 1.11, CI 0.996–1.241) when taken together with NLR2.5 ($p = 0.012$, HR 2.098, CI 1.174–3.75). (Table 5).

Discussion

The main advantage of this study is its prospective nature, which to our knowledge, is one of the firsts to deal with

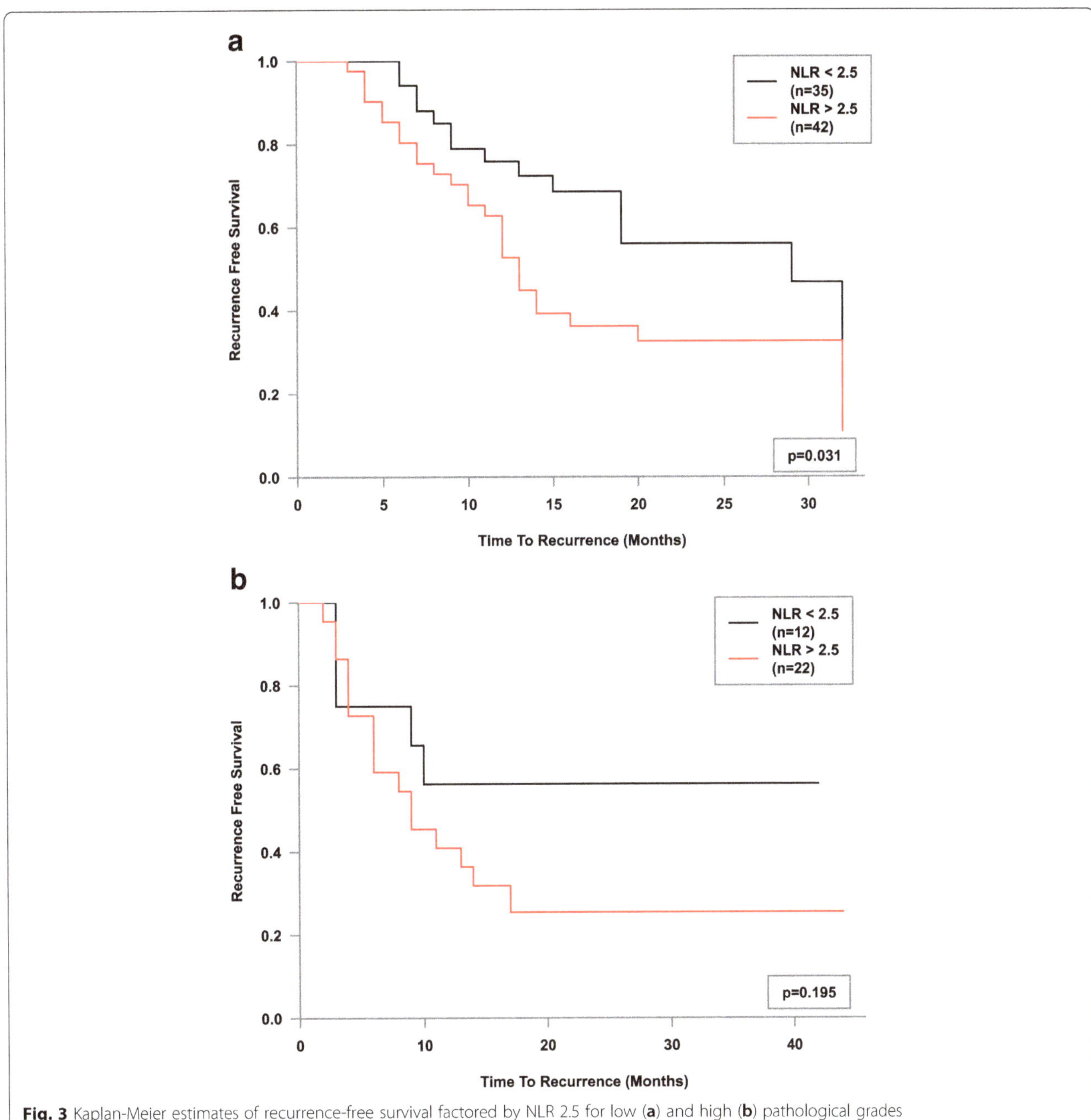

Fig. 3 Kaplan-Meier estimates of recurrence-free survival factored by NLR 2.5 for low (**a**) and high (**b**) pathological grades

NLR as a predictor for NMIBC. Upon diagnosis, NMIBC is initially treated with complete TUR-BT, after which an adjuvant therapy is considered. Based on clinical and pathological factors, patients can be assigned to risk groups, such as the EORTC Score for the assessment of disease recurrence and progression [5]. However, these predictive tools are far from optimal for the individual patient – what is the progression probability cutoff that justifies cystectomy? How aggressive an intra-vesical treatment should be with a 35% risk of recurrence per year? To be able to answer these kinds of questions in a more evidence-based manner, new and novel predictors are a necessity.

In the current study, we prospectively assessed the predictive value of NLR versus and in conjunction to the EORTC score in a group of NMIBC patients. The first main finding for the whole cohort include a statistically significant association between high NLR (> 2.5) and increased probability of recurrence – a finding that manifests in shorter time to recurrence.

In addition, high NLR was consistently associated with worse outcomes in all the sub-groups, although significance was demonstrated only for the Ta Stage, G1 Grade and the BCG treatment group. We believe that given a larger cohort per sub-group, a statistical significance is

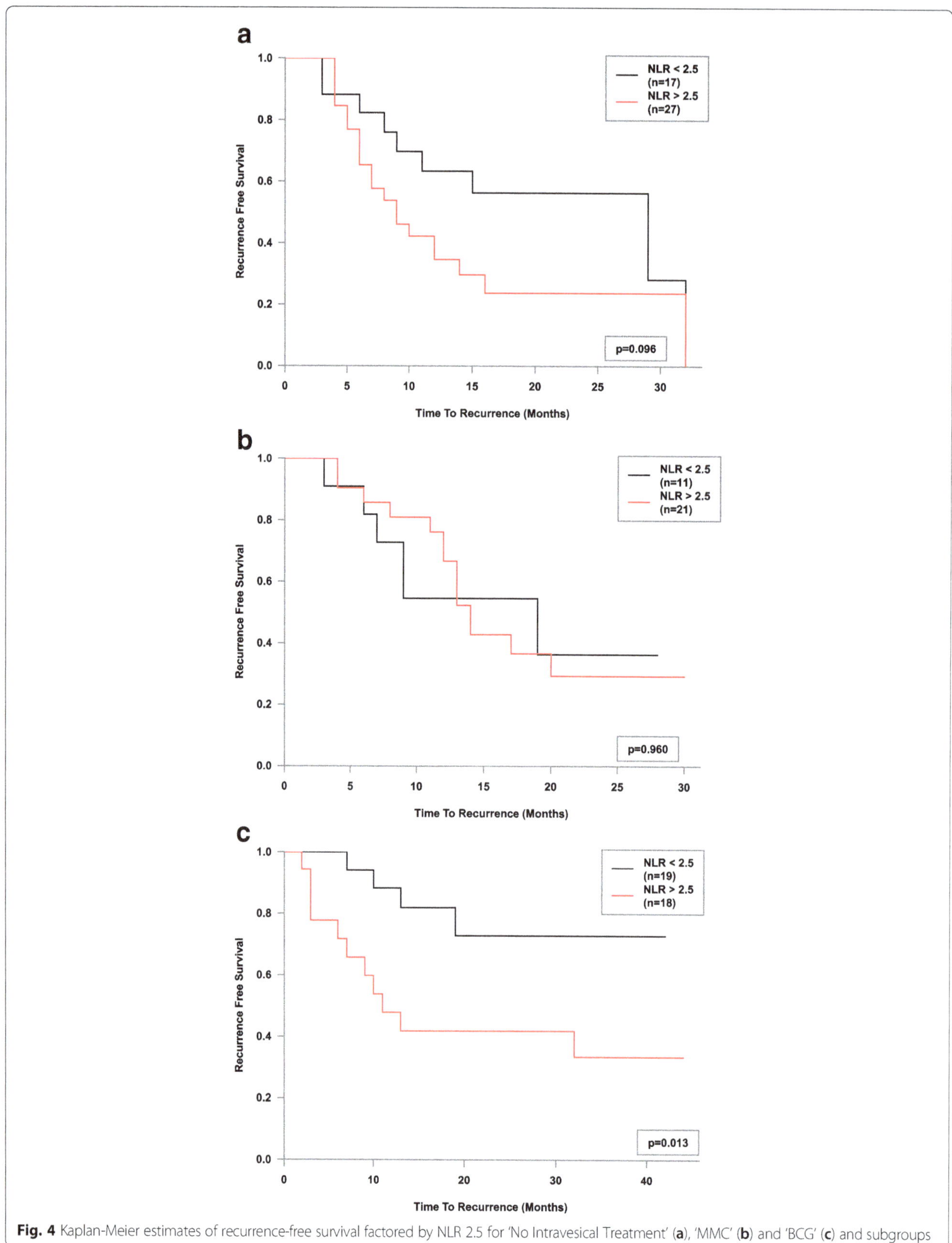

Fig. 4 Kaplan-Meier estimates of recurrence-free survival factored by NLR 2.5 for 'No Intravesical Treatment' (**a**), 'MMC' (**b**) and 'BCG' (**c**) and subgroups

Table 3 Univariate Cox Regression for recurrence using the NLR 2.5 cutoff, stratified by treatment subgroups

			95.0% CI for HR	
Group	*P*-Value	Hazard Ratio	Lower	Upper
Whole Cohort	0.010	2.029	1.185	3.472
No Treatment	0.123	1.866	0.845	4.123
MMC	0.960	1.025	0.392	2.677
BCG	0.023	3.793	1.203	11.956

probable. Nevertheless, the trend is clear – patients with higher NLR presented with worse recurrence-free survival in each stratification. NLR ratio was more significant in patients who received BCG compare to those who received MMC. We may assume that as an immune modulator BCG has better effect in patients with lower NLR. As this is a new finding arising from a prospective study our aim is to keep on analyzing this subgroup in our next prospective study.

The second main finding is the apparent synergistic effect between NLR (> 2.5) and the EORTC score, as the significance of the score increased substantially when calculated alongside the NLR2.5 variable. The EORTC score was used as a measure of reference, as it has been already established for thousands of patients. However, the EORTC score was never designed to be used when BCG intra-vesical treatment is chosen, as was clearly stated in reference [5]. This limitation of the EORTC score matches our results, as this score is undoubtedly significant for the group that received no treatment, but insignificant for whole cohort which includes the BCG treated patients. Luckily, the NLR > 2.5 is specifically significant for the BCG subgroup, in a manner that complements the EORTC score and improves the overall prediction for the whole-cohort.

While the pathophysiology is not yet clear, it has been suggested that the relative neutrophilia increases the number of inflammatory markers that include pro-angiogenic factors (VEGF), growth factors (CXCL8), proteases and anti-apoptotic markers (NF-kB) – all of which support tumor growth and progression. In addition, the lymphocytopenia is suggested to hurt cell-mediated immune response and thus worsening prognosis [16].

Table 4 Univariate Cox Regression for recurrence using the EORTC score, stratified by treatment subgroups

			95.0% CI for HR	
Group	*P*-Value	Hazard Ratio	Lower	Upper
Whole Cohort	0.132	1.085	0.976	1.207
No Treatment	0.024	1.278	1.033	1.580
MMC	0.266	1.128	0.913	1.393
BCG	0.934	1.008	0.841	1.207

Table 5 Multivariate Cox Regression for recurrence using both the EORTC score and NLR 2.5 Cutoff, stratified by treatment subgroups

				95.0% CI for HR	
Group	Variable	*P*-Value	Hazard Ratio	Lower	Upper
Whole Cohort	NLR2.5	0.012	2.098	1.174	3.750
	EORTC	0.058	1.112	0.996	1.241
No Treatment	NLR2.5	0.273	1.673	0.666	4.201
	EORTC	0.039	1.267	1.012	1.587
MMC	NLR2.5	0.640	1.285	0.449	3.682
	EORTC	0.233	1.138	0.920	1.408
BCG	NLR2.5	0.025	3.962	1.193	13.159
	EORTC	0.396	1.086	0.898	1.312

Pretreatment NLR is readily available, and higher values have been shown to correlate with higher stage tumors and adverse treatment outcomes in a wide variety of cancers including malignancies of the gastrointestinal and genitourinary tracts, including urothelial carcinoma of the bladder [6, 7, 12, 13].

Focusing on bladder cancer, several previous studies have evaluated the predictive value of NLR, most of which were conducted on patients undergoing radical cystectomy [9, 17–19]. Based on these studies, NLR may be used in the pre-operative setting to predict tumor invasiveness, or in the post-operative setting, together with pathologic tumor characteristics, to predict outcome. Can et al. found a correlation between muscle invasive disease in TURBT specimens and preoperative NLR > 2.57, patient age, female gender and platelet count, and suggested using NLR > 2.57 in a risk formula which may assist in deciding which patients may benefit from early cystectomy [17]. Similarly, Krane et al. found that patients with a NLR > 2.5 had a significantly higher likelihood of extravesical disease at radical cystectomy, suggesting that they may benefit from neoadjuvant chemotherapy [10]. Finally, Viers et al. found an association between higher pre-operative NLR and significantly increased risk of extravesical tumor extension and lymph node involvement, in a large group of bladder cancer patients undergoing radical cystectomy [9].

Curiously, most of the studies investigating the role of NLR in patients with NMIBC specifically have been retrospective – including our own two previously published articles [12, 13]. To date, only two prospective studies on the matter have been published, after this study's initiation. Favilla et al. further established the predictive value of NLR on recurrence, but did not elaborate regarding the relationship between NLR and the EORTC score [20]. Sebahattin et al. argued that correction for age might alter the results, so a logistic regression analysis (backwards, conditional) of the NLR2.5 and Age as a covariate, was performed. This regression resulted in only NLR2.5 as a significant variable ($p = 0.005$) with Odds ratio of 3.045 (CI 1.392–6.661), meaning that there is an average of at least 3-fold higher probability of recurrence for a person with NLR > 2.5 compared with NLR < 2.5. Age was removed from the model because of insignificance ($p = 0.988$) [21].

Limitations

A prominent limitation dealing with the NLR marker is the volatility of the Neutrophil and Lymphocyte counts. While we did actively exclude patients with hematologic malignances and with active infections, it is possible that some chronic medications or antibiotics affect the NLR value. An argument can be made that this approach might skew results, but as mentioned in the 'Materials' section – we strived to examine the effect of NLR on as much patients as possible, with the intention to generalize, and not marginalize, the NLR usability. We believe that the inclusive cohort in this study (i.e. including a small number of possible antibiotic users) can be regarded more like hurdle rather than a helpful measure, and thus the results are more meaningful. Evidence to this claim can be found on our previous publication, which dealt with a much more 'distilled' cohort [13].

Another limitation of the study is the small cohort per different subgroups. This has resulted in a discrepancy between the literature and our data regarding the known incidence rates of concomitant CIS. A possible explanation can either be attributed to chance, or the notion that many patients with concomitant CIS are discovered already in T2 stage, and thus were not included in this study.

We believe that given a larger cohort per sub-groups such as treatment type or pathological stage, a statistical significance is probable. A larger prospective study may be required to further solidify the place of NLR in predicting disease recurrence in patients with NMIBC and to incorporate it in the current risk calculation tools.

Conclusions

NLR > 2.5 was found to be a significant predictor of disease recurrence and demonstrated high hazard ratio and worse recurrence-free survival in patients with NMIBC, especially in those treated with BCG. Additionally, our data demonstrated statistical evidence that NLR > 2.5 might have an improving effect on the EORTC score's prediction when calculated together. Thus, we propose to consider the incorporation of NLR > 2.5 in the next revisions of the EORTC score.

Abbreviations

AUA: American Urological Association; BCG: Bacillus Calmette–Guérin; CBC: Complete blood count; EORTC: European Organization for Research and Treatment of Cancer; MMC: Mitomycin C; NLR: Neutrophil-to-lymphocyte ratio; NMIBC: Non-muscle invasive bladder cancer; TUR-BT: Trans-urethral resection of bladder tumor

Funding

The study was supported by a grant from: "Technion EVPR Fund - Elias Fund for Medical Research". The grant was purely academic and had no influence on the design, collection, analysis, interpretation or any other aspect of the research.

Authors' contributions

IG project development, data collection, data analysis, manuscript writing. ZB project development, data collection, manuscript writing. ON project development. JR project development, data analysis, manuscript editing. SH project development, data collection, manuscript writing. All authors read and approved the final manuscript.

Competing interests

The authors declare that they have no competing interests.

Author details

[1]Department of Urology, Bnai Zion Medical Center, Faculty of Medicine, Technion - Israel Institute of Technology, Golomb 47, 31048 Haifa, Israel. [2]Department of Mathematics, Technion - Israel Institute of Technology, Haifa, Israel.

References

1. Ferlay J, Soerjomataram I, Dikshit R, Eser S, Mathers C, Rebelo M, et al. Cancer incidence and mortality worldwide: sources, methods and major patterns in GLOBOCAN 2012. Int J Cancer. 2015;136(5):E359–86.
2. Babjuk M, Burger M, Zigeuner R, Shariat SF, van Rhijn BWG, Compérat E, et al. EAU guidelines on non–muscle-invasive Urothelial carcinoma of the bladder: update 2013. Eur Urol. 2013;64(4):639–53.
3. Brausi M, Witjes JA, Lamm D, Persad R, Palou J, Colombel M, et al. A Review of Current Guidelines and Best Practice Recommendations for the Management of Nonmuscle Invasive Bladder Cancer by the International Bladder Cancer Group. J Urol. 2011:2158–67. Available from: http://linkinghub.elsevier.com/retrieve/pii/S002253471104506X.
4. Hidas G, Pode D, Shapiro A, Katz R, Appelbaum L, Pizov G, et al. The natural history of secondary muscle-invasive bladder cancer. BMC Urol. 2013;13:23.
5. Sylvester RJ, van der Meijden APM, Oosterlinck W, Witjes JA, Bouffioux C, Denis L, et al. Predicting recurrence and progression in individual patients with stage ta T1 bladder Cancer using EORTC risk tables: a combined analysis of 2596 patients from seven EORTC trials. Eur Urol. 2006;49(3):466–77 Available from: http://linkinghub.elsevier.com/retrieve/pii/S0302283805008523.
6. Chua W, Charles KA, Baracos VE, Clarke SJ. Neutrophil/lymphocyte ratio predicts chemotherapy outcomes in patients with advanced colorectal cancer. Br J Cancer. 2011;104(8):1288–95.
7. Lee BS, Lee SH, Son JH, Jang DK, Chung KH, Lee YS, et al. Neutrophil-lymphocyte ratio predicts survival in patients with advanced cholangiocarcinoma on chemotherapy. Cancer Immunol Immunother. 2016; 65(2):141–50.
8. Viers BR, Houston Thompson R, Boorjian SA, Lohse CM, Leibovich BC, Tollefson MK. Preoperative neutrophil-lymphocyte ratio predicts death among patients with localized clear cell renal carcinoma undergoing nephrectomy. Urol Oncol Semin Orig Investig. 2014;32(8):1277–84.

9. Viers BR, Boorjian SA, Frank I, Tarrell RF, Thapa P, Karnes RJ, et al. Pretreatment neutrophil-to-lymphocyte ratio is associated with advanced pathologic tumor stage and increased Cancer-specific mortality among patients with Urothelial carcinoma of the bladder undergoing radical cystectomy. Eur Urol. 2014;66(6):1157–64.
10. Krane LS, Richards KA, Kader AK, Davis R, Balaji KC, Hemal AK. Preoperative neutrophil/lymphocyte ratio predicts overall survival and Extravesical disease in patients undergoing radical cystectomy. J Endourol. 2013;27(8):1046–50 Available from: http://online.liebertpub.com/doi/abs/10.1089/end.2012.0606.
11. Gondo T, Nakashima J, Ohno Y, Choichiro O, Horiguchi Y, Namiki K, et al. Prognostic value of Neutrophil-to-lymphocyte ratio and establishment of novel preoperative risk stratification model in bladder cancer patients treated with radical cystectomy. Urology. 2012:1085–91. Available from: https://www.ncbi.nlm.nih.gov/pubmed/22446338.
12. Mano R, Baniel J, Shoshany O, Margel D, Bar-On T, Nativ O, et al. Neutrophil-to-lymphocyte ratio predicts progression and recurrence of non-muscle-invasive bladder cancer. Urol Oncol. 2015;33(2):67.e1–7.
13. Rubinstein J, Bar-On T, Bahouth Z, Mano R, Shoshany O, Baniel J, et al. A mathematical model for predicting tumor recurrence within 24 months following surgery in patients with T1 high-grade bladder cancer treated with BCG immunotherapy. Bladder. 2015;2(2):e18.
14. Montironi R, Lopez-Beltran A. The 2004 WHO classification of bladder tumors: a summary and commentary. Int J Surg Pathol. 2005;13(2):143–53 Available from: http://www.ncbi.nlm.nih.gov/pubmed/15864376.
15. Chang SS, Boorjian SA, Chou R, Clark PE, Daneshmand S, Konety BR, et al. Diagnosis and treatment of non-muscle invasive bladder cancer: AUA/SUO guideline. J Urol. 2016;196(4):1021–9.
16. Paramanathan A, Saxena A. A systematic review and meta-analysis on the impact of pre-operative neutrophil lymphocyte ratio on long term outcomes after curative intent resection of solid tumours. Surg Oncol. 2014: 31–9 Available from: http://www.elsevier.com/locate/suronc%5Cnhttp://ovidsp.ovid.com/ovidweb.cgi?T=JS&PAGE=reference&D=emed12&NEWS=N&AN=2014201553.
17. Can C, Baseskioglu B, Yılmaz M, Colak E, Ozen A, Yenilmez A. Pretreatment parameters obtained from peripheral blood sample predicts invasiveness of bladder carcinoma. Urol Int. 2012;89(4):468–72.
18. Potretzke A, Hillman L, Wong K, Shi F, Brower R, Mai S, et al. NLR is predictive of upstaging at the time of radical cystectomy for patients with urothelial carcinoma of the bladder. Urol Oncol Semin Orig Investig. 2014; 32(5):631–6.
19. Zhang G-M, Zhu Y, Luo L, Wan F-N, Zhu Y-P, Sun L-J, et al. Preoperative lymphocyte-monocyte and platelet-lymphocyte ratios as predictors of overall survival in patients with bladder cancer undergoing radical cystectomy. Tumor Biol. 2015;36(11):8537–43.
20. Favilla V, Castelli T, Urzì D, Reale G, Privitera S, Salici A, et al. Neutrophil to lymphocyte ratio, a biomarker in non-muscle invasive bladder cancer: a single-institutional longitudinal study. Int Braz J Urol. 2016;42(4):685–93.
21. Albayrak S, Zengin K, Tanik S, Atar M, Unal SH, Imamoglu MA, et al. Can the neutrophil-to-lymphocyte ratio be used to predict recurrence and progression of non-muscle-invasive bladder cancer? Kaohsiung J Med Sci. 2016;32(6):327–33. Available from:. https://doi.org/10.1016/j.kjms.2016.05.001.

Emerging concepts and spectrum of renal injury following Intravesical BCG for non-muscle invasive bladder cancer

Azharuddin Mohammed* and Zubair Arastu

Abstract

Background: Intravesical Bacilli Calmette-Guerin (IVBCG) therapy for non-muscle invasive bladder cancer (NMIBC) has long been in use successfully. Albeit rarely, we still face with its safety concerns more than 25 years on since its approval by US Food and Drug Agency in 1990. Local and systemic infection following intravesical BCG is widely reported as compared to immune mediated local or systemic hypersensitivity reactions involving kidneys; acute kidney injury (AKI) and other renal manifestations are well reported but not of chronic kidney disease (CKD).

Case: An interesting case of a female was referred to nephrologists in advanced stages of CKD at an eGFR of 10 ml/min/1.73^2 following IVBCG for NMIBC. Our patient's renal function plateaued when IVBCG was held; and worsened again when reinstilled. It introduces the concept of 'repetitive' immune mediated renal injury presenting as progressive CKD rather than AKI, as is generally reported. Although response was poor, corticosteroids stopped CKD progression to end stage renal disease.

Conclusions: We highlight the need for increased awareness and early recognition of IVBCG renal complications by both urologists and nephrologists in order to prevent progressive and irreversible renal damage. Low incidence of IVBCG renal complications may also be due to under recognition in the era prior to CKD Staging and AKI Network (and AKI e-alerts) that defined AKI as a rise in serum creatinine of ≥26umol/L; hence an unmet need for urgent prospective studies. Major literature review focuses on emerging spectrum of histopathological IVBCG related renal complications and their outcomes.

Keywords: Intravesical bacillus Calmette-Guerin, BCG renal complications, Interstitial nephritis, Granuloma, AKI, CKD, Nephrotic syndrome

Background

Intravesical Bacilli Calmette-Guerin (IVBCG) therapy for non-muscle invasive bladder cancer (NMIBC) has long been in use successfully since 1973. Albeit rarely, we are increasingly facing its renal complications more than 25 years on, since its approval by US Food and Drug Agency in 1990. Renal injury following IVBCG is thought to be due to ascending infection or rarely due to granulomatous interstitial nephritis presenting as acute kidney injury/acute renal failure (AKI/ARF)). Case reports of acute renal injuries such as glomerulonephritis (GN), nephrotic syndrome (NS), rhabdomyolysis and rapidly progressive glomerulonephritis (RPGN) are increasing including fatal consequences in some. However, reports of chronic kidney disease (CKD) are not published, which and may be due to under-recognition. We report here an interesting case of advanced CKD presenting in stage 5 following IVBCG with novel insights into pathological process and guiding management plans.

Case

A 73 year-old Caucasian female referred to Nephrology with an eGFR of 10 ml/min/1.73^2 in June 2016; it was 60 ml/min/1.73^2 in Feb 2015. There was progressive decline of eGFR that dropped to 14 ml/min/1.73^2 in March 2016. There was no history of weight loss, recurrent UTI, new medication use or any autoimmune/vasculitc symptoms. Past medical history included well-controlled hypertension for 4 years and gastro-oesophageal reflux.

* Correspondence: Azharuddin@doctors.org.uk
Royal Shrewsbury Hospital, Mytton Oak Road, Shrewsbury SY3 8XQ, UK

Medications included Lisinopril, Lacidipine and Omeprazole. In November 2014, she had resection of NMIBC staged as high-grade cT1NxMx and receiving scheduled IVBCG (Onco tice12.5 mg) instillations since April 2015. Her IVBCG therapy interrupted due to a national shortage; it recommenced and by the time of referral received 16 instillations until May 2016.

She looked well on examination with BP of 155/69 mmHg and systemic examination was unremarkable with no rash, tender nodules, red eyes or lymphadenopathy. Urine dipstick showed leukocytes ++, protein + and culture showed no growth. Serum creatinine was 357 umol/L (eGFR 10 ml/min/1.73^2). Immunology came negative for ANA, ANCA, Anti GBM, myeloma screen, Hepatitis B and C and Complement levels C3/C4; ultrasound of the kidneys, ureter and bladder was normal. An ultrasound guided renal biopsy performed due to rapidly progressive unexplained decline in kidney function.

Renal biopsy showed interstitial inflammation with moderate lymphocytic infiltration, eosinophil's and a non-caseating granuloma. Background chronic tubular atrophy and some acute changes noted but no tubular inflammatory infiltrate. Immunofluorescence was negative and no AFB demonstrated.

Histological features were suggestive of a 'drug-like' immune mediated hypersensitivity reaction secondary to IVBCG. This was further supported by- patient's ethnicity, absence of previous TB exposure (and current symptoms), any new medications, normal CXR, serum ACE levels, negative Mantoux/TB Interferon assay and negative urine cultures for MTB.

As the last dose of IVBCG was within 6 weeks and acute on chronic biopsy picture, trial of steroids alone commenced (Prednisolone 40 mg daily); aim was to stop further decline in kidney function and buy time for dialysis preparation. It is now increasingly recognised that dialysis patient's outcomes are better who see a nephrologist before dialysis initiation compared to those who don't [1].

Patient responded partially to 6 weeks of steroids; eGFR improved from 10 to 14 ml/min/1.73^2 and then stabilised at 12–13 ml/min/1.73^2 at 9-month follow-up obviating any need for dialysis (Fig. 1). There were no systemic features of BCG infection and repeat cystoscopy showed no recurrence of NMIBC.

Discussion

Urothelial carcinoma is the eleventh most frequent cancer in women with mean age of 60 years and rising incidence in over 50 years [2]. NMIBC accounts for 75–90% of these with poor prognosis in females. Immunotherapy for NMIBC remains the gold standard with efficacy of IVBCG shown to be better than chemotherapy in reducing recurrence, progression and mortality [3]. The total cost for NMIBC is reported to be £32.25(2001–2002) million in UK and $3.7 billion in USA for 2001 [4].

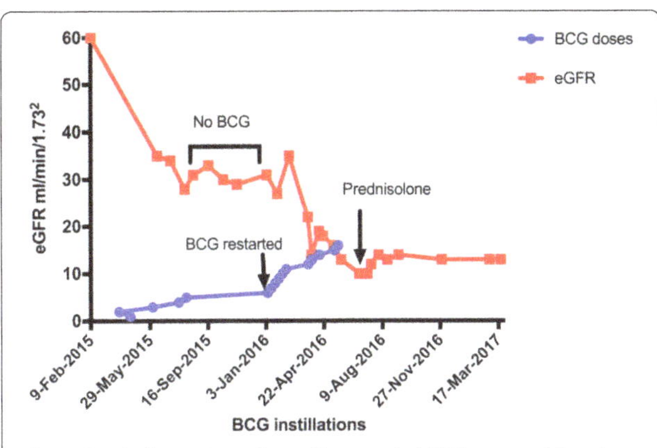

Fig. 1 Graph illustrating effect of intravesical BCG on renal function during treatment and following discontinuation

Use of Intravesical BCG in NMIBC

BCG is a live attenuated vaccine obtained from Mycobacterium bovis. It has been used since the first seminal paper of Morales et al. in 1976 [5, 6]. However, its use increased following FDA approval in 1990 providing more data on its safety and efficacy over the last quarter of a century.

Dose

Practice patterns vary but standard regimen of IVBCG for high-grade NMIBC is induction (6 consecutive weekly doses) with 1–3 years maintenance (3 consecutive weekly doses) at 3, 6, 12, 18, 24, 30, and 36 months.

Mechanism

Mechanism of action is unknown but local immune response following phagocytosis of BCG antigen is well recognised. Antitumor effect and cytotoxicity is mediated via cytokine release and soluble factors such as TNF- α, IFN- γ and NO [7].

Adverse effects

IVBCG is generally well tolerated albeit minor self-limiting adverse effects in 10–50% patients that includes flu-like symptoms, malaise and local bladder irritability causing dysuria, frequency and urgency. They occur 4–6 h after instillation and between 3 and 7 doses of IVBCG and do not require any treatment. However, fatality reports due to systemic reaction raised concerns on its established safety profile [8, 9]. Early IVBCG years witnessed haematogenous spread (lungs, liver, kidney, peritoneum, prostate and testis) after traumatic/non-traumatic catheterisation; consequent infection and DIC rarely caused multi organ failure and death [9–12]. Lately, increasing publications noticed on immune complications such as hypersensitivity, anaphylactoid purpura, Henoch Schönlein Purpura (HSP) and glomerular and tubulo-interstitial injuries [13, 14]. We exclusively review here renal complications of IVBCG.

Reported spectrum of renal injury following IVBCG since 1990 is listed above (Table 1) and the data summarised below:

- **Asymptomatic renal granuloma (*n* = 4):** Incidentally detected on follow-up imaging and seem to show favourable prognosis. Granuloma resolved with Anti-Tuberculous therapy (ATT) in one case and required nephro-ureterectomy in another due to left renal pelvic tumour. However, recent case series managed conservatively for 2 years showed no systemic features or progression [15, 16].
- **AKI due to interstitial nephritis with/without granuloma (*n* = 8):** This is the commonest presentation reported with elevated serum creatinine levels. Analysis of these cases highlights following:
    - Biopsies showed significant interstitial inflammation with moderate fibrosis; granulomas seen in only 50%.
    - Therapies involved prednisolone alone and pulsed methylprednisolone with/without ATT.
    - Outcome: Three (37.5%) patients were able to come off dialysis with above regimes; rest showed partial recovery.
- **AKI with Glomerulonephritis (*n* = 2):** In one case, mild renal dysfunction was associated with hypertension, haematuria and proteinuria. It responded well to steroids and ATT. Another case from Japan recently reported RPGN with fatal outcome in an elderly male [17]. Importance of history of recent IVBCG use was emphasised as well as fatal infection risk following immunosuppression and plasma exchange amongst elderly.
- **Nephrotic syndrome – Membranous nephropathy (*n* = 1):** This is the only case reported to date in adults. Although malignancy and infection associated nephrotic syndrome is well known, authors reported this case to be due to IVBCG. Remission achieved with prednisolone 80 mg daily and ACEi after a month, and maintained at 6 months [18].
- **AKI with Haemolytic uremic syndrome, Rhabdomyolysis and Multiorgan Failure (*n* = 1):** Patient developed multi organ failure after the eighth standard dose and died despite maximum intensive care management and plasma exchange. It calls for increased clinician awareness of rare but serious IVBCG complications.

Renal toxicity

Incidence

Reliable data on incidence of IVBCG renal toxicity is lacking due to various patient and treatment related factors discussed below. Under-recognition is probably significant prior to CKD Staging (using eGFR) and AKI Network era that defined AKI as a rise in serum creatinine of ≥26umol/L. A large study (*N* = 2602) by Lamm et al. in 1992 reported 2 cases (0.1%) of renal abscess, seen only with Connaught strain of BCG [19]. Manufacturers of one BCG strain stated 9% renal toxicity in their study arm (*N* = 112) with 1.8% in ≥ Grade 3 cancer [9].

Patient factors

This is the second case of renal failure in females, which could be due to gender differences of NMIBC, M: F ratio of 3:1. High environmental and industrial carcinogen exposure in men like aromatic amines in cigarette smoke, dye and rubber industry may also explain this difference.

Trauma, UTI and site

Traumatic catheterization and concurrent cystitis are well known factors for high-risk of serious adverse events and a close monitoring can reduce toxicity. Upper tract urothelial carcinoma and evidence of vesicoureteric reflux are other important factors to consider [20].

Strain type

Repeated culture and attenuation of Mycobacterium Bovis produces BCG strains of variable immunogenicity, virulence and toxicity, which limits obtaining absolute comparative toxicity data for all strains reliably. Renal abscess seen with Connaught strain [19]. Most BCG strains cause renal toxicity including Pasteur, Onco Tice, Connaught, and Tokyo strains [15, 16, 21–24].

Dose

Toxicity reported to be dose dependent in addition to strain specific. Analyses of cases show no correlation of severity of kidney injury to number of instillations with an exception of rare fatality after eight instillations [8] (Table 1). It becomes a hard clinical choice to limit BCG instillations when no reliable alternatives to radical cystectomy are available that reduce recurrence and progression of NMIBC and maintain functional urinary bladders.

Repetitive injury

Almost all renal injury cases reported AKI *during or after* administration of standard or higher doses. Interestingly, our case shows that there might be a window of opportunity when interrupting therapy could lead to stabilization of renal function. A national shortage of IVBCG interrupted patient's therapy; renal function trend during this period demonstrated that eGFR

Table 1 Clinical spectrum of renal presentations, treatment and their outcome following Intravesical BCG

Year/ Ref	Age	Sex	Clinical Presentation	Initial SCr(mg/dL)	BCG Strain	BCG Instillations	Renal Histology	Granuloma	Treatment	Recovery	Last SCr(mg/dL)
1991 [21]	70	M	VH, Raised Cr	3	Pasteur	11	Interstitial epitheloid granulomas	Yes	I + P	Partial	1.8
1991 [21]	70	M	ARF	5.4	Pasteur	18	Interstitial nephritis with mesangial IgM and C3 deposits	No	I + E + P	Poor Died	Off HD; CrCl 10
1991 [21]	48	M	Hematuria and Proteinuria	1.3	Pasteur	9	Diffuse mesangial proliferation with subendothetial deposits of IgG + C3 and moderate interstitial fibrosis;	No	I + R	Complete	
2000 [8]	72	M	ARF- HUS, Rhabdomyolysis	3.8	?	8	No biopsy as patient too unwell	N/A	Pl.Ex, HD	None Died	–
2000 [25]	67	M	UTI		?		Renal caseating granulomas	Yes	I + R + Pip	Complete	–
2001 [14]	57	F	UTI	–	Tokyo	5	–	NA	Pulse CS	Complete	–
2001 [14]	76	M	UTI	–	Tokyo	6	–	NA	Pulse CS	Complete	–
2005 [22]	72	M	ARF	2.9	Tice	9	Acute tubulointersttial nephritis. Mesangial proliferation + focal segmental changes;IF-ve	No	I + R + P	Partial	1.9
2006 [23]	72	F	ARF	3.1	Connaught	5	Diffuse Interstitial Nephritis +2 non-necrotising Granulomas; IF nonspecific IgM + C3	Yes	Pred alone	Complete	1.3
2007 [24]	76	M	ARF	6.5	?	10	Diffuse and severe interstitial nephritis	No	MP, Pred	Partial	3.4
2007 [18]	54	M	Nephrotic Syndrome	Normal	?	12	Membranous glomerulonephritis - IgM, C3 and IgG+	No	Pred alone	Complete Remission	Normal
2013 [12]	76	M	AKI	7.9	?	10	Tubulointerstitial nephritis with moderate eosinophilic infiltrate	No	Oral MP, ATT, HD	Partial	Off HD; 2.5
2015 [15]	52	M	Surveillance CT	1.2	Onco Tice	18	Necrotising granuloma with no interstitial inflammation; IF not done;	Yes	ATT	Complete	1.2
2015 [16]	68	M	VH	–	OncoTice	18	Non-necrotising granulomas	Yes	None	Complete	–
2015 [16]	74	M	NVH	–	OncoTice	9	Chronic Granulomatous Interstitial Nephritis	Yes	None	Complete	–
2017 [17]	80	M	AKI-RPGN HSP	3.6	Connaught	8	IgA-Fibrinoid necrosis + 20% crescents Mesangial IgA. Skin- HSP vasculitis	No	MP, Pred Pl.Ex, HD	Partial Died	Off HD; 2.8
Present	73	F	Advanced CKD5	4	OncoTice	16	Interstitial nephritis with granuloma and acute/chronic tubular damage, IF negative	Yes	Pred alone	Poor	3.3

AAT Antituberculous Therapy, *AKI* Acute Kidney injury, *ARF* Acute renal failure, *CS* Corticosteroids, *E* Ethambutol, *HD* Hemodialysis, *HSP* Henoch ≈Schönlein Purpura, *HUS* Haemolytic Uremic Syndrome, *IgA* Immunoglobulin A, *I* Isoniazid, *MP* Methyl Prednisolone, *NVH* Non-Visible Haematuria, *Pip* Piperacillin, *Pl.Ex* Plasma Exchange, *Pred* Prednisolone, *P* Pyrazinamide, *R* Rifampicin, *SCr* Serum creatinine, *VH* Visible Haematuria, *RPGN* Rapidly Progressive Glomerulonephritis, *UTI* Urinary Tract Infection

plateaued. More intriguing was a decline in renal function again following readministration of IVBCG suggesting a cumulative dose related repetitive injury that could present as CKD rather than a one-hit process causing AKI (13, 14, 17–19)Fig 1. Therefore, early recognition of renal dysfunction during IVBCG treatment is vital.

Granuloma

Presence of renal granuloma in the context of IVBCG requires comprehensive patient evaluation for infectious, autoimmune and non-infectious causes such as sarcoidosis and medications. Case series analysis ($n = 15$) show that although the median numbers of instillations in granulomatous cases were non-significantly higher, serum creatinine at presentation was lower and had no fatalities compared to non-granulomatous presentation (Table.2, Fig 2). This suggests complex immune-pathological mechanisms for renal injury that depends on strain virulence, toxicity and host response, which may already be low in this age group. However, as the data is limited formal conclusions cannot be drawn or generalised, highlighting need for urgent prospective studies.

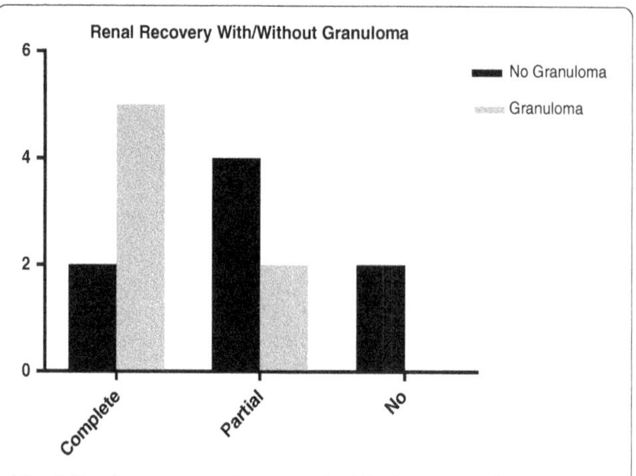

Fig. 2 Renal outcome in Intravesical BCG related granulomatous and non-granulomatous renal disease

- Good response to corticosteroids can obviate dialysis dependence even in late stages; partial response can avert an unplanned dialysis as seen in our case.

Key messages

- Spectrum of renal injury following IVBCG can present:
  - After standard doses
  - Without any constitutional symptoms
  - Early or late stages (of AKI/CKD) requiring dialysis.
- Cumulative toxicity with repetitive doses needs consideration for preventing avoidable progressive renal damage.
- Renal biopsy even in late stages can guide management, prognosis and exclude malignancy in uncertain cases.

Conclusion

- Majority of patients do benefit from IVBCG; nevertheless, rarely it causes a spectrum of immune mediated renal injuries that include granulomatous/non-granulomatous interstitial nephritis, glomerulonephritis, nephrotic syndrome and systemic (and local) hypersensitivity reactions.
- A decline in kidney function, haematuria and proteinuria during BCG treatment, in the absence of identifiable causes, should prompt suspicion of treatment related renal complication and an early

Table 2 Demographics and clinical differences between Intravesical BCG related granulomatous and non-granulomatous disease

	No. Granuloma ($n = 8$)	Granuloma ($n = 7$)	p =
Gender n = (M, F)	8, 0	5, 2	NA
Age (Years)	72 (58–76)	70 (67–73)	0.48
No. of Instillations	9.5 (8.25–11.5)	13.5 (8–18)	0.40
BCG Strains	Pas, Tice, Conn	Pas, Onc Tice, Conn	
Peak creatinine (mg/dL)	4.6 (1.9–6.4)	3 (1.7–3.8)	0.28
Required HD (n=)	3	0	
Death ($n = 3$)			
17 -day	1		
32-day	1		
1-year	1		
Recovery (n = 15)			–
Partial/None	6	2	–
Complete	2	5	

nephrology referral considered for further evaluation and consideration of renal biopsy.
- Risk of AKI with/without CKD (rarely advanced renal failure) would need to be included in the IVBCG Patient Information Leaflets (and Consent Forms) with a plan for scheduled renal function monitoring for occurrence of AKI during and up to 90 days after therapy as per standard practice.
- Urgent prospective observational studies can help assess the true incidence of IVBCG renal toxicity using the newer AKIN based AKI e-alerts and CKD Staging.

Abbreviations
AKI: Acute Kidney injury; AKIN: Acute Kidney Injury Network; ARF: Acute Renal Failure; ATT: Antituberculous therapy; BCG: QBacilli Calmette-Guerin; CKD: Chronic Kidney Disease; CS: Corticosteroids; DIC: Disseminated Intravascular Coagulation; eGFR: estimated Glomerular Filtration Rate; HD: Hemodialysis; HSP: Henoch Schonlein Purpura; HSP: Henoch Schönlein Purpura; HUS: Hemolytic Uremic Syndrome; MP: Methyl Prednisolone; MTB: Mycobacterium Tuberculosis; NMIBC: Non Muscle invasive Bladder Cancer; NS: Nephrotic Syndrome; NVH: Non-Visible Hematuria; Pl.Ex: Plasma Exchange; RPGN: Rapidly Progressive Glomerulonephritis; UTI: Urinary tract Infection; VH: Visible Hematuria

Acknowledgements
None.

Funding
None.

Authors' contributions
AM discovered the case and treated patient. AM and ZA carried out literature research, participated in design and drafting of the case. All authors actively contributed to the case and read and approved the final manuscript. AM is the corresponding author. All authors read and approved the final manuscript.

Competing interests
The authors declare that they have no competing interests.

References
1. Gillespie BW, Morgenstern H, Hedgeman E, et al. Nephrology care prior to end-stage renal disease and outcomes among new ESRD patients in the USA. Clin Kidney J. 2015;8(6):772–80.
2. Lucca I, Klatte T, Fajkovic H, de Martino M, Shariat SF. Gender differences in incidence and outcomes of urothelial and kidney cancer. Nat Rev Urol. 2015;12(10):585–592.
3. Kamat AM, Flaig TW, Grossman HB, Konety B, Lamm D, O'Donnell MA, et al. Expert consensus document: consensus statement on best practice management regarding the use of intravesical immunotherapy with BCG for bladder cancer. Nat Rev Urol. 2015;12(4):225–35.
4. Boustead GB, Fowler S, Swamy R, et al. Stage, grade and pathological cancer in the UK: British Association of Urological Surgeons (BAUS) urological tumour registry. BJU Int. 2014;113:924–30.
5. Morales A, Eidinger D, Bruce AW. Intracavitary bacillus Calmette-Guerin in the treatment of superficial bladder tumors. J Urol. 1976;116(2):180–3.
6. Lamm DL. Efficacy and safety of bacille Calmette-Guérin immunotherapy in superficial bladder cancer. Clin Infect Dis. 2000;31(Suppl 3):S86–90.
7. Redelman-Sidi G, Glickman MS, Bochner BH. The mechanism of action of BCG therapy for bladder cancer–a current perspective. Nat Rev Urol. 2014; 11(3):153–62.
8. Peyrière H, Klouche K, Béraud JJ, Blayac JP, Hillaire-Buys D. Fatal systemic reaction after multiple doses of intravesical bacillus Calmette-Guérin for polyposis. Ann Pharmacother. 2000;34(11):1279–82.
9. Vaccineshoppe.com. TheraCys. Full Prescribing Information. [Online]. 2015. Available at: https://www.vaccineshoppe.com/image.cfm?doc_id=12635&image_type=product_pdf
10. Gonzalez OY, Musher DM, Brar I, Furgeson S, Boktour MR, Septimus EJ, et al. Spectrum of bacille Calmette-Guérin (BCG) infection after intravesical BCG immunotherapy. Clin Infect Dis. 2003;36(2):140–8.
11. Elzein F, Albogami N, Saad M, El Tayeb N, Alghamdi A, Elyamany G. Disseminated Mycobacterium Bovis infection complicating Intravesical BCG instillation for the treatment of superficial transitional cell carcinoma of the bladder. Clin Med Insights Case Rep. 2016;9:71–3.
12. Mat O, Kada R, Phillipart P, et al. Late and reversible kidney-lung failure after intra-bladder BCG therapy. Open Journal of Nephrology. 2013:120–3.
13. Hirayama T, Matsumoto K, Tsuboi T, Fujita T, Satoh T, Iwamura M, et al. Anaphylactoid purpura after intravesical therapy using bacillus Calmette-Guerin for superficial bladder cancer. Hinyokika Kiyo. 2008;54(2):127–9.
14. Shimasaki N, Yamasaki I, Kamada M, Syuin T. Two cases of successful treatments with steroid for local and systemic hypersensitivity reaction following intravesical instillation of bacillus Calmette-Guerin. Hinyokika Kiyo. 2001;47(4):281–4.
15. Bhat S, Srinivasa Y, Paul F. Asymptomatic renal BCG granulomatosis: an unusual complication of intravesical BCG therapy for carcinoma urinary bladder. Indian J Urol. 2015;31(3):259–61.
16. Al-Qaoud T, Brimo F, Aprikian AG, Andonian S. BCG-related renal granulomas managed conservatively: a case series. Can Urol Assoc J. 2015; 9(3–4):E200–3.
17. Tsukada H, Miyakawa H. Henoch Schönlein Purpura nephritis associated with Intravesical bacillus Calmette-Guerin (BCG) therapy. Intern Med. 2017;56:541–4.
18. Singh NP, Prakash A, Kubba S, Ganguli A, Agarwal SK, Dinda AK, et al. Nephrotic syndrome as a complication of intravesical BCG treatment of transitional cell carcinoma of urinary bladder. Ren Fail. 2007;29(2):227–9.
19. Lamm DL, van der Meijden PM, Morales A, Brosman SA, Catalona WJ, Herr HW, et al. Incidence and treatment of complications of bacillus Calmette-Guerin intravesical therapy in superficial bladder cancer. J Urol. 1992;147(3):596–600.
20. Ristau BT, Tomaszewski JJ, Ost MC. Upper tract urothelial carcinoma: current treatment and outcomes. Urology. 2012;79(4):749–56.
21. Modesto A, Marty L, Suc JM, Kleinknecht D, de Frémont JF, Marsepoil T, et al. Renal complications of intravesical bacillus Calmette-Guérin therapy. Am J Nephrol. 1991;11(6):501–4.
22. Fry A, Saleemi A, Griffiths M, Farrington K. Acute renal failure following intravesical bacille Calmette-Guérin chemotherapy for superficial carcinoma of the bladder. Nephrol Dial Transplant. 2005;20(4):849–50.
23. Kennedy SE, Shrikanth S, Charlesworth JA. Acute granulomatous tubulointerstitial nephritis caused by intravesical BCG. Nephrol Dial Transplant. 2006;21(5):1427–9.
24. Manzanera Escribano MJ, Morales Ruiz E, Odriozola Grijalba M, Gutierrez Martínez E, Rodriguez Antolín A, Praga TM. Acute renal failure due to interstitial nephritis after intravesical instillation of BCG. Clin Exp Nephrol. 2007;11(3):238–40.
25. Numao N, Goto S, Suzuki S. A case of renal tuberculosis following bacillus Calmette-Guerin instillation therapy for bladder cancer. Hinyokika Kiyo. 2000; 46(2):109–11.

24

Influence of sildenafil on blood oxygen saturation of the obstructed bladder

Jeroen R Scheepe[1*], Arjen Amelink[2], Katja P Wolffenbuttel[1] and Dirk J Kok[1]

Abstract

Background: Blood oxygen saturation (BOS) is decreased in a low-compliant, overactive obstructed bladder. The objective of this study is to determine the effect of Sildenafil (SC) on bladder function and BOS) in an in vivo animal model of bladder outlet obstruction.

Methods: Thirty-two guinea pigs; sham operated (n = 8), sham operated + SC (n = 8), urethrally obstructed (n = 8) and urethrally obstructed + SC (n = 8) were studied during an 8 week period. BOS of the bladder wall was measured by differential path-length spectroscopy (DPS) before obstruction, at day 0, and at week 8. The bladder function was evaluated by urodynamic studies every week.

Results: Before surgery and after sham operation all study parameters were comparable. After sham operation, bladder function and BOS did not change. In the obstructed group the urodynamic parameters were deteriorated and BOS was decreased. In the group obstruction + SC, bladder compliance remained normal and overactivity occurred only sporadic. BOS remained unchanged compared to the sham group and was significantly higher compared to the obstruction group.

Conclusions: In an obstructed bladder the loss of bladder function is accompanied by a significant decrease in BOS. Treatment of obstructed bladders with SC yields a situation of high saturation, high bladder compliance and almost no overactivity. Maintaining the microcirculation of the bladder wall might result in better bladder performance without significant loss of bladder function. Measurement of BOS and interventions focussing on tissue microcirculation may have a place in the evaluation / treatment of various bladder dysfunctions.

Keywords: Bladder dysfunction, Bladder outlet obstruction, Guinea pig, Hypoxia, PDE5 inhibitor

Background

There is growing evidence that ischemia of the bladder wall contributes to the initiation of bladder dysfunction. Several studies have shown effects in obstructed bladder that can be interpreted as long term results of hypoxia [1]. Furthermore, there is an increasing interest in the nitric oxide (NO) pathway as a potential pharmacological target to treat lower urinary tract symptoms.

Phosphodiesterase 5 (PDE5) is involved in the NO pathway and it has been immunolocalized both in the detrusor muscle cells and in the vascular endothelium [2]. PDE5 inhibitors were found to improve several functional aspects of bladder dysfunction in human and animal studies [2-10]. The mechanisms behind this have not been fully elucidated yet, but it can be assumed that PDE5 inhibitors influence detrusor muscle cell action directly but also indirectly through enhancement of tissue microcirculation of the bladder tissue [11]. In a previous study we have shown in a Guinea pig model of bladder outlet obstruction (BOO) that the oxygen saturation is significantly lower in the obstructed bladder compared to sham operated bladder, both during the voiding and filling phase [12].

The objective of this study is to investigate the effect of the PDE5 inhibitor Sildenafil citrate (SC), which enhances tissue microcirculation, on bladder function and blood oxygen saturation (BOS) *in vivo* in an animal model of bladder outlet obstruction.

* Correspondence: j.scheepe@erasmusmc.nl
[1]Department of Urology and Pediatric Urology, Erasmus Medical Center Rotterdam, Sophia Children's Hospital, Rotterdam, The Netherlands
Full list of author information is available at the end of the article

Methods

Animals and study design

Animal experiments were approved by the Erasmus Medical Center animal ethics committee. Furthermore, the experiments were conducted according to the ARRIVE guidelines.

Thirty-two immature male albino Guinea pigs (Hartley strain) weighing approximately 250 g were used. Sixteen animals were urethrally obstructed and 8 of them received daily s.c. injections with sildenafil citrate (SC) (10 mg/kg b.w./day). The other 8 animals received saline only. Another group of 16 animals were sham operated and also divided into two groups: plus SC (n = 8) and plus saline (n = 8). All 32 animals were followed for 8 weeks. Urodynamic investigations were performed before surgery and at weeks 2,3,4,5,6,7 and 8. DPS measurements were performed at day 0 before surgery (n = 32) and 8 weeks after sham operation (n = 16) or obstruction (n = 16).

Experimental model, surgical procedures and DPS measurements

The Guinea pig model for partial bladder outlet obstruction (BOO) as described by Kok and Wolffenbuttel et al. [13,14] was used.

Obstruction and sham operation were done using ketamine/xylazine anesthesia. The peritoneal cavity was accessed via a lower vertical midline abdominal incision. A silver jeweler jump ring with an internal diameter of 2.2 mm was placed around the bladder neck above the prostate and left there (obstructed group) or removed (sham operated group). A glass fiber probe was then placed directly on the body of the bladder for BOS measurements. At the day of sacrifice a similar midline incision was made to allow probe access to measure BOS of the bladder wall, as described below, during multiple filling/voiding cycles. Intravesical pressure was measured simultaneously. The flow rate was not measured during DPS measurements but each DPS measurement sequence was preceded by a complete urodynamic investigation, including flow rate measurement. After the final DPS measurement the animal was sacrificed and the bladder was removed en bloc in order to determine the bladder weight.

Urodynamics

Urodynamic investigations were performed at week 0 (before the obstruction/sham operation and first DPS measurement sequence), week 2, 3, 4, 5, 6, 7 and at week 8 (before the second DPS measurement sequence). For each measurement the animals were anesthetized using ketamine (43 mg/kg i.m.) and xylazine (0.9 mg/kg i.m.). Through a 24-gauge suprapubic catheter bladder pressure was measured and the bladder was filled continuously with sterile saline at a rate of 0.23 ml per minute. Flow rate was measured with an ultrasound transducer (T106 small animal Flow meter, Transonic Systems, Ithaca, NY) around the penis.

From the urodynamic data we calculated:

- 1) Number of overactive contractions (NOC): Number of overactive contractions (>10 cm H_2O) that occur during 1 filling cycle. The average NOC of all cycles during 1 urodynamic investigation is reported.
- 2) Maximum voiding pressure (P_{max} in cm H_2O): Average P_{max} of all voids during 1 urodynamic investigation is reported.
- 3) Contractility (W_{max} in W/m^2): Relation between pressure and flow during a voiding according to Griffiths et al. [15]. The average W_{max} for all voidings during 1 urodynamic investigation is reported.
- 4) The maximal flow rate (Q_{max} in ml/sec): Highest absolute value of the flow during voiding.
- 5) Bladder compliance (ml/cm H2O) was defined as the relationship between change in bladder volume and the change in bladder pressure in the filling phase. Care was taken that pressure values obtained during these periods were not influenced by a nearby voiding or overactive contraction.

Differential path-length spectroscopy (DPS)

Blood oxygenation of the bladder wall was measured *in vivo* by differential path-length spectroscopy (DPS) using glass-fibers at the 2 time points where the bladder was accessible. During concomitant bladder pressure measurement the probe was placed in gentle contact with the serosal surface of the anterior bladder wall. To avoid artefacts caused by pressing the probe too hard to the bladder wall the probe was regularly repositioned. The experimental setup used for DPS measurements and the DPS data analysis routine was previously described in detail by Amelink et al. [16,17]. Complete sessions consisted of a few hundred to more then a thousand single DPS measurements. During voiding, up to 10 DPS measurements and during filling, up to hundreds of DPS measurements could be performed. The average saturation was calculated when at least 5 measurement points were available.

Statistics

We tested the significance of changes at the 2 time points in the obstructed and sham operated groups with the paired Student t test. Differences between the obstructed and sham operated groups were tested with the unpaired Student t test.

Results

Loss of animals

Two animals from the obstruction group with saline developed bladder stones and had to be removed from the study.

In all SC treated animals the urodynamic investigation at week 5 was not performed due to organizational problems.

Urodynamic data and BOS before operation

Before obstruction or sham operation there were no statistically significant differences between the 4 groups concerning contractility (±3 W/m^2), overactivity (no unstable contractions) and maximum voiding pressure (<30 cm H_2O) (Figures 1, 2 and 3). The average value for bladder compliance was higher in the two SC treated groups but this difference was not significant (Figure 4). Flow rate was comparable in all 4 groups (data not shown).

The BOS of the bladder during filling averaged between 92% and 95% in the four groups (Figure 5). The complete range was moved slightly to higher values in the two SC treated groups but all differences between the groups were not statistically significant. During voiding the average BOS ranged from 84% to 94% in the 4 groups. The individual BOS values showed more variation, ranging from 62% to 98% (Figure 5).

Urodynamic data and BOS after sham operation

In both the sham + saline and sham + SC group the maximum voiding pressure, compliance, contractility and overactivity did not change during the 8 week follow-up. A few unstable contractions were found in some animals from both groups at weeks 4 and 8. No differences were found between both groups except for a statistically significant increase in contractility at week 8 in the sham + SC group (Figure 1). At week 8 BOS was comparable between both groups and unchanged from the values at day 0 (Figure 6).

Urodynamic data and BOS after obstruction

In the *obstruction + saline group* bladder compliance was significantly lower compared to both day 0 and to the corresponding value in the sham + saline group from week 2 up until week 8. Maximum voiding pressure increased compared to day 0 and to the sham + saline group, reaching significance at weeks 3,4,6,7 and 8. Bladder overactivity was present from week 2 onwards. Bladder contractility was higher compared to day 0 and to the sham + saline group, reaching significance at weeks 2,3,6,7 and 8. The average value for BOS decreased significantly both in the filling and voiding phase. The lower limit of individual voids was 12% (Figure 6).

In the *obstruction + SC group* compliance remained comparable to the values at day 0 and to the values in both sham groups. Compared to the obstruction + saline group the compliance was significantly higher at weeks 2,3,6,7 and 8. The maximum voiding pressure was similar to the obstruction + saline group and significantly higher compared to day 0 and to the sham groups. Contractility was increased significantly compared to day 0 and to both sham groups and even compared to the obstruction + saline group (weeks 3,4,6,7 and 8). Overactivity was found throughout the 8 week follow-up but was significantly lower as compared to the obstruction + saline group.

BOS did not decrease in the obstruction + SC group after 8 weeks of obstruction. It was significantly higher compared to the obstruction + saline group. The lowest individual value was 71% (Figure 6).

Bladder weight

The average bladder weights of the sham + saline group and obstruction + saline group was 0.75 ± 0.07. and 1.64 ± 0.36 grams, respectively ($p < 0.04$). Treatment of the obstructed animals with SC resulted in a significant lesser

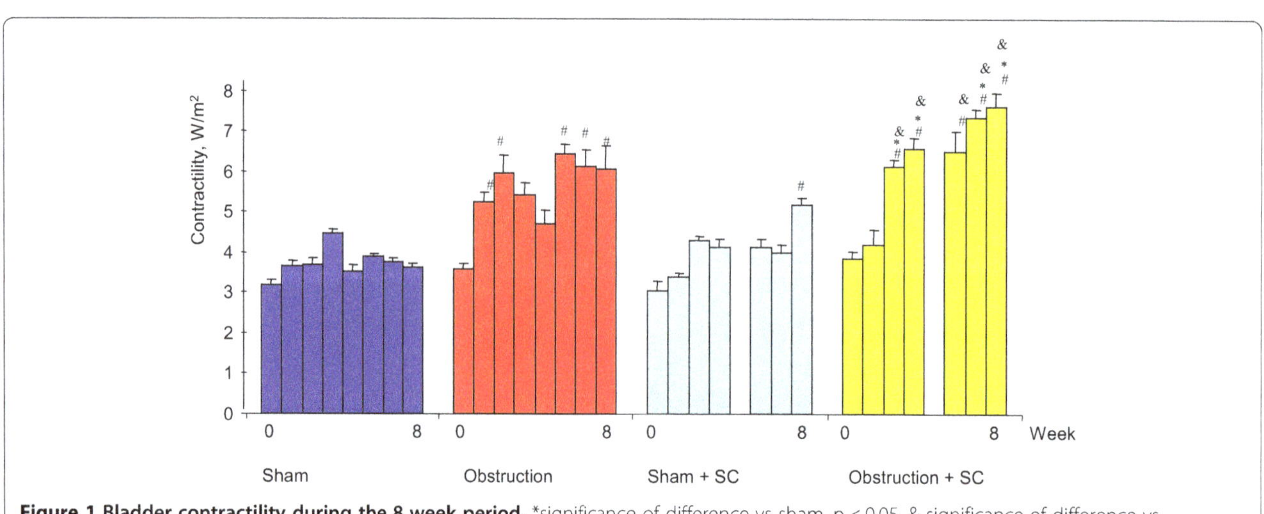

Figure 1 Bladder contractility during the 8 week period. *significance of difference vs sham, $p < 0.05$, & significance of difference vs obstruction, *significance of difference versus sham + sildenafil.

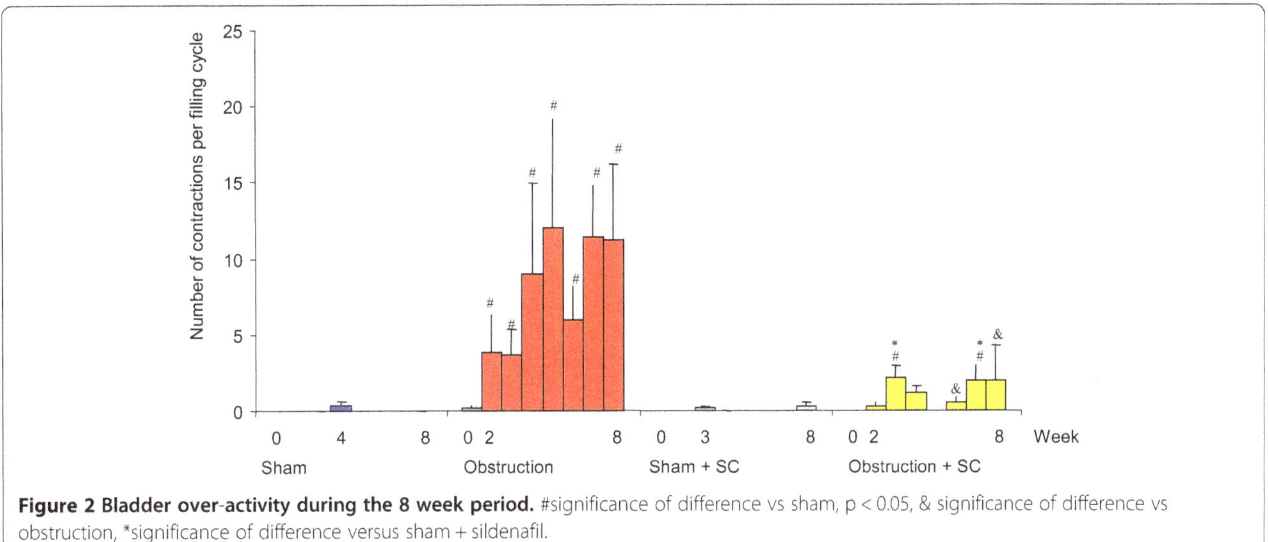

Figure 2 Bladder over-activity during the 8 week period. #significance of difference vs sham, $p < 0.05$, & significance of difference vs obstruction, *significance of difference versus sham + sildenafil.

increase of bladder weight (0.91 ± 0.1 gr.). The bladder weight of the sham + SC group was lower (0.55 ± 0.03) compared to the sham + saline group.

Discussion

During bladder filling the saturation in the normal Guinea pig bladder is around 90%. At the end of bladder filling and during voiding there is a marked decrease in saturation. Shortly after voiding the saturation returns to its high pre-voiding value.

The obstructed bladder is characterized by a significantly lower saturation both during voiding and filling. This decrease in saturation is more pronounced when detrusor overactivity occurs during the filling phase [12].

In contrast, in Guinea pigs with BOO treated with SC the bladder saturation both during filling and voiding remains as high as in the sham operated animals. This maintenance of a high saturation level is accompanied by normal bladder compliance and less overactivity. Maintaining bladder compliance and damping detrusor overactivity might be explained by direct smooth muscle cell action of the PDE5 inhibitor SC. However, the maximum voiding pressure and the contractility of SC-treated obstructed bladder increase at least as much as in the saline treated obstructed bladder. This phenomenon can not be explained by a direct muscle relaxing effect of SC alone. Possibly the maintenance of an almost normal bladder function in animals with BOO treated with SC is an effect of enhanced bladder microcirculation rather then a direct effect on muscle cells. Obstructed bladders treated with SC have a higher saturation level.. Muscle cells acting aerobically can produce force more efficiently than the

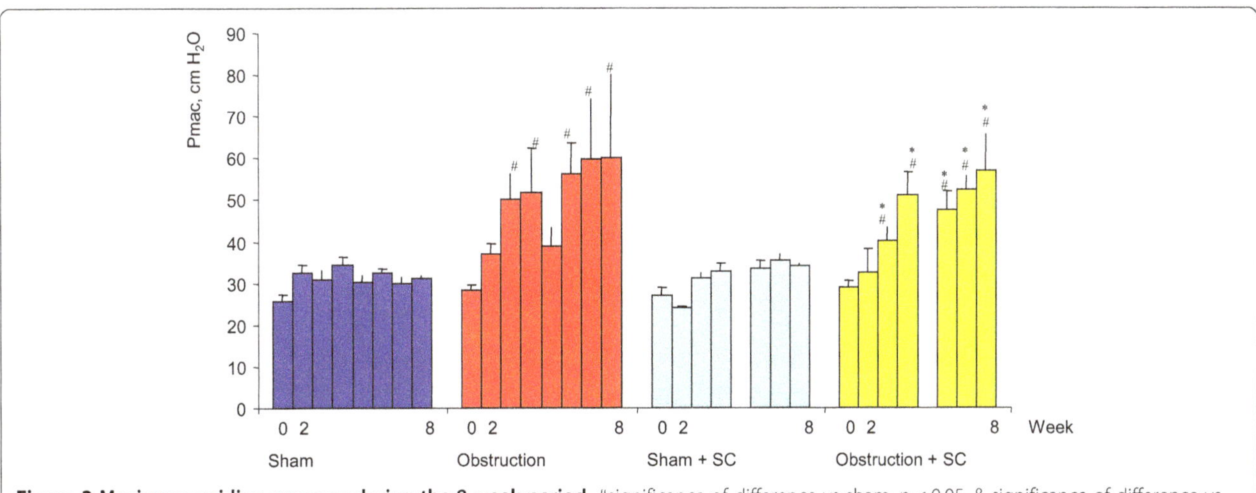

Figure 3 Maximum voiding pressure during the 8 week period. #significance of difference vs sham, $p < 0.05$, & significance of difference vs obstruction, *significance of difference versus sham + sildenafil.

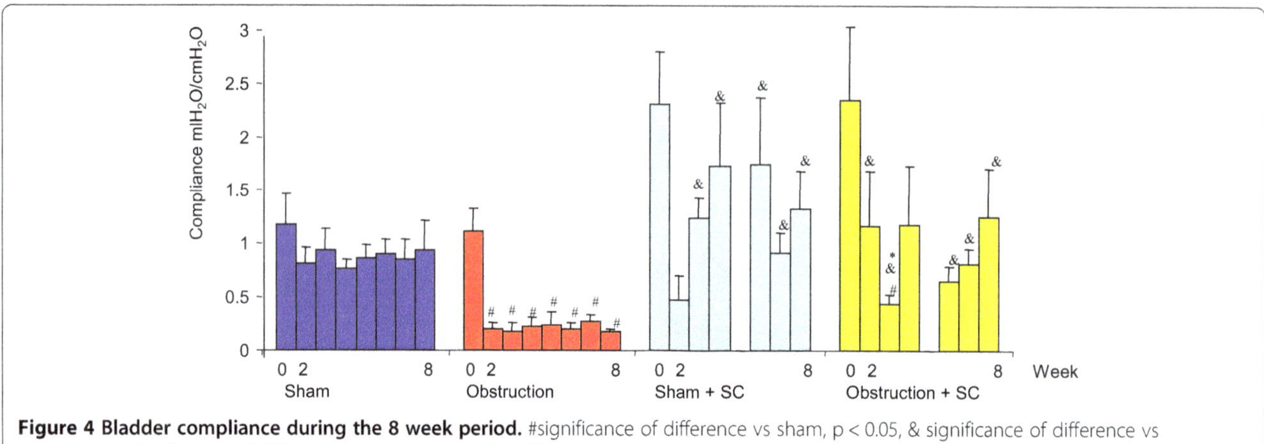

Figure 4 Bladder compliance during the 8 week period. #significance of difference vs sham, $p < 0.05$, & significance of difference vs obstruction, *significance of difference versus sham + sildenafil.

same amount of muscle cells acting under anaerobic circumstances. As a consequence, the increased contractility and voiding pressure that are needed to overcome the obstruction need less muscle mass and the bladder wall increases less in size resulting in less muscle hypertrophy. This may partly explain the better compliance and the lower bladder weight that was observed in the SC treated obstructed bladder. Low saturation may excite nerve endings in the bladder wall, leading to overactivity and higher muscle tone. Maintenance of a high saturation could prevent this nerve action and may result in better bladder compliance. In support of this is our finding that SC treated obstructed bladder shows less overactivity.

Similar effects of PDE5 inhibitors on bladder function have been found with *in vitro* muscle strip tests in a rat model of BOO [18,19]. The carbachol induced contractile force of bladder strips tested *in vitro* is reduced by BOO. Vardenafil treatment during the obstructive period diminishes this in vitro loss of carbachol induced contractility [18]. Muscle strips from sham operated rats that received vardenafil showed an increased contractility as compared to normal rat bladder strips [19]. In our experiments, we noticed a trend for increased contractility of the whole bladder in the sildenafil treated sham operated animals but this was only significant at week 8. This might be explained by a slight increase of bladder saturation during detrusor contraction. Furthermore, in the sildenafil treated sham operated animals the bladder weight was lower compared to sham + saline group. Thus, possibly the unobstructed bladder also benefits from optimal saturation.

In our experimental setup we did not determine a tissue marker for hypoxia such as glycogen or hypoxia-inducible factor 1 (HIF-1). In a previous study we demonstrated that the presence of glycogen deposits in the bladder wall correlates well with loss of bladder function in both Guinea pigs and humans [20,21]. Furthermore, we demonstrated in another study [12] that the glycogen content of the bladder wall was increased in obstructed Guinea pigs in comparison with sham operated animals. The same study revealed a good correlation between DPS measurements and glycogen deposits in the bladder wall. Therefore, we did not expect any further relevant information from tissue markers in this experimental setup and determination of glycogen deposits were not done on a regular basis.

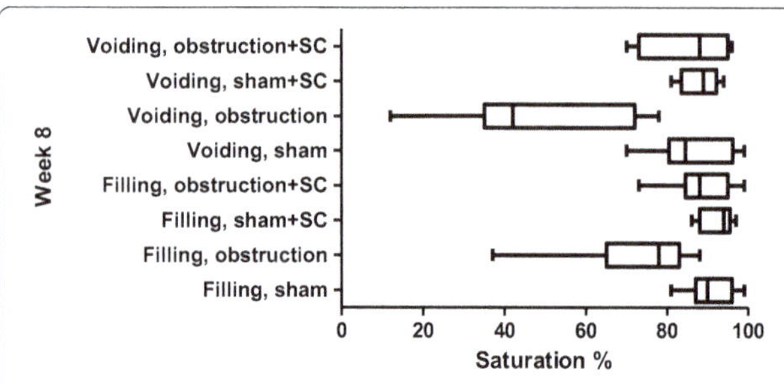

Figure 5 The % saturation during filling and voiding before sham/obstructive surgery. The bars represent the lowest, highest and average value.

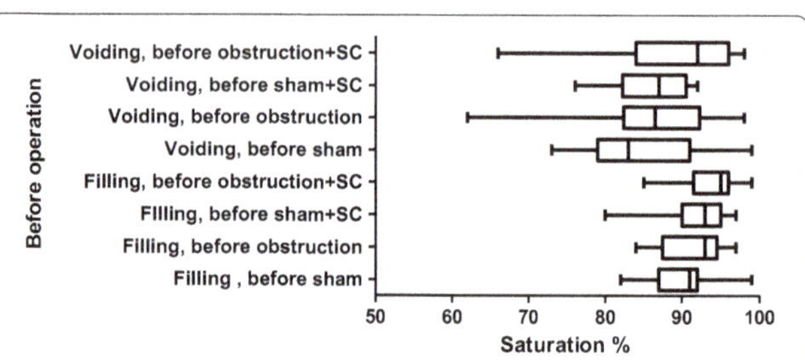

Figure 6 The % saturation during filling and voiding 8 weeks after sham/obstructive surgery. The bars represent the lowest, highest and average value.

There is evidence that oxidative stress is a key feature in the initiation and progression of voiding dysfunction [1]. Although the data are preliminary, they correlate with a mechanism where bladder dysfunction in BOO is initiated by bladder pressure related ischemia and reperfusion injury. With the present model it is not obvious if the effect is just a matter of better flow due to vessels smooth muscle relaxation or due to preservation of microvasculature or stimulation of angiogenesis. Future experiments with DPS-measurements of blood volume per cross-sectional area and measurements of vessel diameters might answer these questions.

The mechanism of increased pressure and overactivity reducing saturation that in turn reduces bladder function by impeding aerobic muscle action and by excitation of bladder nerves poses a self enhancing loop. Direct actions on the saturation part in this loop like with the PDE5 inhibitor sildenafil citrate used here may disrupt this loop and thereby might prevent the loss of bladder function that otherwise occurs.

Conclusions

In a normal bladder BOS is high in the filling phase and drops slightly during voiding. In an obstructed bladder the loss of bladder function is accompanied by a significant decrease in BOS during voiding and filling. Treatment of obstructed bladders with SC maintains normal BOS during filling and voiding resulting in high bladder compliance and less DO. This supports the hypothesis that maintaining the microcirculation of the bladder wall results in better bladder performance without significant loss of bladder function. Measurement of BOS and interventions focussing on tissue microcirculation may have a place in the evaluation/treatment of various bladder dysfunctions.

Abbreviations

BOO: Bladder outlet obstruction; BOS: Blood oxygen saturation; DPS: Differential path-length spectroscopy; NOC: Number of overactive contractions; PDE5: Phosphodiesterase 5; SC: Sildenafil citrate.

Competing interests

The authors declare that they have no competing interests.

Authors' contributions

JRS participated in de conception and design of the study, and performed acquisition and analysis of the data, and performed drafting of the manuscript. AA performed acquisition and analysis of the data, and participated in critical revision of the manuscript. KPW performed acquisition of the data and participated in critical revision of the manuscript. DJK participated in de conception and design of the study, and performed acquisition and analysis of the data. All authors read and approved the final manuscript.

Acknowledgements

Part of the study was supported by a grant from the Pfizer "OAB-LUTS" program, grant nr GA6166206.

Author details

[1]Department of Urology and Pediatric Urology, Erasmus Medical Center Rotterdam, Sophia Children's Hospital, Rotterdam, The Netherlands. [2]Department of Radiation Oncology, Center for Optical Diagnostics and Therapy, Erasmus Medical Center, Rotterdam, The Netherlands.

References

1. Brading A, Pessina F, Esposito L, Symes S: **Effects of metabolic stress and ischaemia on the bladder, and the relationship with bladder overactivity.** *Scand J Urol Nephrol* 2004, **215**(Suppl):84–92.
2. Filippi S, Morelli A, Sandner P, Fibbi B, Mancina R, Marini M, Gacci M, Vignozzi L, Vannelli GB, Carini M, Forti G, Maggi M: **Characterization and functional role of an androgen-dependent phosphodiesterase-5 activity in bladder.** *Endocrinology* 2007, **148:**1019–1029.
3. Speakman MJ: **PDE5 inhibitors in the treatment of LUTS.** *Curr Pharm Des* 2009, **15**(30):3502–3505.
4. Yanai Y, Hashitani H, Hayase M, Sasaki S, Suzuki H, Kohri K: **Role of nitric oxide/cyclic GMP pathway in regulating spontaneous excitations in detrusor smooth muscle of the guinea-pig bladder.** *Neurourol Urodyn* 2008, **27**(5):446–453.
5. Mulhall JP, Guhring P, Parker M, Hopps C: **Assessment of the impact of Sildenafil citrate on lower urinary tract symptoms in men with erectile dysfunction.** *J Sex Med* 2006, **51:**662–667.
6. Qiu Y, Kraft P, Craig EC, Liu X, Haynes-Johnson D: **Identification and functional study of phosphodiesterases in rat urinary bladder.** *Urol Res* 2001, **29:**388–392.
7. Beamon CR, Mazar C, Salkini MW, Phull HS, Comiter CV: **The effect of Sildenafil citrate on bladder outlet obstruction: a mouse model.** *BJU Int* 2009, **104**(2):252–256.
8. Gacci M, Del Popolo G, Macchiarella A, Celso M, Vittori G, Lapini A, Serni S, Sandner P, Maggi M, Carini M: **Vardenafil improves urodynamic parameters in men with spinal cord injury: resultes from a single dose, pilot study.** *J Urol* 2007, **178:**2040–2043.
9. Sairam K, Kulinskaya E, McNicholas TA, Boustead GB, Hanbury DC: **Sildenafil influences lower urinary tract symptoms.** *BJU Int* 2002, **90:**836–839.
10. Nomiya M, Burmeister DM, Sawada N, Campeau L, Zarifpour M, Keys T, Peyton C, Yamaguchi O, Andersson KE: **Prophylactic effect of tadalafil on bladder function in a rat model of chronic bladder ischemia.** *J Urol* 2013, **189:**754–761.
11. Oger S, Behr-Roussel D, Gorny D, Lebret T, Validire P, Cathelineau X, Alexandre L, Giuliano F: **Signalling pathways involved in sildenafil-induced relaxation of human bladder dome smooth muscle.** *Br J Pharmacol* 2010, **160:**1135–1143.
12. Scheepe JR, Amelink A, de Jong BWD, Wolffenbuttel KP, Kok DJ: **Changes in bladder wall blood oxygen saturation in the overactive obstructed bladder.** *J Urol* 2011, **186**(3):1128–1133.
13. Kok DJ, Wolffenbuttel KP, Minekus JP, van Mastrigt R, Nijman JM: **Changes in bladder contractility and compliance due to urethral obstruction: a longitudinal follow-up of guinea pigs.** *J Urol* 2000, **164**(3):1021–1024.
14. Wolffenbuttel KP, Kok DJ, Minekus JP, van Koeveringe GA, van Mastrigt R, Nijman JM: **Urodynamic follow-up of experimental urethral obstruction in individual guinea pigs.** *Neurourol Urodyn* 2001, **20**(6):699–713.
15. Griffiths DJ, Constantinou CE, van Mastrigt R: **Urinary bladder function and its control in healthy females.** *Am J Physiol* 1986, **251:**R225–R230.
16. Amelink A, Kaspers OP, Sterenborg HJCMHJ, Van Der Wal JE, Roodenburg JL, Witjes MJ: **Non-invasive measurement of the morphology and physiology of oral mucosa by use of optical spectroscopy.** *Oral Oncol* 2008, **44:**65–71.
17. Amelink A, Kok DJ, Sterenborg HJ, Scheepe JR: **In vivo measurement of bladder wall oxygen saturation using optical spectroscopy.** *J Biophotonics* 2011, **4**(10):715–720.
18. Matsumoto S, Hanai T, Uemura H, Levin RM: **Effects of chronic treatment with vardenafil, a phosphodiesterase 5 inhibitor, on female rat bladder in a partial bladder outlet obstruction model.** *BJU Int* 2009, **103:**987–990.
19. Matsumoto S, Hanai T, Uemura H: **Chronic treatment with a PDE5 inhibitor increases contractile force of normal bladder in rats.** *Int Urol and Nephrol* 2010, **42:**53–56.

20. de Jong BW, Wolffenbuttel KP, Scheepe JR, Kok DJ: **The detrusor glycogen content of a de-obstructed bladder reflects the functional history of that bladder during PBOO.** *Neurourol Urodyn* 2008, **27**(5):454–460.
21. Scheepe JR, de Jong BW, Wolffenbuttel KP, Arentshorst ME, Lodder P, Kok DJ: **The effect of oxybutynin on structural changes of the obstructed guinea pig bladder.** *J Urol* 2007, **178:**1807–1812.

Clinical significance of *CDH13* promoter methylation as a biomarker for bladder cancer

Feng Chen[†], Tao Huang[†], Yu Ren, Junjun Wei, Zhongguan Lou, Xue Wang, Xiaoxiao Fan, Yirun Chen, Guobin Weng and Xuping Yao[*]

Abstract

Background: Methylation of the tumor suppressor gene H-cadherin (*CDH13*) has been reported in many cancers. However, the clinical effect of the *CDH13* methylation status of patients with bladder cancer remains to be clarified.

Methods: A systematic literature search was performed to identify eligible studies in the PubMed, Embase, EBSCO, CKNI and Wanfang databases. The pooled odds ratio (OR) and the corresponding 95 % confidence interval (95 % CI) was calculated and summarized.

Results: Nine eligible studies were included in the present meta-analysis consisting of a total of 1017 bladder cancer patients and 265 non-tumor controls. A significant association was found between *CDH13* methylation levels and bladder cancer (OR = 21.71, $P < 0.001$). The results of subgroup analyses based on sample type suggested that *CDH13* methylation was significantly associated with bladder cancer risk in both the tissue and the urine (OR = 53.94, $P < 0.001$; OR = 7.71, $P < 0.001$; respectively). A subgroup analysis based on ethnic population showed that the OR value of methylated *CDH13* was higher in Asians than in Caucasians (OR = 35.18, $P < 0.001$; OR = 8.86, $P < 0.001$; respectively). The relationships between *CDH13* methylation and clinicopathological features were also analyzed. A significant association was not observed between *CDH13* methylation status and gender ($P = 0.053$). Our results revealed that *CDH13* methylation was significantly associated with high-grade bladder cancer, multiple bladder cancer and muscle invasive bladder cancer (OR = 2.22, $P < 0.001$; OR = 1.45, $P = 0.032$; OR = 3.42, $P < 0.001$; respectively).

Conclusion: Our study indicates that *CDH13* methylation may play an important role in the carcinogenesis, development and progression of bladder cancer. In addition, *CDH13* methylation has the potential to be a useful biomarker for bladder cancer screening in urine samples and to be a prognostic biomarker in the clinic.

Keywords: *CDH13* methylation, Bladder cancer, Screening, Biomarker

Abbreviations: CDH13, H-cadherin; CI, Confidence interval; MIBC, Muscle invasive bladder cancer; OR, Odds ratio; TCC, Transitional cell carcinoma; TNM, Tumor/node/metastasis.

Background

Human bladder cancer is the most common urinary system malignancy in the world. According to global cancer statistics, approximately 74,000 cases of bladder cancer will be diagnosed in the USA in 2015, leading to an estimated 16,000 deaths [1]. Bladder cancer consists of three histological and pathological types: urothelial carcinoma, squamous cell carcinoma and adenocarcinoma. Urothelial carcinoma, also known as transitional cell carcinoma (TCC), is the most common type, accounting for 90 % of all bladder cancer cases [2, 3]. Clinically, studies have shown that non-muscle invasive bladder cancer (stages Ta – T1) accounts for approximately 70–80 % of all cases, with the remainder being characterized as muscle invasive bladder cancer (stages T2–T4). Furthermore, 10–30 % of non-muscle invasive bladder cancer (NMIBC) will progress to muscle invasive bladder cancer (MIBC) [4, 5]. MIBC patients

* Correspondence: yxp4815415@163.com
[†]Equal contributors
Laboratory of Kidney Carcinoma, Ningbo urology & Nephrology Hospital, Ningbo 315040, Zhejiang, China

have a much worse outcome with regards to tumor recurrence and progression, with a 5-year survival rate of 25–60 % [6–8]. Thus, additional noninvasive biomarkers for the prediction and diagnosis of bladder cancer are needed in the clinic.

Epigenetic changes are early and frequent events in cancer that play an important role in carcinogenesis. DNA methylation is the most common epigenetic alteration in human cancers [9–11]. The detection of aberrantly methylated genes can be used as a diagnostic or prognostic biomarker for human cancers, especially when the aberrant methylation silences tumor suppressor genes [12–14]. The *CDH13* gene, located on 16q24, encodes a protein that belongs to the cadherin family [15]. *CDH13*, a tumor suppressor gene (TSG), is also called H-cadherin or T-cadherin and plays a pivotal role in cell–cell adhesion [16]. The expression of *CDH13* in human tumor cells can inhibit their invasive potential and markedly reduce their proliferation [17–19]. *CDH13* promoter methylation has been reported in some human cancers including bladder cancer [16].

However, the association between *CDH13* promoter methylation and bladder cancer remains to be clarified. In this study, a meta-analysis was conducted to evaluate the effect of *CDH13* methylation on the clinicopathological features of patients with bladder cancer.

Methods

Search strategy

A systemic literature search for studies published prior to November 16, 2015 was conducted in the PubMed, Embase, EBSCO, CKNI and Wanfang databases without any language restrictions. The following keywords and search terms were used: (CDH13 OR cadherin 13 OR H-cadherin OR T-cadherin) AND (bladder cancer OR bladder tumor OR bladder carcinoma OR bladder neoplasm) AND (methylation OR epigenetic silencing). The reference lists of the retrieved articles and reviews were then manually searched to identify potentially relevant studies.

Inclusion criteria

The eligible studies met the following criteria: 1) the patients were diagnosed with bladder cancer based on histopathology; 2) *CDH13* methylation was evaluated in different types of samples, such as tissue, serum, plasma and urine; 3) regarding control samples by cystoscopy and histopathological confirmation, tissue samples belonged to normal tissues, while fluid samples such as serum, plasma or urine were from healthy individuals or patients with benign urological diseases; 4) the studies showed the associations between *CDH13* methylation and clinicopathological parameters, including gender (male vs female), cancer tumor/node/metastasis (TNM) stage (T2/T4 vs Ta/T1), grade (grade 3 vs grade1/2) or tumor number (multiple vs single); 5) the methylation frequency of the *CDH13* gene was sufficient for the case-control or cohort studies; 6) the studies were published in English or Chinese. The studies that were excluded did not meet our inclusion criteria. When the authors published more than one paper using the same sample data, either the most recent study or the study using the largest sample size was selected. The current meta-analysis was reported based on the Preferred Reporting Items for Systematic Reviews and Meta-Analysis (PRISMA) statement.

Data extraction

The following pieces of information from the eligible studies were collected: first author surname, year of publication, ethnicity, histological type, types of samples, detection method, number of samples, clinicopathological parameters, gender, stage, grade, tumor number, frequency of *CDH13* methylation, etc. As a control group, our meta-analysis used non-cancerous samples including non-cancerous diseases of the bladder and normal healthy tissue, according to each individual study in the original literature. Of these studies, a tumor stage of ≤ 1 was defined as early stage, a tumor stage of ≥ 2 was defined as advanced stage, a tumor grade of ≤ 2 was defined as low-grade, and a tumor grade of 3 was defined as high-grade. The final eligible studies were independently assessed by two reviewers for the current meta-analysis.

Data analysis

The analysis was conducted using STATA 12.0 (Stata Corporation) to evaluate the relationships between *CDH13* methylation and bladder cancer via the pooled odds ratio (OR) and the corresponding 95 % confidence interval (95 % CI). The frequency of *CDH13* methylation was analyzed according to various cancer characteristics. A statistical test for heterogeneity was performed based on the chi-square test and Q statistic [20]. If substantial heterogeneity ($I^2 \geq 50$ % or $p < 0.1$) was observed, a random-effects model was used to calculate the parameters. Otherwise, a fixed effects model assuming a lack of heterogeneity was used [21, 22]. Egger's test was used to evaluate for possible publication bias [23]. A p value of less than 0.05 was considered statistically significant.

Results

Study characteristics

The search method described above obtained 49 potentially relevant articles. We carefully reviewed the titles, abstracts and full-texts of the articles. In total, 9 published studies (English, 7; Chinese, 2) met the inclusion criteria of the present meta-analysis [24–32] and

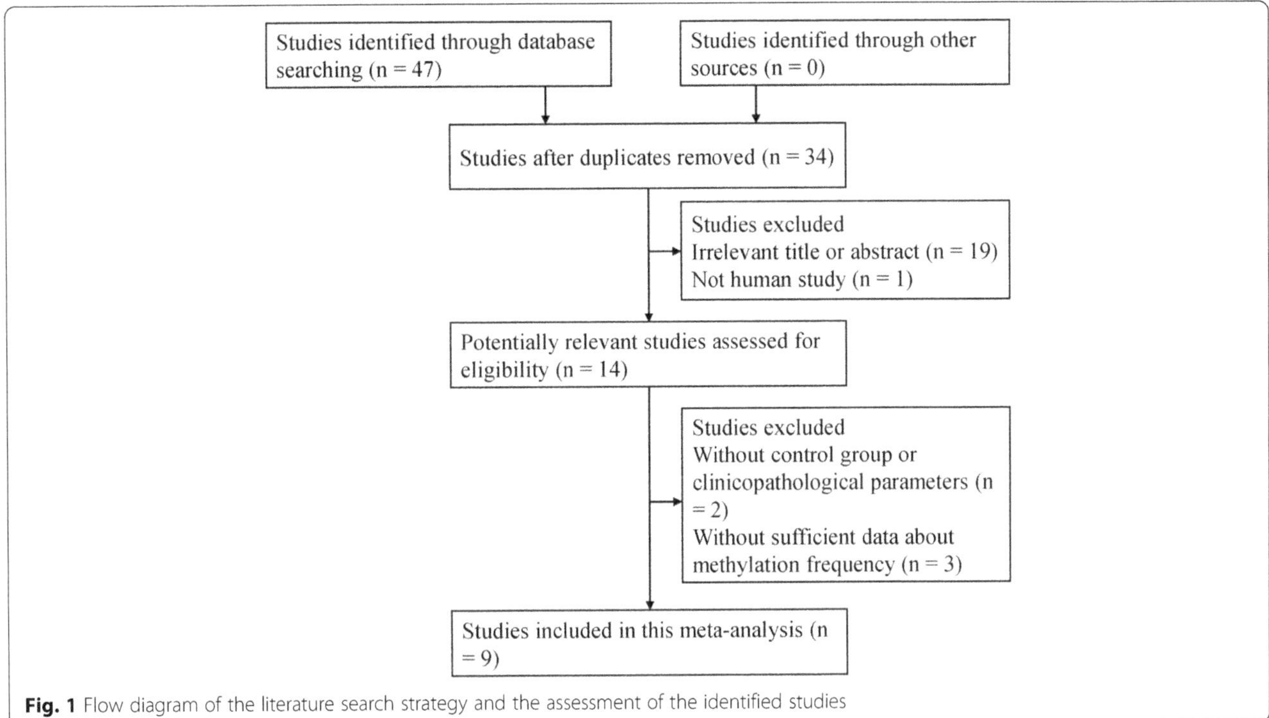

Fig. 1 Flow diagram of the literature search strategy and the assessment of the identified studies

included 1017 bladder cancer patients and 265 controls, as shown in Fig. 1. Of these studies, 8 studies assessed the association between *CDH13* methylation and bladder cancer risk, 5 studies evaluated the relationship between *CDH13* methylation and gender, 5 studies explored the association between *CDH13* methylation and tumor number, 4 studies reported the tumor grade (grade 3 vs grade 1-2), and 5 studies evaluated the effect of clinical stage (T2-T4 vs Ta-T1). The main characteristics of the included studies were presented in Table 1.

CDH13 methylation and the risk of bladder caner

The heterogeneity among the studies was not significant ($p = 0.495$ and $I^2 = 0.0$ %), and therefore, the fixed effects model was used. The OR value of *CDH13* methylation in bladder cancer patients compared with non-tumor controls was 21.71 (95 % CI: 9.83–47.94, $P < 0.001$) (Fig. 2); this analysis included 920 bladder cancer patients and 265 controls. Subgroup analyses were performed to investigate the difference in *CDH13* methylation according to sample type (tissue and urine) and ethnicity (Caucasians and Asians) (Table 2). The results showed that the pooled OR value for the tissue group was higher than that of the urine group (OR = 53.94, 95 % CI = 12.83–226.87, $P < 0.001$; OR = 7.71, 95 % CI = 2.65–22.39, $P < 0.001$; respectively). The subgroup analysis according to ethnic populations revealed that the OR value of methylated *CDH13* in Asians was higher than in Caucasians

Table 1 Basic characteristics of the studies included in the current meta-analysis

					Methylation %		Number		Gender		Grade		Stage		Tumor number	
First author	Year	Ethnicity	Method	Sample	Case	Control	Cases	Controls	Male	Female	3	1-2	≥2	≤1	Multiple	Single
Maruyama et al.	2001	Caucasians	MSP	Tissue	29.9 %	-	97	-	-	-	65	32	-	-	-	-
Meng et al.	2007	Asians	MSP	Urine	15.2 %	0 %	92	30	-	-	-	-	27	65	-	-
Yu et al.	2007	Asians	MSP	Urine	16.7 %	0 %	132	30	-	-	-	-	-	-	-	-
Cabello et al.	2011	Caucasians	*	Urine	27.1 %	6 %	96	50	-	-	36	60	18	78	-	-
Agundez et al.	2011	Caucasians	*	Tissue	62.6 %	0 %	91	10	82	9	-	-	-	-	44	47
Lin et al.	2011	Asians	MSP	Serum	30.7 %	0 %	127	41	88	39	31	96	49	78	74	53
Lin et al.	2012	Asians	MSP	Tissue	35.3 %	0 %	133	43	94	39	37	96	48	85	82	51
Lin et al.	2013	Asians	MSP	Tissue	60.6 %	0 %	71	23	49	22	-	-	32	39	43	28
Lin et al.	2014	Asians	MSP	Tissue	44.9 %	0 %	178	38	124	54	-	-	-	-	76	102

MSP methylation-specific polymerase chain reaction, "-" indicates data not available
*indicates MS-MLPA (Methylation-Specific Multiplex Ligation-Dependent Probe Amplification)

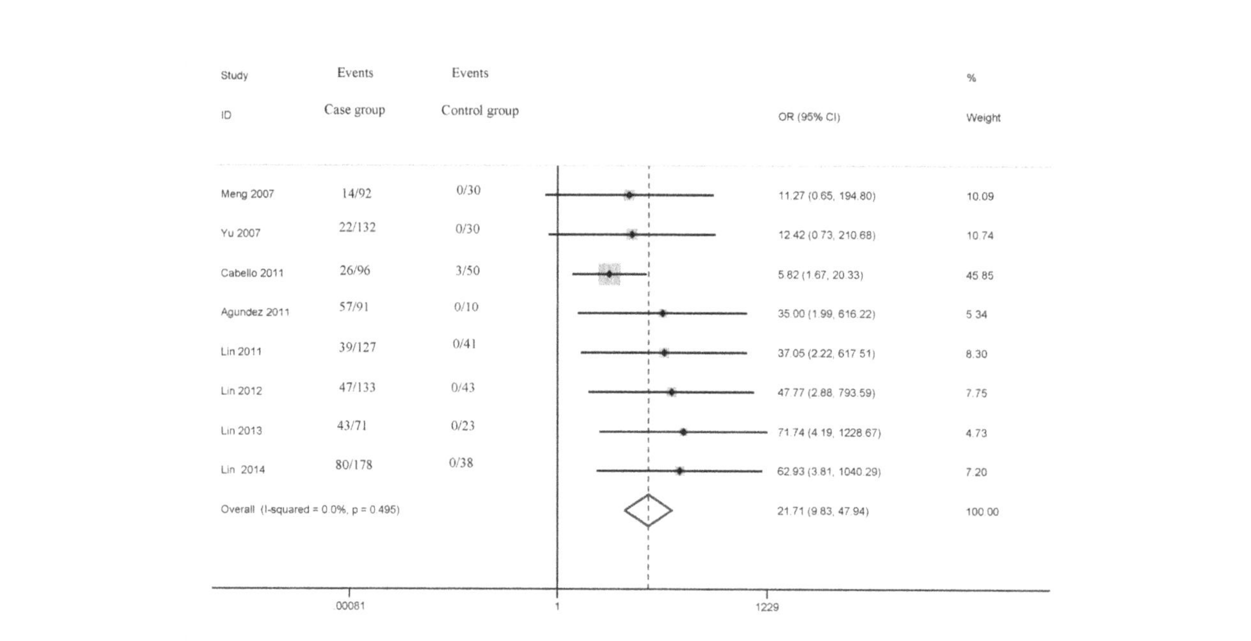

Fig. 2 Forest plot of the association between *CDH13* methylation and bladder cancer from a fixed-effects model, including 8 studies with 920 bladder cancer patients and 265 controls, OR = 21.71, 95 % CI: 9.83–47.94, *P* < 0.001

(OR = 35.18, 95 % CI = 11.20–110.55, *P* < 0.001; OR = 8.86, 95 % CI = 2.91–27.03, *P* < 0.001; respectively).

The relationships between *CDH13* methylation and clinicopathological features

The associations between *CDH13* methylation and clinicopathological features were analyzed, as shown in Table 3. The analyses of *CDH13* methylation and gender, tumor grade and tumor number used the random effects model, while a fixed effects model was used for tumor stage. A significant association was not found between *CDH13* methylation and gender in the 5 studies analyzed (OR = 1.46, 95 % CI = 0.99–2.15, *P* = 0.053), which included 437 male patients and 163 female patients (Fig. 3). The pooled OR from 5 studies including 174 advanced bladder cancer patients and 345 early stage bladder cancer patients indicated that *CDH13* methylation was significantly higher in advanced stage tumors than in early stage tumors (OR = 3.42, 95 % CI = 1.72–6.80, *P* < 0.001) (Fig. 4). Results from 4 studies comparing a total of 169 high-grade patients and 284 low-grade patients showed that *CDH13* methylation was significantly associated with high-grade bladder cancer (OR = 2.22, 95 % CI = 1.72–6.80, *P* < 0.001) (Fig. 5). Results from 5 studies analyzing a total of 319 bladder cancer patients with multiple tumors and 281 bladder cancer patients with single tumors demonstrated that methylated *CDH13* was significantly associated with patients harboring multiple tumors (OR = 1.45, 95 % CI = 1.03–2.04, *P* = 0.032) (Fig. 6).

Table 2 Summary of the relationship between *CDH13* methylation and bladder cancer

	Studies	Overall OR (95 % CI)	I^2; p	*P* value	Cases	Controls	p (Egger's test)
Total	8	21.71 (9.83–47.94)	0.0 %; 0.495	<0.001	920	265	0.008
Material:							
Urine	3	7.71 (2.65–22.39)	0.0 %; 0.831	<0.001	320	110	
Tissue	4	53.94 (12.83–226.87)	0.0 %; 0.986	<0.001	473	114	
Race:							
Caucasians	2	8.86 (2.91–27.03)	24.0 %; 0.251	<0.001	187	60	
Asians	6	35.18 (11.20–110.55)	0.0 %; 0.903	<0.001	733	205	

CDH13 H-cadherin, *OR* odds ratio, *CI* confidence interval

Table 3 The correlations between *CDH13* methylation and clinicopathological features

	Studies	Overall OR (95 % CI)	I^2; p	*P* value	p (Egger's test)	Patients	
Gender						Male	Female
	5	1.46 (0.99–2.15)	0.0 %; 0.496	0.053	0.085	437	163
Grade						High-grade	Low-grade
	4	2.22 (1.43–3.43)	0.0 %; 0.641	<0.001	0.613	169	284
Stage						MIBC	NMIBC
	5	3.42 (1.72–6.80)	59.0 %; 0.045	<0.001	0.279	174	345
Number						Multiple	Single
	5	1.45 (1.03–2.04)	0.0 %; 0.779	0.032	0.038	319	281

MIBC muscle invasive bladder cancer (stages T2–T4), *NMIBC* non-muscle invasive bladder cancer (stages Ta – T1), *low-grade* tumor grade ≤ 2, *high-grade* tumor grade of 3

Significant heterogeneity was found in relation to tumor stage in cancer ($I^2 = 59.0$ %, $p = 0.045$). Thus, a sensitivity analysis by omitting a single study was carried out to assess the stability of the pooled OR. When we removed this study by Lin 2011 et al. [25], the heterogeneity was significantly decreased, with the absence of heterogeneity ($I^2 = 14.7$ %, $p = 0.318$). However, the pooled OR of *CDH13* promoter methylation was not significantly changed (OR = 2.75, 95 % = 1.71–4.44, $P < 0.001$), suggesting the stability of our analyses.

Publication bias

Egger's test was performed to assess for publication bias of the included studies (Tables 2 and 3). Egger's

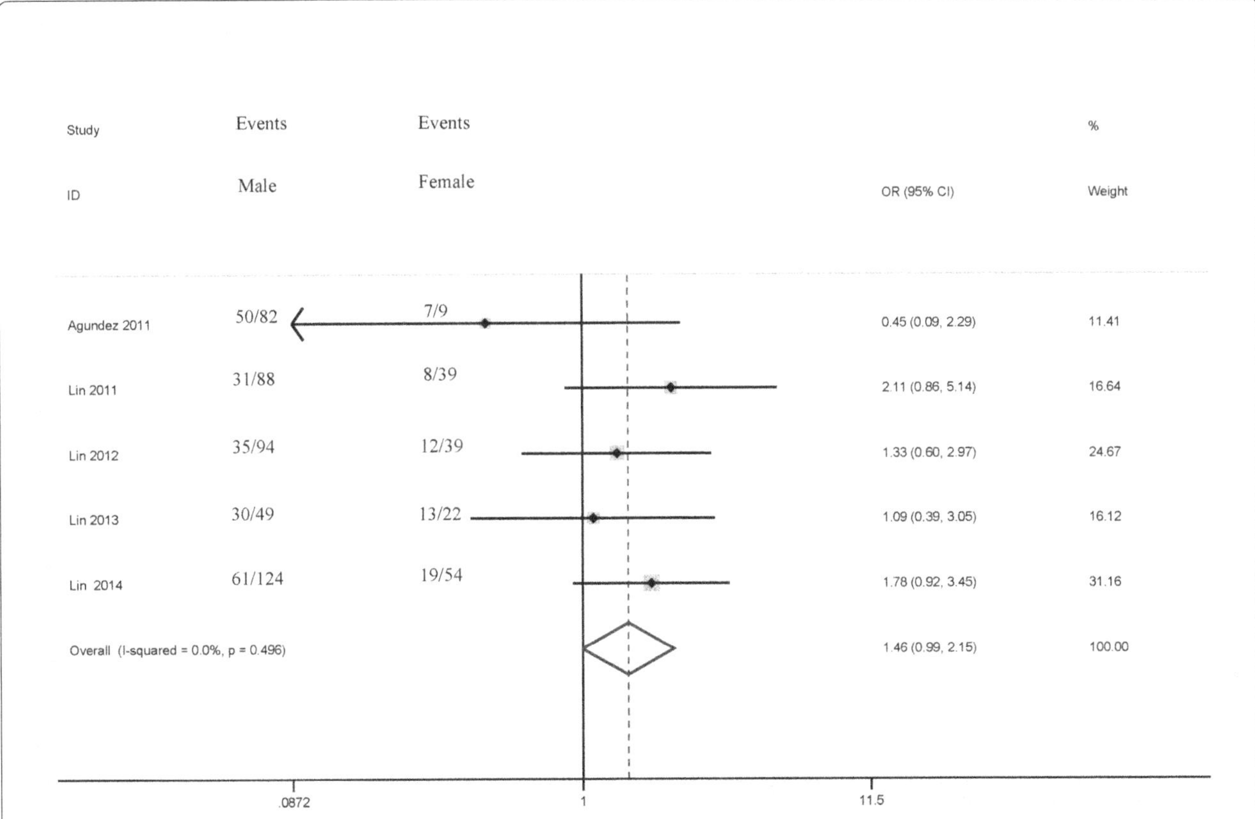

Fig. 3 Forest plot of the association between *CDH13* methylation and gender from a fixed-effects model, including 5 studies with 437 male patients and 163 female patients, OR = 1.46, 95 % CI = 0.99–2.15, *P* = 0.053

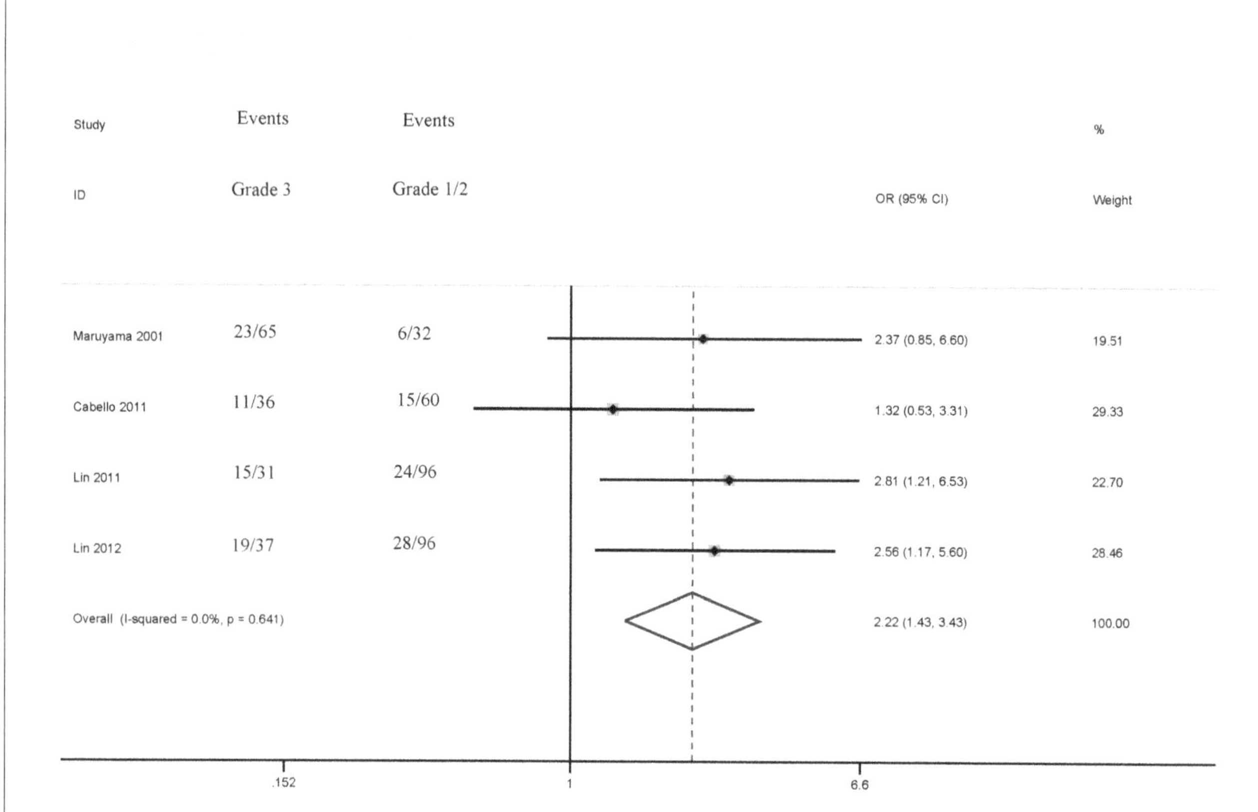

Fig. 4 Forest plot of the association between *CDH13* methylation and tumor grade from a fixed-effects model, including 4 studies with 169 high-grade patients and 284 low-grade patients, OR = 2.22, 95 % CI = 1.72–6.80, $P < 0.001$

test provided strong statistical evidence for a publication bias in the comparison between *CDH13* methylation of bladder cancer patients and non-tumor controls ($p = 0.008$). The relatively small number of control samples (265 controls versus 920 bladder cancer patients) may cause publication bias. Egger's test indicated a lack of publication bias in the current analysis of *CDH13* methylation status and clinicopathological features ($p > 0.05$). Egger's funnel plot of the publication bias test for *CDH13* methylation was shown in Additional file 1: Table S1.

Discussion

DNA methylation in the blood, sputum, urine, feces, and other bodily fluids can be used as a non-invasive biomarker for the early detection of various cancers [12, 33, 34]. Aberrant methylation of the *CDH13* gene has been reported in many cancers, including non-small cell lung cancer [35], breast cancer [36], gastric cancer [37], and colorectal carcinoma [38]. However, the potential of *CDH13* gene methylation to be a biomarker for bladder cancer has not yet been evaluated. The methylation rate of *CDH13* gene was relatively lower in non-tumor control samples, with a mean methylation frequency of 1.1 % in this study. The findings of the current study showed that *CDH13* promoter methylation was significantly higher in bladder cancer patients than in non-tumor control samples (OR = 21.71, $P < 0.001$), suggesting that the methylation of *CDH13* may be involved in the development of bladder cancer. No significant heterogeneity was observed in cancer vs. controls ($p = 0.495$ and $I^2 = 0.0$ %), indicating the reliability of our results. In addition, the result of a subgroup analysis based on sample type suggested that the *CDH13* methylation status was significant in both tissue and urine samples (OR = 53.94, $P < 0.001$; OR = 7.71, $P < 0.001$; respectively), indicating that the detection of *CDH13* methylation has the potential to be a non-invasive biomarker in the urine, which may aid in the early screening for and the diagnosis of bladder cancer. The OR value in Asians (OR = 35.18, $P < 0.001$) was significantly higher than in Caucasians (OR = 8.86, $P < 0.001$), which revealed that *CDH13* methylation may be a relatively more important risk factor among Asian populations.

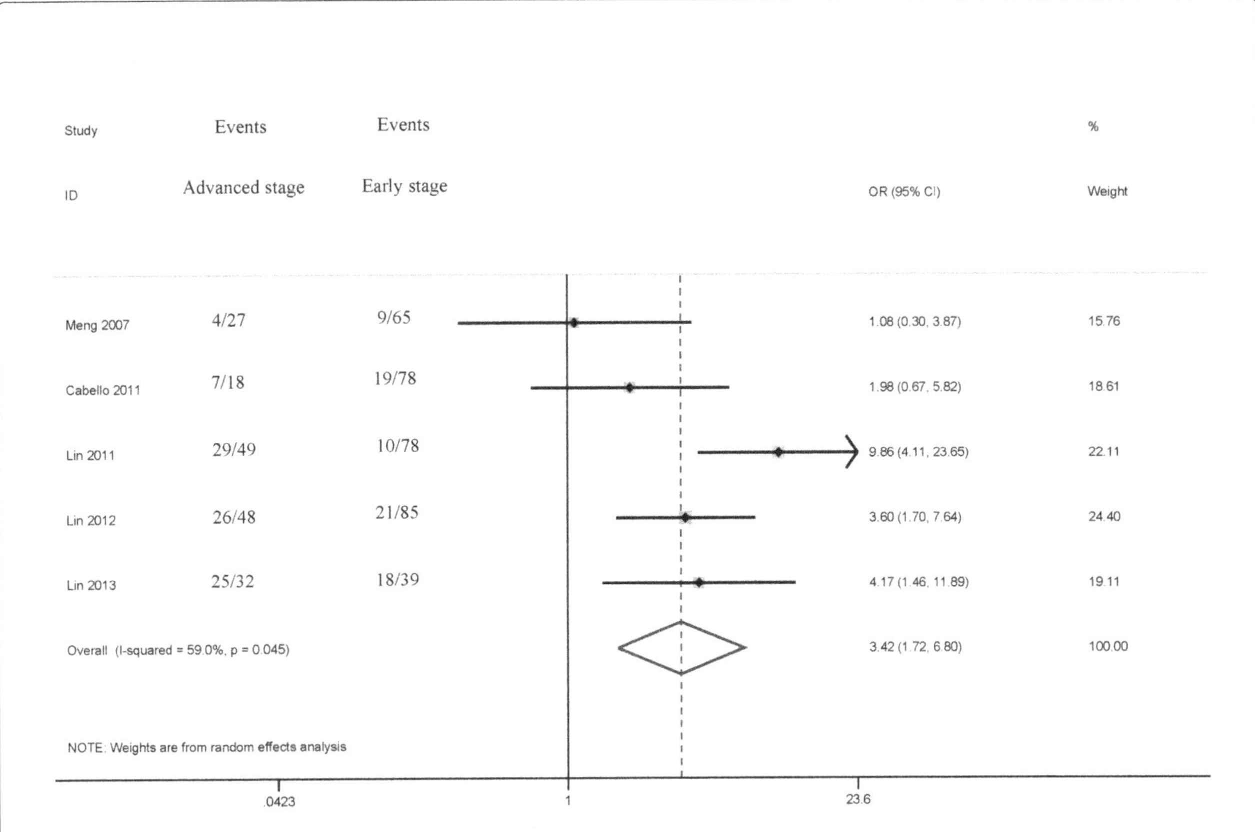

Fig. 5 Forest plot of the correlation between *CDH13* methylation and tumor stage from a random-effects model, including 5 studies with 174 advanced bladder cancer patients and 345 early stage bladder cancer patients, OR = 3.42, 95 % CI = 1.72–6.80, $P < 0.001$

In addition, we conducted meta-analyses to determine the correlations between *CDH13* methylation and clinicopathological characteristics. The results showed that the *CDH13* methylation status was not associated with gender (OR = 1.46, 95 % CI = 0.99–2.15, $P = 0.053$). The levels of methylated *CDH13* were significantly higher in muscle invasive bladder cancer (stages T2–T4) than in non-muscle invasive bladder cancer (stages Ta – T1) (OR = 3.42, $P < 0.001$). *CDH13* methylation status was significantly associated with high-grade (grade 3) bladder cancer (OR = 2.22, $P < 0.001$). The levels of methylated *CDH13* were significantly higher in bladder cancer consisting of multiple tumors than in bladder cancer consisting of a single tumor (OR = 1.45, $P = 0.032$). Patients with multiple tumors, high-grade bladder cancer, or muscle invasive bladder cancer are characterized by a high incidence of recurrence and progression and a poorer outcome [39, 40]. Our findings indicated that *CDH13* promoter methylation was a very useful biomarker that can predict the recurrence of bladder cancer.

Some limitations of the current meta-analysis should be considered. First, the inclusion of articles published only in English and Chinese might lead to a selection bias. Second, the primary ethnic population of the patients in the current study was Asian, while only two studies involving Caucasians were involved in this meta-analysis. Other ethnicities, such as Africans, were limited. Third, due to the limitation of eligible studies in fluid samples, we did not further evaluate the diagnostic capacity of *CDH13* promoter methylation for patients with non-muscle invasive bladder cancer. Thus, more studies based on urine and blood samples are very essential to evaluate whether *CDH13* promoter methylation can become a noninvasive biomarker for the detection and diagnosis of non-muscle invasive bladder cancer in the future. Therefore, additional studies incorporating larger sample sizes are required to confirm our results in the future.

Conclusion

Our study indicates that *CDH13* methylation may play a key role in the initiation and progression of bladder cancer, especially among Asian populations. In addition, *CDH13* methylation has the potential to become a useful

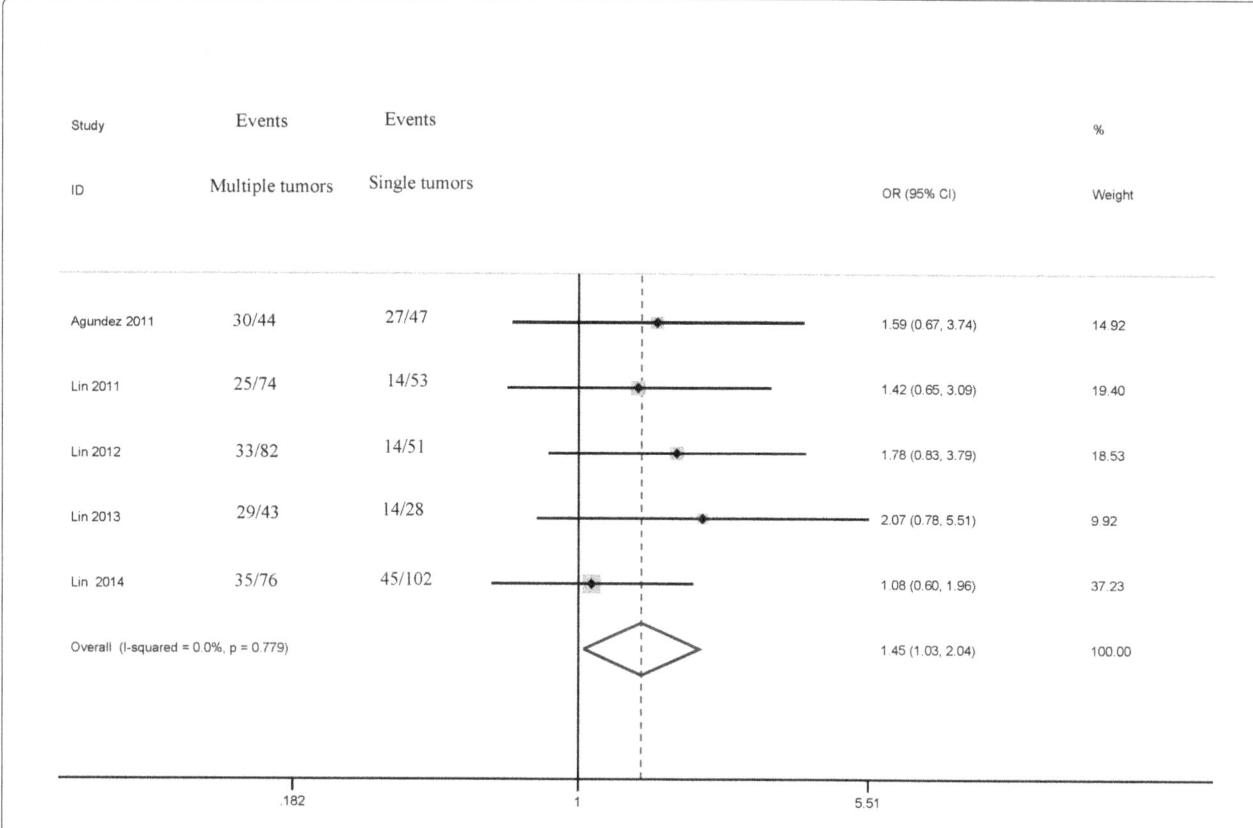

Fig. 6 Forest plot of the correlation between *CDH13* methylation and tumor number form a fixed-effects model, including 5 studies with 319 bladder cancer patients with multiple tumors and 281 bladder cancer patients with single tumors, OR = 1.45, 95 % CI = 1.03–2.04, *P* = 0.032

biomarker for the clinical screening of bladder cancer in the urine. *CDH13* methylation may also be a prognostic biomarker for patients with tumor progression.

Acknowledgements
This research was supported by grants from the Ningbo Natural Science Foundation "2009A610115 and 2009A610143".

Authors' contributions
FC and XY contributed to the conception, design and final approval of the submitted manuscript. FC, TH, YR, JW, ZL, XW, XF, YC and GW contributed to the completion of article analysis the data extraction and the calculation and design of the figures and tables. All the authors approved the final manuscript.

Competing interests
The authors declare that they have no competing interests.

References

1. Siegel RL, Miller KD, Jemal A. Cancer statistics, 2015. CA Cancer J Clin. 2015;65:5–29.
2. Fleshner NE, Herr HW, Stewart AK, Murphy GP, Mettlin C, Menck HR. The national cancer data base report on bladder carcinoma. The american college of surgeons commission on cancer and the american cancer society. Cancer. 1996;78:1505–13.
3. Kantor AF, Hartge P, Hoover RN, Fraumeni Jr JF. Epidemiological characteristics of squamous cell carcinoma and adenocarcinoma of the bladder. Cancer Res. 1988;48:3853–5.
4. Gierth M, Burger M. Bladder cancer. Progress in defining progression in nmibc. Nat Rev Urol. 2013;10:684–5.
5. Jacobs BL, Lee CT, Montie JE. Bladder cancer in 2010: How far have we come? CA Cancer J Clin. 2010;60:244–72.
6. Black PC, Dinney CP. Bladder cancer angiogenesis and metastasis–translation from murine model to clinical trial. Cancer Metastasis Rev. 2007;26:623–34.
7. Herr HW, Dotan Z, Donat SM, Bajorin DF. Defining optimal therapy for muscle invasive bladder cancer. J Urol. 2007;177:437–43.
8. Shariat SF, Karakiewicz PI, Palapattu GS, Lotan Y, Rogers CG, Amiel GE, et al. Outcomes of radical cystectomy for transitional cell carcinoma of the bladder: A contemporary series from the bladder cancer research consortium. J Urol. 2006;176:2414–22.
9. Ghavifekr Fakhr M, Farshdousti Hagh M, Shanehbandi D, Baradaran B. DNA methylation pattern as important epigenetic criterion in cancer. Genet Res Int. 2013;2013:317569.
10. Delpu Y, Cordelier P, Cho WC, Torrisani J. DNA methylation and cancer diagnosis. Int J Mol Sci. 2013;14:15029–58.
11. Ma X, Wang YW, Zhang MQ, Gazdar AF. DNA methylation data analysis and its application to cancer research. Epigenomics. 2013;5:301–16.
12. Shivapurkar N, Gazdar AF. DNA methylation based biomarkers in non-invasive cancer screening. Curr Mol Med. 2010;10:123–32.
13. Kim YK, Kim WJ. Epigenetic markers as promising prognosticators for bladder cancer. Int J Urol. 2009;16:17–22.
14. Paluszczak J, Baer-Dubowska W. Epigenetic diagnostics of cancer–the application of DNA methylation markers. J Appl Genet. 2006;47:365–75.

15. Takeuchi T, Ohtsuki Y. Recent progress in t-cadherin (cdh13, h-cadherin) research. Histol Histopathol. 2001;16:1287–93.
16. Andreeva AV, Kutuzov MA. Cadherin 13 in cancer. Genes Chromosomes Cancer. 2010;49:775–90.
17. Kuphal S, Martyn AC, Pedley J, Crowther LM, Bonazzi VF, Parsons PG, et al. H-cadherin expression reduces invasion of malignant melanoma. Pigment Cell Melanoma Res. 2009;22:296–306.
18. Lee SW, Reimer CL, Campbell DB, Cheresh P, Duda RB, Kocher O. H-cadherin expression inhibits *in vitro* invasiveness and tumor formation *in vivo*. Carcinogenesis. 1998;19:1157–9.
19. Lee SW. H-cadherin, a novel cadherin with growth inhibitory functions and diminished expression in human breast cancer. Nat Med. 1996;2:776–82.
20. Zintzaras E, Ioannidis JP. Hegesma: Genome search meta-analysis and heterogeneity testing. Bioinformatics. 2005;21:3672–3.
21. Higgins JP, Thompson SG, Deeks JJ, Altman DG. Measuring inconsistency in meta-analyses. BMJ. 2003;327:557–60.
22. DerSimonian R. Meta-analysis in the design and monitoring of clinical trials. Stat Med. 1996;15:1237–48.
23. Egger M, Davey Smith G, Schneider M, Minder C. Bias in meta-analysis detected by a simple, graphical test. BMJ. 1997;315:629–34.
24. Lin YL, Xie PG, Ma JG. Aberrant methylation of cdh13 is a potential biomarker for predicting the recurrence and progression of non muscle invasive bladder cancer. Med Sci Monit. 2014;20:1572–7.
25. Lin YL, Sun G, Liu XQ, Li WP, Ma JG. Clinical significance of cdh13 promoter methylation in serum samples from patients with bladder transitional cell carcinoma. J Int Med Res. 2011;39:179–86.
26. Lin YL, Liu XQ, Li WP, Sun G, Zhang CT. Promoter methylation of h-cadherin is a potential biomarker in patients with bladder transitional cell carcinoma. Int Urol Nephrol. 2012;44:111–7.
27. Agundez M, Grau L, Palou J, Algaba F, Villavicencio H, Sanchez-Carbayo M. Evaluation of the methylation status of tumour suppressor genes for predicting bacillus calmette-guerin response in patients with t1g3 high-risk bladder tumours. Eur Urol. 2011;60:131–40.
28. Cabello MJ, Grau L, Franco N, Orenes E, Alvarez M, Blanca A, et al. Multiplexed methylation profiles of tumor suppressor genes in bladder cancer. J Mol Diagn. 2011;13:29–40.
29. Yu J, Zhu T, Wang Z, Zhang H, Qian Z, Xu H, et al. A novel set of DNA methylation markers in urine sediments for sensitive/specific detection of bladder cancer. Clin Cancer Res. 2007;13:7296–304.
30. Maruyama R, Toyooka S, Toyooka KO, Harada K, Virmani AK, Zochbauer-Muller S, et al. Aberrant promoter methylation profile of bladder cancer and its relationship to clinicopathological features. Cancer Res. 2001;61:8659–63.
31. Meng J, Yu J, Zhu T, Zhang H, Xu H, Wang W, et al. Detection of bladder cancer by accessing DNA methylation state in urine sediments. Tumor. 2007;27:374–8.
32. Lin Y, Guan T, Xiang D, Sun G, Wu G, Wang H. The clinical significance of the promoter methylation of CDHI3 gene in bladder cancer. Int J Urol Nephrol. 2013;33:174–7.
33. Kristiansen S, Nielsen D, Soletormos G. Methylated DNA for monitoring tumor growth and regression: How do we get there? Crit Rev Clin Lab Sci. 2014;51:149–59.
34. Qureshi SA, Bashir MU, Yaqinuddin A. Utility of DNA methylation markers for diagnosing cancer. Int J Surg. 2010;8:194–8.
35. Drilon A, Sugita H, Sima CS, Zauderer M, Rudin CM, Kris MG, et al. A prospective study of tumor suppressor gene methylation as a prognostic biomarker in surgically resected stage i to iiia non-small-cell lung cancers. J Thorac Oncol. 2014;9:1272–7.
36. Moelans CB, de Groot JS, Pan X, van der Wall E, van Diest PJ. Clonal intratumor heterogeneity of promoter hypermethylation in breast cancer by ms-mlpa. Mod Pathol. 2014;27:869–74.
37. Tahara T, Maegawa S, Chung W, Garriga J, Jelinek J, Estecio MR, et al. Examination of whole blood DNA methylation as a potential risk marker for gastric cancer. Cancer Prev Res (Phila). 2013;6:1093–100.
38. Konishi K, Watanabe Y, Shen L, Guo Y, Castoro RJ, Kondo K, et al. DNA methylation profiles of primary colorectal carcinoma and matched liver metastasis. PLoS One. 2011;6:e27889.
39. Lopez-Beltran A. Bladder cancer: Clinical and pathological profile. Scand J Urol Nephrol Suppl. 2008;42:95-109.
40. Dalbagni G. The management of superficial bladder cancer. Nat Clin Pract Urol. 2007;4:254–60.

Permissions

All chapters in this book were first published in UROLOGY, by BioMed Central; hereby published with permission under the Creative Commons Attribution License or equivalent. Every chapter published in this book has been scrutinized by our experts. Their significance has been extensively debated. The topics covered herein carry significant findings which will fuel the growth of the discipline. They may even be implemented as practical applications or may be referred to as a beginning point for another development.

The contributors of this book come from diverse backgrounds, making this book a truly international effort. This book will bring forth new frontiers with its revolutionizing research information and detailed analysis of the nascent developments around the world.

We would like to thank all the contributing authors for lending their expertise to make the book truly unique. They have played a crucial role in the development of this book. Without their invaluable contributions this book wouldn't have been possible. They have made vital efforts to compile up to date information on the varied aspects of this subject to make this book a valuable addition to the collection of many professionals and students.

This book was conceptualized with the vision of imparting up-to-date information and advanced data in this field. To ensure the same, a matchless editorial board was set up. Every individual on the board went through rigorous rounds of assessment to prove their worth. After which they invested a large part of their time researching and compiling the most relevant data for our readers.

The editorial board has been involved in producing this book since its inception. They have spent rigorous hours researching and exploring the diverse topics which have resulted in the successful publishing of this book. They have passed on their knowledge of decades through this book. To expedite this challenging task, the publisher supported the team at every step. A small team of assistant editors was also appointed to further simplify the editing procedure and attain best results for the readers.

Apart from the editorial board, the designing team has also invested a significant amount of their time in understanding the subject and creating the most relevant covers. They scrutinized every image to scout for the most suitable representation of the subject and create an appropriate cover for the book.

The publishing team has been an ardent support to the editorial, designing and production team. Their endless efforts to recruit the best for this project, has resulted in the accomplishment of this book. They are a veteran in the field of academics and their pool of knowledge is as vast as their experience in printing. Their expertise and guidance has proved useful at every step. Their uncompromising quality standards have made this book an exceptional effort. Their encouragement from time to time has been an inspiration for everyone.

The publisher and the editorial board hope that this book will prove to be a valuable piece of knowledge for researchers, students, practitioners and scholars across the globe.

List of Contributors

Hiroaki Kobayashi, Eiji Kikuchi, Takahiro Maeda, Nobuyuki Tanaka, Akira Miyajima, Ken Nakagawa and Mototsugu Oya
Department of Urology, Keio University School of Medicine, 35 Shinanomachi, Shinjuku-ku, Tokyo 160-8582, Japan

Shuji Mikami
Division of Diagnostic Pathology, Keio University School of Medicine, 35 Shinanomachi, Shinjuku-ku, Tokyo 160-8582, Japan

Shunichiro Nomura, Yasutomo Suzuki, Ryo Takahashi, Ryoji Kimata, Tsutomu Hamasaki, Go Kimura and Yukihiro Kondo
Departments of Urology, Nippon Medical School, 1-1-5 Sendagi, Bunkyo-ku, Tokyo 113-8603, Japan

Mika Terasaki, Akira Shimizu and Yasuhiro Terasaki
Analytic Human Pathology, Nippon Medical School, 1-1-5 Sendagi, Bunkyo-ku, Tokyo 113-8603, Japan

Hiromitsu Negoro and Osamu Ogawa
Department of Urology, Kyoto University Graduate School of Medicine, Kyoto, Japan

Nobuyuki Nishikawa
Department of Urology, Kyoto University Graduate School of Medicine, Kyoto, Japan
Department of Cell Physiology, Nagoya City University Graduate School of Medical Sciences, Nagoya, Japan

Masaaki Imamura
Department of Urology, Kyoto University Graduate School of Medicine, Kyoto, Japan
Department of Urology, Otsu Red Cross Hospital, Otsu, Japan

Rie Yago, Mari Suzuki and Kazunari Tanabe
Department of Urology, Tokyo Women's Medical University, Tokyo, Japan

Yuichiro Yamazaki
Department of Urology, Kanagawa Children's Medical Centre, Yokohama, Japan

Yoshinobu Toda
Department of Clinical Laboratory Science, Tenri Health Care University, Tenri, Japan

Akihiro Kanematsu
Department of Urology, Hyogo College of Medicine, Nishinomiya, Japan

Yongquan Wang, Zhiyong Xiong, Zhansong Zhou and Gensheng Lu
Center of Urology, Southwest Hospita, Third Militar, Medical University, 400038 Chongqing, China

Wei Gong
Department of Biochemistry and Molecular Biology, College of Basic Medical Sciences, Third Military Medical University, 400038 Chongqing, China

Guoqing Chen, Limin Liao and Di Miao
Department of Urology, China Rehabilitation Research Center, Beijing 100068, China
Department of Urology, Capital Medical University, Beijing, China
Center of Neural Injury and Repair, Beijing Institute for Brain Disorders, Beijing, China

Gustav Andersson, Christoffer Wennersten, Alexander Gaber, Karolina Boman, Björn Nodin and Karin Jirström
Department of Clinical Sciences, Oncology and Pathology, Lund University, Skåne University Hospital, Lund 221 85, Sweden

Mathias Uhlén
Science for Life Laboratory, Royal Institute of Technology, Stockholm 171 21, Sweden
School of Biotechnology, AlbaNova University Center, Royal Institute of Technology, Stockholm 106 91, Sweden

Ulrika Segersten and Per-Uno Malmström
Department of Surgical Sciences, Uppsala University, Uppsala 751 85, Sweden

Firas Aljabery and Staffan Jahnson
Department of Urology, Linköping University Hospital, Linköping, Sweden
Department of Clinical and Experimental Medicine, Faculty of Health Sciences, Linköping University, Linköping, Sweden

Gunnar Lindblom and Susann Skoog
Department of Radiology, Linköping University Hospital, Linköping, Sweden

Ivan Shabo and Hans Olsson
Department of Clinical and Experimental Medicine, Faculty of Health Sciences, Linköping University, Linköping, Sweden

Johan Rosell
Regional Cancer Center Southeast Sweden, County Council of Östergötland, Linköping, Sweden

Vivien Gardner, Joel Vetter and Gerald L Andriole
Division of Urologic Surgery, Department of Surgery, Washington University School of Medicine, 4960 Children's Place, St Louis, MO 63110, USA

Henry Lai
Division of Urologic Surgery, Department of Surgery, Washington University School of Medicine, 4960 Children's Place, St Louis, MO 63110, USA
Department of Anesthesiology, Washington University School of Medicine, 4960 Children's Place, St Louis, MO 63110, USA

David Burmeister, Bimjhana Bishwokarma, Tamer AbouShwareb, Maja Herco and Karl-Erik Andersson
Wake Forest Institute for Regenerative Medicine, 391 Technology Way, Winston-Salem, NC 27101, USA

George Christ
Wake Forest Institute for Regenerative Medicine, 391 Technology Way, Winston-Salem, NC 27101, USA
Departments of Biomedical Engineering and Orthopaedic Surgery, and Laboratory of Regenerative Therapeutics, University of Virginia, 415 Lane Road, Charlottesville, VA 22908, USA

John Olson and Josh Tan
Wake Forest Department of Biomolecular Imaging, Medical Center Blvd, Winston-Salem, NC 27157, USA

Hongzhou Cai, Ting Xu and Qing Zou
Department of Urologic Surgery, Affiliated Cancer Hospital of Jiangsu Province of Nanjing Medical University, Nanjing, China

Bin Yu and Zicheng Xu
Department of Urologic Surgery, Affiliated Cancer Hospital of Jiangsu Province of Nanjing Medical University, Nanjing, China
Department of Urology, First Affiliated Hospital of Nanjing Medical University, Nanjing, China

Min Gu
Department of Urology, First Affiliated Hospital of Nanjing Medical University, Nanjing, China

Jin Zhou
Department of Hospital Infection Control, Affiliated Cancer Hospital of Jiangsu Province of Nanjing Medical University, Nanjing, China

Naim B Farah
department of surgery, section of Uro-oncology, King Hussein Cancer Center, Amman, Jordan

Rami Ghanem
Section of Uro-oncology, King Hussein Cancer Center, Amman, Jordan

Mahmoud Amr
Department of Surgical oncology, Amman, Jordan

Jong-hyun Yun
Department of Urology, Soonchunhyang University Gumi Hospital, Soonchunhyang University School of Medicine, Gumi, South Korea

Jae Heon Kim
Department of Urology, Soonchunhyang University Hospital, Soonchunhyang University School of Medicine, Seoul, South Korea

Suyeon Park
Department of Biostatistics, Soonchunhyang University Hospital, Seoul, South Korea

Changho Lee
Department of Urology, Soonchunhyang University Cheonan Hospital, Soonchunhyang University School of Medicine, 31 Soonchunhyang 6 gil, Dongnam-Gu, Cheonan, Chungcheongnam-do 330-721, South Korea

Ajay Gopalakrishna, Thomas A. Longo, Joseph J. Fantony and Brant A. Inman
Division of Urology, Duke University Medical Center, Durham, NC 27710, USA

Richmond Owusu
Department of Urology, University of California San Diego, San Diego, CA, USA

Wen-Chi Foo and Rajesh Dash
Department of Pathology, Duke University Medical Center, Durham, NC, USA

Ronaldo Alvarenga Álvares
SARAH Network of Rehabilitation Hospitals, Unit Belo Horizonte, Minas Gerais, Av Amazonas 5953, Gameleira 30510-000, Brazil

Ivana Duval Araújo and Marcelo Dias Sanches
Federal University of Minas Gerais - UFMG, Rua Alfredo Balena, 190, 30130-100, Brazil

Jun Liu, Jian Cao and Xiaokun Zhao
Department of Urology, 2nd xiangya Hospital, Central South University, NO.139 Middle Renmin Road, 410011 Changsha, Hunan, China

Yiming Wang and Limin Liao
Department of Urology, China Rehabilitation Research Center, 10 Jiaomen Beilu, Beijing 100068, Fentai District, China
Department of Urology of Capital Medical University, Center of Neural Injury and Repair, Beijing Institute for Brain Disorders, 10 Youanmenwai Xitoutiao, Beijing 100069, Fentai District, China

Joseph A. Hypolite and Anna P. Malykhina
Division of Urology, Department of Surgery, University of Colorado Denver, Anschutz Medical Campus, 12700 E 19th Ave. Mail Stop C317, Aurora, CO 80045, USA

A. Ivchenko, R.-H. Bödeke, C. Neumeister and A. Wiedemann
Department of Urology, Evangelisches KrankenhausWitten gGmbH, UniversityWitten/ Herdecke, Pferdebachstrasse 27, 58455 Witten, Germany
Department of Statistics, Institute of Medical Informatics, University Clinic Giessen, Rudolf-Buchheim-Strasse 6, 35392 Gießen, Germany
Department of Medical Science/Clinical Research, Dr. R. Pfleger GmbH, Dr.-Robert-Pfleger-Strasse 12, 96052 Bamberg, Germany

Zhaohui Chen
Advanced Clinical Biosystems Research Institute, Cedars-Sinai Medical Center, Los Angeles, CA, USA

Jayoung Kim
Department of Surgery, Cedars-Sinai Medical Center, 8700 Beverly Blvd, Los Angeles, CA 90048, USA
Department of Biomedical Sciences, Cedars-Sinai Medical Center, 8700 Beverly Blvd, Los Angeles, CA 90048, USA
Department of Medicine, University of California, Los Angeles, CA, USA

Yoshihiro Komohara and Chaoya Ma
Department of Cell Pathology, Graduate School of Medical Sciences, Kumamoto University, Kumamoto 860-8556, Japan

Takanobu Motoshima
Department of Cell Pathology, Graduate School of Medical Sciences, Kumamoto University, Kumamoto 860-8556, Japan
Department of Urology, Graduate School of Medical Sciences, Kumamoto University, Kumamoto, Japan

Arni Kusuma Dewi
Department of Cell Pathology, Graduate School of Medical Sciences, Kumamoto University, Kumamoto 860-8556, Japan
Department of Anatomy Histology, Faculty of Medicine Airlangga University, Surabaya, Indonesia

Yoshiaki Kawano, Wataru Takahashi and Motohiro Takeya
Department of Urology, Graduate School of Medical Sciences, Kumamoto University, Kumamoto, Japan

Masatoshi Eto
Department of Urology, Graduate School of Medical Sciences, Kumamoto University, Kumamoto, Japan
Department of Urology, Graduate School of Medical Sciences, Kyushu University, Fukuoka, Japan

Hirotsugu Noguchi, Sohsuke Yamada and Toshiyuki Nakayama
Department of Pathology and Cell Biology, School of Medicine, University of Occupational and Environmental Health, Kitakyushu, Japan

Shohei Kitada and Naohiro Fujimoto
Department of Urology, School of Medicine, University of Occupational and Environmental Health, Kitakyushu, Japan

Yoshinao Oda
Department of Anatomic Pathology, Graduate School of Medical Sciences, Kyushu University, Fukuoka, Japan

Masaaki Sugimoto
Department of Anatomic Pathology, Graduate School of Medical Sciences, Kyushu University, Fukuoka, Japan
Department of Urology, Graduate School of Medical Sciences, Kyushu University, Fukuoka, Japan

Marvin J. Van Every
Department of Urology, Gundersen Health System, 1900 South Ave, La Crosse, WI 54601, USA

Garrett Dancik
Department of Mathematics and Computer Science, Eastern Connecticut State University, 83 Windham Street, Willimantic, CT 06226, USA

Venki Paramesh
Department of Cardiothoracic Surgery, Gundersen Health System, 1900 South Ave, La Crosse, WI 54601, USA

Grzegorz T. Gurda
Department of Pathology, Gundersen Health System, 1900 South Ave, La Crosse, WI 54601, USA
Gundersen Medical Foundation, 1300 Badger Street, La Crosse, WI 54601, USA

David R. Meier, Steven E. Cash, Craig S. Richmond and Sunny Guin
Gundersen Medical Foundation, 1300 Badger Street, La Crosse, WI 54601, USA

Nobuhiro Kushida, Yohei Kawashima, Hidenori Akaihata, Junya Hata, Kei Ishibashi, Ken Aikawa and Yoshiyuki Kojima
Department of Urology, Fukushima Medical University School of Medicine, 1, Hikarigaoka, Fukushima 960-1295, Japan

Osamu Yamaguchi
Division of Bioengineering and LUTD Research, Nihon University School of Engineering, Nihon University, 1, Nakagawara, Tokusada, Tamura, Koriyama 963-8642, Japan

Itamar Getzler, Zaher Bahouth, Ofer Nativ and Sarel Halachmi
Department of Urology, Bnai Zion Medical Center, Faculty of Medicine, Technion - Israel Institute of Technology, Golomb 47, 31048 Haifa, Israel

Jacob Rubinstein
Department of Mathematics, Technion - Israel Institute of Technology, Haifa, Israel

Azharuddin Mohammed and Zubair Arastu
Royal Shrewsbury Hospital, Mytton Oak Road, Shrewsbury SY3 8XQ, UK

Jeroen R Scheepe, Katja P Wolffenbuttel and Dirk J Kok
Department of Urology and Pediatric Urology, Erasmus Medical Center Rotterdam, Sophia Children's Hospital, Rotterdam, The Netherlands

Arjen Amelink
Department of Radiation Oncology, Center for Optical Diagnostics and Therapy, Erasmus Medical Center, Rotterdam, The Netherlands

Feng Chen, Tao Huang, Yu Ren, Junjun Wei, Zhongguan Lou, Xue Wang, Xiaoxiao Fan, Yirun Chen, Guobin Weng and Xuping Yao
Laboratory of Kidney Carcinoma, Ningbo urology & Nephrology Hospital, Ningbo 315040, Zhejiang, China

Index

www.ingramcontent.com/pod-product-compliance
Lightning Source LLC
Chambersburg PA
CBHW082018190326
41458CB00010B/3226